FIFTH EDITION

LANGE Q&A™

INTERNAL MEDICINE

Yashesh Patel, MD, MSc, FRCPC
Assistant Professor
University of Toronto
Division of General Internal Medicine
Mount Sinai Hospital
Toronto, Ontario
Canada

 Medical

New York Chicago San Francisco Lisbon London Madrid Mexico City Milan
New Delhi San Juan Seoul Singapore Sydney Toronto

Lange Q&A: Internal Medicine, Fifth Edition

1 2 3 4 5 6 7 8 9   QDB/QDB   14 13 12 11

ISBN 978-0-07-170346-8
MHID 0-07-170346-2

Notice

This book was set in Palatino by Glyph International.
The editors were Kirsten Funk and Cindy Yoo.
The production supervisor was Sherri Souffrance.
Project management was provided by Harleen Chopra, Glyph International.
The cover designer was the Gazillion Group.
Quad/Graphics was printer and binder.

This book is printed on acid-free paper.

Library of Congress Cataloging-in-Publication Data

Patel, Yashesh R., author.
  Lange Q & A. Internal medicine / Yashesh Patel, MD, MSc, FRCPC.—Fifth Edition.
    p. ; cm.
  Lange Q and A. Internal medicine
  Internal medicine
  Includes bibliographical references and index.
  ISBN-13: 978-0-07-170346-8 (pbk. : alk. paper)
  ISBN-10: 0-07-170346-2 (pbk. : alk. paper)   1. Internal medicine—Examinations, questions, etc.   I. Title.   II. Title: Lange Q and A. Internal medicine.   III. Title: Internal medicine.
  [DNLM: 1. Internal Medicine—Examination Questions. WB 18.2]
  RC58.G59   2011
  616.0076—dc22
                                                                    2010050552

Contents

Student Reviewers

Adam Darnobid
Fourth Year Medical Student
SUNY Upstate Medical University
Class of 2009

Edward Gould
Fourth Year Medical Student
SUNY Upstate Medical University
Class of 2009

Justin Penn, MD
Internal Medicine Resident
University of Rochester
Class of 2008

Preface

The practice of internal medicine requires both breadth and depth of knowledge. To acquire mastery of the subject requires extensive reading and clinical experience. The knowledge base is also constantly expanding and changing as medicine enters the era of molecular biology and large randomized clinical trials. This book provides a review of the major content areas in internal medicine by presenting a wide variety of typical examination questions along with referenced answers.

The fifth edition of the book is enhanced by more in-depth clinical vignettes and answers that reflect the current knowledge and practice in internal medicine. There are also new images to complement the questions. In a departure from previous editions, I have tried to reference most of the questions with content from the 17th edition of *Harrison's Principles of Internal Medicine*. This textbook is familiar to most learners and easily assessable for further reading.

The content has been organized to reflect the areas tested on Step 2CK of the United States Medical Licensing Examination (USMLE Step 2CK). The format of the questions is modeled after the format used on the USMLE, making it an ideal study guide for individuals preparing for licensing examinations. While the chapters are organized by organ system to facilitate thorough review of relevant content, also included is a comprehensive practice test that mimics the random question order of a typical examination.

The questions and answers reflect the increasing growth of knowledge in the field of internal medicine. As a result, reviewing the answer explanations gives the reader a "mini review" of basic concepts and pathophysiology in internal medicine, allowing the reader to approach clinical problems in an appropriate manner. Answer explanations discuss not only the correct answer, but why the other answers are incorrect.

I hope that you find this review helpful in your studies.

Yashesh Patel, MD, MSc, FRCPC

Acknowledgments

I would like to thank the countless medical students and residents who teach me and compel me to learn every day. This book would not be possible without the stimulation and learning that I receive from them every day. Thanks also to Kirsten Funk at McGraw-Hill for all her advice and help in guiding this revision.

Yashesh Patel, MD, MSc, FRCPC

CHAPTER 1

Cardiology
Questions

DIRECTIONS (Questions 1 through 61): For each of the questions in this section select the one lettered answer that is the best response in each case.

1. A 62-year-old man with coronary artery disease (CAD) presents to the emergency room with symptoms of feeling faint. The symptoms started earlier in the day and are more prominent when he is standing up. He reports no chest pain or dyspnea and is otherwise well. Medical history includes type 2 diabetes, dyslipidemia, and hypertension. His medications are atenolol, metformin, atorvastatin, and ramipril.

   On physical examination, blood pressure is 125/70 mm Hg, heart rate is 56/min and irregular. Heart sounds S1 and S2 are normal, the lungs are clear, and he is alert and oriented. The electrocardiogram (ECG) shows Wenckebach type atrioventricular (AV) block. **Which of the following are you most likely to see on the ECG?**

   (A) progressive PR shortening
   (B) progressive lengthening of the PR interval
   (C) tachycardia
   (D) dropped beat after progressive lengthening of the PR interval
   (E) fixed 2:1 block

2. A 72-year-old woman is seen in the office for routine follow-up. She had a pacemaker inserted 4 years ago for symptomatic bradycardia because of AV nodal disease. She is clinically feeling well and has not experienced any angina, dyspnea on exertion, or syncope. Her past medical history also includes chronic stable angina and hypertension. Medications are atenolol, fosinopril, and hydrochlorothiazide.

   Physical examination is normal except for a pacemaker in the left upper chest. Her ECG shows normal sinus rhythm at a rate of 68/min but no pacemaker spikes. Her pacemaker only functions when the ventricular rate falls below a preset interval. **Which of the following best describes her pacemaker function?**

   (A) asynchronous
   (B) atrial synchronous
   (C) ventricular synchronous
   (D) ventricular inhibited
   (E) atrial sequential

3. A 42-year-old man is brought to the emergency department 7 days after an open cholecystectomy complaining of sudden onset shortness of breath (SOB) and chest pain. The pain does not radiate, is sharp in quality, and gets worse with inspiration. He reports no fever, cough, or sputum production and was well up until today.

   On physical examination, blood pressure is 145/86 mm Hg, pulse is 120/min, respirations 24/min, and oxygen saturation of 97%.

The heart sounds are normal, the lungs clear on auscultation, and there is no chest-wall tenderness on palpation. The surgical site is clean and not inflamed, and the abdomen soft and not tender. The left calf diameter is larger than the right. Pulmonary embolism is clinically suspected. **Which of the following is the most common ECG finding of pulmonary embolism?**

(A) a deep S wave in lead I

(B) depressed ST segments in leads I and II

(C) prominent Q wave in lead I, and inversion of T wave in lead III

(D) sinus tachycardia

(E) clockwise rotation in the precordial leads

4. A 63-year-old woman is brought to the emergency department after developing symptoms of exertional chest discomfort and one episode of transient loss of consciousness. She noticed non-radiating retrosternal chest discomfort starting 3 weeks ago, and today while out walking with her daughter started feeling lightheaded and transiently lost consciousness. There was no seizure activity or incontinence noted and she made a full recovery within minutes.

The physical examination shows a blood pressure of 150/80 mm Hg, heart rate is 88/min and regular. On cardiac auscultation S1 is normal, S2 is soft, and there is a 3/6 systolic ejection murmur with radiation to the carotids. The carotid upstroke is diminished, lungs are clear, and there are no focal neurological deficits. **Which of the following is the most likely diagnosis?**

(A) mitral stenosis

(B) mitral insufficiency

(C) aortic stenosis

(D) aortic insufficiency

(E) tricuspid stenosis

5. A 42-year-old man is seen in the clinic with a 1-week history of fever and chills. He reports no localizing symptoms for the fever and there is no recent travel history. His past medical history is significant for congenital valvular heart disease which has been asymptomatic, and he is not on any medications.

On examination he appears unwell; blood pressure is 120/70 mm Hg, heart rate is 100/min, and there is a 3/6 pansystolic murmur at the apex that radiates to the axilla and a soft S1 sound. His lungs are clear, abdomen is soft but there are petechiae on his conjunctival sac, linear hemorrhages under a few fingernails, and painful, tender, and erythematous nodules on some of the distal fingertips. **Which of the following is the most responsible mechanism for these physical findings?**

(A) direct bacterial invasion

(B) immune response

(C) vascular phenomena

(D) valvular damage

(E) preexisting cardiac dysfunction

6. A 73-year-old man is seen in the office for routine follow-up appointment. Medical history includes paroxysmal atrial fibrillation, hypertension, dyslipidemia, and type 2 diabetes. His medications are amiodarone, enalapril, diltiazem, atorvastatin, and warfarin.

On physical examination, blood pressure is 135/80 mm Hg, heart rate is 72/min regular, the heart sounds are normal, there is a S4, and the lungs are clear. **Which of the following drugs mediates its effect by interfering with movement of calcium through the *slow channel*?**

(A) enalapril

(B) diltiazem

(C) atorvastatin

(D) amiodarone

(E) warfarin

7. A 67-year-old man presents to his local emergency department with anterior chest discomfort radiating down his left arm and associated sweating and shortness of breath. His ECG reveals an anterior myocardial infarction (MI)

and he receives thrombolytic therapy since primary angioplasty is not available at this center. Three days later, he develops chest pain that is made worse by lying down and better with sitting up. The pain is sharp in quality and non-radiating. It is also different from the pain associated with his MI, and sublingual nitroglycerine has no effect.

On physical examination, blood pressure is 145/80 mm Hg, heart rate is 100/min and regular. Heart sounds are normal except for a biphasic rub heard best at the apex. The lungs are clear to auscultation, and the remaining exam is normal. His ECG shows evolving changes from the anterior infarction but new PR-segment depression and 1-mm ST-segment elevation in all the limb leads. **Which of the following is the most likely diagnosis?**

(A) reinfarction
(B) pulmonary embolus
(C) viral infection
(D) post-MI pericariditis
(E) dissecting aneurysm

8. **Which of the following best describes the effect of calcium ions on the myocardium?**

(A) positively inotropic
(B) negatively inotropic
(C) positively chronotropic
(D) negatively chronotropic
(E) excitation contraction uncoupling

9. A 22-year-old primagravida woman develops hypertension at 32 weeks. She reports no vision change, headache, shortness of breath, or abdominal symptoms. Her pregnancy is uneventful until now. She has no significant past medical history and is not on any medications except vitamins.

On examination the blood pressure is 160/100 mm Hg, heart rate is 100/min, and the rest of the examination is normal except for 1+ pedal edema. Her complete blood count, liver enzymes, and electrolytes are normal. The urinalysis is positive for proteinuria. **Which of the following is true for this type of hypertension?**

(A) improves in the third trimester
(B) leads to large-birth-weight babies
(C) should be controlled with medications
(D) spares the placenta
(E) spares maternal kidney function

10. A 61-year-old man is evaluated in the emergency department for chest pain with radiation to his neck. He is having an anterior ST-elevation MI and is admitted to the coronary care unit after undergoing primary angioplasty which resolved his symptoms. The following day, he develops bradycardia but no symptoms of chest pain or shortness of breath. His medications are clopidogrel, aspirin, metoprolol, and ramipril.

On physical examination, his blood pressure is 126/84 mm Hg, pulse is 50/min, and on cardiac auscultation the heart sounds are normal, with no extra sounds or rubs. His ECG has changed from one obtained post angioplasty. **Which of the following ECG findings is the best indication for this patient to receive a pacemaker?**

(A) persistent bradycardia
(B) second-degree AV block Mobitz type I
(C) first-degree AV block
(D) new right bundle branch block
(E) left bundle branch block (LBBB) and second-degree AV block Mobitz type II

11. An 18-year-old woman is seen in clinic for symptoms of shortness of breath on exertion. Her past health history is noncontributory except for an appendectomy at the age of 8. She reports of no recent cough, sputum, wheeze, or chest discomfort.

On physical examination, she appears well. The blood pressure is 120/70 mm Hg, heart rate is 80/min and regular, and respiratory rate is 12/min. Auscultation of the heart reveals an increased intensity of the pulmonary component of the second heart sound. The lungs are clear and the remaining physical is normal. Her CXR is shown in Figure 1–1. **Which of the following explanations is the most likely cause of her dyspnea?**

Figure 1–1.

(A) pulmonary stenosis
(B) aortic stenosis
(C) MI
(D) pulmonary hypertension
(E) systemic hypertension

12. A 22-year-old woman is evaluated in the emergency department because of symptoms of prolonged palpitations. She complains of no associated chest discomfort, shortness of breath, or lightheadedness. The palpitations have occurred twice before, but they always stopped spontaneously after 5 minutes, and she cannot

associate them with any triggers. The past health history is negative and she is not on any medications.

On physical examination, the blood pressure is 110/70 mm Hg, heart rate is 160/min and regular. The heart and lung examinations are normal, and the ECG is shown in Figure 1–2. The heart rate abruptly changes to 72/min after applying carotid sinus pressure. **Which of the following is the most likely diagnosis?**

(A) sinus tachycardia
(B) paroxysmal atrial fibrillation
(C) paroxysmal atrial flutter
(D) paroxysmal supraventricular tachycardia (PSVT)
(E) paroxysmal ventricular tachycardia

13. A 73-year-old man is seen in the office for assessment of new-onset chest pain and shortness of breath on exertion. The pain is described as retrosternal pressure and non-radiating. Medical history includes hypertension, type 2 diabetes and dyslipidemia. His medications are atenolol, metformin, glyburide, and simvastatin.

On examination, the blood pressure is 140/90 mm Hg, heart rate is 60/min and cardiac auscultation reveals a murmur. On his ECG the rhythm is sinus and there is left axis deviation with voltage enlargement consistent with left ventricular hypertrophy. He is sent for a coronary angiogram and it reveals noncritical stenosis of the coronary arteries. **This occurs most frequently with which of the following valvular heart diseases?**

(A) mitral stenosis
(B) mitral insufficiency
(C) pulmonary stenosis
(D) aortic stenosis
(E) aortic insufficiency

14. An 82-year-old woman presents to the emergency department with new-onset syncope. She was walking at the time and reported no prodrome prior to the event. After a brief episode of disorientation lasting less than a minute she was back to her baseline. Lately

Figure 1–2. (Reproduced, with permission, from Fuster V et al, *Hurst's the Heart*, 11th ed. New York: McGraw-Hill, 2004:819.)

she has noticed shortness of breath on exertion but no chest discomfort.

Physical examination reveals a blood pressure of 110/95 mm Hg, heart rate of 80/min, and a harsh systolic ejection murmur heard best at the base of the heart and radiating to both carotids. The carotid pulse is late in peaking and diminished in volume. **Auscultation of the second heart sound at the base might reveal which of the following findings?**

(A) it is accentuated

(B) it is diminished

(C) it is normal in character

(D) it is widely split due to delayed ventricular ejection

(E) it shows fixed splitting

15. A 69-year-old woman is brought to the emergency department complaining of easy fatigue and one episode of syncope. She was feeling well until the day of presentation and reports no chest pain, fever, cough, or shortness of breath. Her past medical history is significant for angina, hypertension, and dyslipidemia. Medications include metoprolol, amlodipine, and atorvastatin.

On physical examination, the blood pressure is 110/80 mm Hg, heart rate is regular at 56/min, and inspection of the jugular venous pressure (JVP) reveals irregular large *a* waves. The ECG (see Figure 1–3) has fixed PP and RR intervals but varying PR intervals. **Which of the following conditions is this most likely caused by?**

(A) surgical removal of an atrium

(B) independent beating of atria and ventricles

(C) a re-entry phenomenon

(D) a drug effect of amlodipine

(E) a heart rate under 60 beats/min

Figure 1–3. (Reproduced, with permission, from Fuster V et al, *Hurst's the Heart*, 11th ed. New York: McGraw-Hill, 2004:904.)

16. A 57-year-old man presents to the emergency department with a 1-day history of chest pain and shortness of breath. An ECG is diagnostic for an evolving anterior MI, and treatment is initiated with aspirin, metoprolol, and heparin. His post MI course is complicated by the development of heart failure. **Nitroglycerin would be a useful first medication under which circumstances?**

(A) severe pulmonary congestion, blood pressure 80 mm Hg systolic

(B) clear lungs, blood pressure 120 mm Hg systolic

(C) clear lungs, blood pressure 80 mm Hg systolic

(D) clear lungs, blood pressure 160 mm Hg systolic

(E) moderate pulmonary congestion, blood pressure 130 mm Hg systolic

17. A 28-year-old man presents to the hospital feeling unwell for weeks with new symptoms of fever, chills, and night sweats. He reports no cough, sputum, or dysuria, and his past medical history is negative for important co-morbidities. He is not taking any medications.

   Pertinent findings on physical examination are a blood pressure of 120/70 mm Hg heart rate of 100/min, and temperature of 38.5°C. The heart sounds are normal but there is a 3/6 systolic murmur. The lungs are clear, the abdomen is nontender, and his peripheral exam is normal. He is admitted to the hospital for further investigations, and two days later the blood cultures are positive for *viridans group streptococci* in multiple sets. **Which of the following cardiac lesions has the highest risk of developing endocarditis?**

(A) ventricular septal defect

(B) atrial septal defect, secundum type

(C) mitral valve prolapse with regurgitation

(D) pure mitral stenosis

(E) asymmetric septal hypertrophy

18. A 47-year-old woman presents to the emergency department with symptoms of new-onset transient right arm weakness and word-finding difficulty lasting 3 hours. She is also experiencing exertional dyspnea, and had a syncopal event 1 month ago. Her medical history is only remarkable for 2 uneventful pregnancies, and she is not taking any medications.

   Physical examination reveals normal vital signs, and no residual focal neurological deficits. The ECG and CT brain are normal but an echocardiogram reveals a cardiac tumor in the left atrium, it is pendunculated, and attached to the endocardium. **Which of the following is the most likely cause of this lesion?**

(A) myxoma
(B) sarcoma
(C) rhabdomyoma
(D) fibroma
(E) lipoma

19. A 72-year-old woman comes to the emergency department complaining of palpitations and dyspnea. The symptoms started suddenly and there is no associated chest pain, fever, or light-headedness. Her past medical history includes hypertension, dyslipidemia, and osteoarthritis. Her medications are enalapril, hydrochlorothiazide, simvastatin, and acetaminophen.

Her ECG shows new-onset atrial flutter with a ventricular rate of 150/min. She is hemodynamically stable with a blood pressure of 155/90 mm Hg, but is experiencing palpitations. The jugular venous pressure and heart sounds are normal. There are no murmurs, and the lungs are clear. **Which of the following drugs is the best intravenous choice for controlling the heart rate?**

(A) diltiazem
(B) lidocaine
(C) aminophylline
(D) magnesium
(E) atropine

20. Several of the older patients in your practice intend to pursue exercise programs. They have no cardiac symptoms, but some do have vascular risk factors such as diabetes or hypertension. **In these patients, which of the following best describes exercise electrocardiography?**

(A) it is an invasive procedure
(B) it is contraindicated in patients over 65 years of age
(C) it detects latent disease
(D) it has a morbidity of approximately 5%
(E) it is used in pulmonary embolism

21. A 58-year-old man is undergoing cardiac catheterization for evaluation of chest pain symptoms. He is worried about the risks, and as part of obtaining informed consent, you advise him about the risks and benefits of the procedure. **Which of the following best describes coronary angiography?**

(A) it is contraindicated in the presence of cyanosis
(B) it is considered noninvasive
(C) it is generally performed with cardiopulmonary bypass
(D) it may cause renal failure
(E) it requires carotid artery puncture

22. A 23-year-old man develops sharp left-sided chest pain and presents to the office for evaluation. The pain does not change with respiration but is aggravated by lying down and relieved by sitting up. He reports having flu like illness 1 week prior to presentation with fevers, chills, and myalgias. He is otherwise well with no other symptoms or significant past medical history.

On physical examination, the blood pressure is 130/75 mm Hg, heart rate is 92/min, and cardiac auscultation reveals a friction rub heard at the lower left sternal border, unaffected by respiration. The lungs are clear and the remaining physical examination is normal. **Which of the following is the most likely cause for his symptoms?**

(A) rheumatic fever
(B) tuberculosis (TB)
(C) herpes simplex virus
(D) MI
(E) coxsackievirus

23. A 72-year-old woman with angina and heart failure undergoes right and left cardiac catheterization. **The pulmonary capillary "wedge" pressure is an approximation of the pressure in which of the following structures?**

(A) pulmonary artery (PA)

(B) pulmonary vein

(C) left atrium

(D) right atrium

(E) vena cava

24. A 58-year-old man with hypertension is brought to the emergency room after sudden-onset chest pain that radiates to his back and arms. The pain does not change with deep inspiration, and he reports no fever, cough, or sputum. His only medication is losartan.

On physical examination he is in moderate distress with a blood pressure of 160/90 mm Hg in the left arm and 120/70 mm Hg in the right arm. Cardiac examination reveals a soft second heart sound and a murmur of aortic insufficiency. His ECG shows sinus tachycardia but no acute ischemic changes, and the chest x-ray (CXR) is shown in Figure 1–4. **Which of the following is the most appropriate next step in confirming the diagnosis?**

Figure 1–4.

(A) coronary angiography

(B) transthoracic echocardiography

(C) computerized tomography (CT) chest

(D) exercise stress test

(E) cardiac troponin level

25. A 25-year-old woman is evaluated in the office for symptoms of gradual but progressive exertional dyspnea. She has been well with no prior health history. Presently she reports no cough, sputum, wheezing, or pleuritic chest discomfort symptoms.

On examination, the blood pressure is 110/70 mm Hg, heart rate is 88/min, and auscultation of the heart reveals a normal S1 but fixed splitting of her second heart sound and a 3/6 systolic ejection murmur heard best over the left sternal border. An echocardiogram confirms the presence of an atrial septal defect. **Which of the following is the best physiologic explanation for her condition?**

(A) pulmonary blood flow is greater than systemic blood flow

(B) pulmonary blood flow is less than systemic blood flow

(C) pulmonary blood flow is equal to systemic blood flow

(D) the left ventricle is enlarged

(E) the systemic blood pressure is elevated

26. A 19-year-old man comes to his doctor's office complaining of chest discomfort on exertion. There is no history of chest trauma, respiratory symptoms, constitutional symptoms, or cocaine use. The discomfort is described as chest heaviness radiating to his arms and neck which exertion, and relieved with rest. He has no prior medical illnesses, and there is no family history of premature CAD.

His physical examination is entirely normal as is the ECG and CXR. **Which of the following is the most likely diagnosis?**

(A) mitral stenosis

(B) coronary artery aneurysm

(C) coarctation

(D) atrial septal defect

(E) Werner syndrome

27. A 65-year-old woman presents to the office complaining of progressive shortness of breath on exertion. She reports no chest pain, cough, or wheeze, and otherwise feels well. There is no history of overt blood loss, change in bowel habits, or weight loss. Her past medical history is significant only for cholecystitis, and a remote wrist fracture after a fall.

On examination the only pertinent physical findings are a blood pressure of 120/50 mm Hg, a soft S2, and a diastolic and systolic murmur heard best at the left sternal border. There is also a rapidly rising, forceful carotid pulse that collapses quickly. **Which of the following is the most likely diagnosis?**

(A) mitral stenosis
(B) mitral regurgitation
(C) aortic stenosis
(D) aortic regurgitation
(E) coarctation of the aorta

28. A 63-year-old woman on digoxin for chronic atrial fibrillation experiences fatigue, nausea, and anorexia. Her symptoms started gradually about 1 week ago. She notes no chest pain, palpitations, fever, or shortness of breath. Her past medical history is significant for heart failure, type 2 diabetes, and chronic kidney disease.

On physical examination her pulse is regular at 50 beats/min, blood pressure is 130/80 mm Hg, and the heart sounds, chest, and abdominal examinations are normal. On the ECG, no P waves are visible and the QRS complexes are narrow and regular. (See Figure 1–5.) Her complete blood count (CBC) and electrolytes are normal except for an increase in her urea and creatinine twice over baseline. **Which of the following is the most appropriate management step?**

(A) an increase in digitalis dose
(B) complete cessation of digitalis
(C) withdrawal of digitalis for one dose
(D) addition of a beta-blocker
(E) addition of a calcium channel blocker

Figure 1–5.

29. A 47-year-old man presents to the emergency department complaining of progressive swelling in his feet and abdomen, and shortness of breath on exertion. Physical examination confirms the presence of edema, ascites, and hepatosplenomegaly. Inspection of the jugular venous pulse reveals a markedly elevated venous pressure with a deep y descent. The cardiac silhouette on the chest x-ray is normal. **Which of the following etiologies is not a possible explanation for this syndrome?**

    (A) rheumatic fever
    (B) TB
    (C) unknown cause
    (D) previous acute pericarditis
    (E) neoplastic involvement of the pericardium

30. A 65-year-old man presents to the emergency department after developing symptoms of palpitations and dizziness. The symptoms started suddenly and were not associated with any chest pain or shortness of breath. There is no prior history of palpitations, and his past medical history is significant for hypertension and dyslipidemia. His medications are losartan and atorvastatin.

    On physical examination he appears unwell, the blood pressure is 80/50 mm Hg and the heart rate is 150/min and regular. His ECG shows a "saw-toothed" pattern of P waves, but no ischemic changes. (See Figure 1–6.) **Which of the following procedures is most appropriate in converting him back to sinus rhythm?**

    (A) carotid sinus pressure
    (B) gagging procedures
    (C) Valsalva maneuver
    (D) eyeball compression
    (E) electrical cardioversion

Figure 1–6. (Reproduced, with permission, from Fuster V et al, *Hurst's the Heart*, 11th ed. New York: McGraw-Hill, 2004:843.)

31. A 63-year-old woman presents to the emergency department with symptoms of palpitations. The symptoms started suddenly with no associated chest pain or shortness of breath. Her physical examination is normal except for a rapid heart rate at 150/min and blood pressure of 120/74 mm Hg. Her ECG shows a narrow complex tachycardia with atrial flutter waves. **Which of the following is the most likely mechanism of this arrhythmia?**

    (A) atrial asystole
    (B) atrial bigeminy
    (C) right atrial macro-reentry
    (D) AV nodal re-entry
    (E) accessory pathway

32. A 62-year-old man presents to the office for assessment of symptoms of shortness of breath. The symptoms are worse with exertion and he notes difficulty lying down. He reports no chest pain or palpitations but his feet are swollen. His past medical history includes hypertension and type 2 diabetes, for which he is taking ramipril, amlodipine, and metformin.

    On physical examination, the blood pressure is 125/84 mm Hg, heart rate is 100/min. The jugular venous pressure is 8 cm above the sternal angle, with a third heart sound, pedal edema, and bibasilar crackles on auscultation of the lungs. **Which one of the following may be implicated in fluid retention for this condition?**

    (A) decreased renin
    (B) increased aldosterone
    (C) increased estrogen
    (D) increased growth hormone
    (E) decreased vasopressin

33. A 73-year-old man comes to the office for follow up 3 months after an anterior MI. He is clinically feeling well, and has no further angina symptoms since his hospitalization. His medications are clopidogrel, aspirin, ramipril, metoprolol, and atorvastatin.

    On physical examination, the blood pressure is 110/70 mm Hg and heart rate is 64/min. The jugular venous pressure is normal; the apical impulse is diffuse and displaced to the left. The heart sounds are normal with no S3, and the lungs are clear. His ECG shows Q waves in the anterior leads with persistent ST-segment elevation. (See Figure 1–7.) **The current ECG is most compatible with which of the following diagnosis?**

    (A) ventricular aneurysm
    (B) hibernating myocardium
    (C) acute infarction
    (D) silent infarction
    (E) early repolarization

34. A 79-year-old man presents to the office for evaluation of a recent episode of syncope while getting up to go to the bathroom in the middle of the night. He reports no symptoms of chest pain, palpitations, or lightheadedness prior to the event. His medications are tamsulosin, ramipril, and hydrochlorothiazide.

    On physical examination, he has a slow upstroke in his carotid pulse and a diamond-shaped systolic murmur at the base. His chest is clear. **Which of the following findings is his echocardiogram most likely to reveal?**

    (A) mitral regurgitation
    (B) stenosis of the proximal ascending aorta
    (C) aortic regurgitation
    (D) normal cardiac valves
    (E) aortic stenosis

Figure 1–7.

35. A 49-year-old man is evaluated in the office for cardiac risk factor assessment. He is active with no cardiorespiratory symptoms, but his father had a MI at the age of 55 years. His past medical history is negative for type 2 diabetes, hypertension, and he does not smoke.

   His physical examination including blood pressure and cardiac exam are entirely normal. Fasting lipids and glucose are ordered as screening tests. **Which lipid pattern suggests the lowest risk for CAD?**

   (A) total cholesterol 215 mg/dL, high-density lipoprotein (HDL) cholesterol 28 mg/dL

   (B) total cholesterol 215 mg/dL, HDL cholesterol 43 mg/dL

   (C) total cholesterol 180 mg/dL, HDL cholesterol 29 mg/dL

   (D) total cholesterol 202 mg/dL, HDL cholesterol 45 mg/dL

   (E) total cholesterol 225 mg/dL, HDL cholesterol 40 mg/dL

36. A 16-year-old boy is found to have hypertension on routine evaluation. He has no symptoms of shortness of breath or chest discomfort, but occasionally on exertion notes that his legs get tired easily. He has no other past medical history.

   On physical examination, the blood pressure in his arms is 140/90 mm Hg (bilaterally). Measurement of the blood pressure in his legs is 20mm Hg lower than in the arms. The remaining physical examination is normal. **Which of the following is the most likely diagnosis?**

   (A) aortic insufficiency

   (B) coarctation of the aorta

   (C) normal variant

   (D) ventricular aneurysm

   (E) severe juvenile diabetes

37. A 79-year-old man comes to the office for re-assessment of his blood pressure. He has had hypertension for 40 years, and takes numerous medications. For most of this time the blood pressure was well controlled until the past 5 years when he has required multiple medication changes.

    On physical examination, the blood pressure is 155/90 mm Hg in the right arm and 160/90 mm Hg in the left arm. The cardiac apex is displaced and sustained and heart sounds are normal except for an accentuated S2 and S4. His lungs are clear and remaining exam is normal. His CXR reveals cardiomegaly. **Which of the following findings is most likely on his ECG?**

    (A) clockwise rotation of the electrical axis
    (B) rSR' pattern in V1
    (C) right axis deviation
    (D) high-voltage QRS complexes in V5 and V6
    (E) prolonged PR interval in the limb leads

38. A 59-year-old woman presents to the emergency department with progressive shortness of breath, inability to lay down at night, and swelling in her feet. She has no prior history of heart failure but does have poorly controlled hypertension, dyslipidemia, and angina. Medications are aspirin, ramipril, metoprolol, and atorvastatin. She volunteers that her adherence to medications and follow-up appointments is poor.

    On physical examination, the blood pressure is 165/95 mm Hg, heart rate is 100/min, and the jugular venous pressure is 10 cm above the sternal angle. The heart sounds are normal; there is an S3 and 2+ pedal edema. The lungs have bibasilar crackles up to the mid chest. **Urinalysis and urine biochemistry is most likely to show which of the following?**

    (A) decreased urinary sodium content
    (B) low urine specific gravity
    (C) increased urinary chloride content
    (D) red blood cell (RBC) casts
    (E) proteinuria

39. A 76-year-old woman presents to the office for evaluation of symptoms of weight loss, anxiety, and palpitations. The symptoms started 1 month ago, and are involuntary. She has no prior history of anxiety or palpitations and her only medical history is hypertension for which she is taking losartan.

    On examination, the blood pressure is 120/70 mm Hg, heart rate is 100/min and regular. On auscultation the heart sounds are normal and the lung clear. There is a thyroid goiter, warm skin, and a fine tremor in her hands. **Which of the following is the most likely cardiac finding?**

    (A) prolonged circulation time
    (B) decreased cardiac output
    (C) paroxysmal atrial fibrillation
    (D) pericardial effusion
    (E) aortic insufficiency

40. A 72-year-old woman is found to have an irregular pulse rate at a routine clinic visit. She is experiencing no new symptoms at rest or on exertion. Her past medical history includes hypertension, osteoarthritis, and dyslipidemia.

    On physical examination, the blood pressure is 135/85 mm Hg, heart rate is approximately 72/min and irregular. The heart sounds reveal an irregular S1 and normal S2 with no audible murmurs. The jugular venous pressure is normal and the lungs are clear. On the ECG, there are no P waves and an irregular RR interval at a rate of 70/min. (See Figure 1–8.) On her previous ECG from 4 years ago she was in sinus rhythm. **Which of the following is the most appropriate next step in management?**

    (A) cardioversion
    (B) antiarrhythmic therapy
    (C) beta-blocker
    (D) anticoagulation
    (E) aspirin

Figure 1–8.

41. A 47-year-old woman is seen in the emergency department for accelerated hypertension (blood pressure 210/105 mm Hg). She notes frequent headaches for the past month but no chest pain, shortness of breath, vision changes, or limb weakness. Her past medical history is negative except for hypertension during her first pregnancy. Family history is also positive for both parents and a brother who have hypertension.

On physical examination, the blood pressure is 210/105 mm Hg in both arms, the heart rate is 88/min, and the patient is alert and oriented. The heart sounds reveal a S4, the lungs are clear and there are no focal neurological deficits. **Which of the following findings are most likely on examination of the fundii? (See Figure 1–9.)**

(A) retinitis obliterans
(B) cotton wool spots
(C) retinal detachment
(D) optic atrophy
(E) foveal blindness

Figure 1–9. (Reproduced, with permission, from Kasper DL et al, *Harrison's Principles of Internal Medicine*, 16th ed. New York: McGraw-Hill, 2005:168.)

42. A 32-year-old man presents to the office for routine evaluation. He has no symptoms but has noticed some new "nodules" on his legs. The nodules are not tender or painful, and there is no history of injury to the site. On physical examination there are lumps on his Achillis tendon, as well as yellow lesions around his eyes, and pigmentation of his iris.

(See Figure 1–10 a and b.) **Which of the following is the most likely diagnosis?**

Figure 1–10. (Reproduced, with permission, from Wolff K and Johnson RA, *Fitzpatrick's Color Atlas & Synopsis of Clinical Dermatology*, 5th ed. New York: McGraw-Hill, 2005:447, 449.)

(A) familial hyperlipidemia

(B) diabetes

(C) myxedema

(D) chronic renal disease

(E) an inherited defect of glycogen utilization

43. A 22-year-old woman presents to the office with symptoms of sharp chest pain that is made worse with lying down especially on her left side. One week prior to the onset of symptoms she had "flu" like illness with fevers, chills, and myalgias. Her past medical history is negative and she is not taking any medications.

On physical examination, the blood pressure is 130/80 mm Hg with no pulsus paradoxus, and heart rate 100/min. The heart sounds are normal but there is a pericardial rub heard best at the apex in the left lateral decubitus position, the lungs are clear and there is no peripheral edema. **Which of the following features determines the patient's clinical course and prognosis?**

(A) specific gravity of the fluid

(B) presence or absence of blood in the fluid

(C) presence or nature of any underlying disease

(D) cellular count of the fluid

(E) viscosity of the fluid

44. A 65-year-old man comes to the office with symptoms of postural hypotension with dizziness. These are new symptoms for him and he reports no chest pain, shortness of breath, or palpitations. His past medical history is significant for type 2 diabetes, hypertension, and dyslipidemia. Medications include hydrochlorothiazide, ramipril metformin, and insulin.

On physical examination, his blood pressure is 110/80 mm Hg supine and 85/70 mm Hg standing (after 2 minutes), the pulse rate remains the same at 80/min. The jugular venous pressure is 3 cm above the sternal angle and the heart sounds are normal. **Which of the following is the most likely diagnosis?**

(A) thyrotoxicosis

(B) consequence of diuretic therapy

(C) venous varicosities

(D) complication of diabetes mellitus (DM)

(E) essential hypotension

45. A 22-year-old woman is seen in the clinic for follow up on the results of a recently performed echocardiogram. She was originally seen for an annual health assessment and on cardiac examination an abnormality was detected which prompted the echocardiogram. She otherwise is well and has no cardiac or respiratory symptoms. The echocardiogram reveals mitral valve prolapse. **Which of the following is the most common physical finding in this condition?**

(A) diastolic rumble

(B) absent first heart sound

(C) diastolic click

(D) aortic regurgitation

(E) late systolic murmur

46. A 56-year-old man presents to the emergency department because of symptoms of persistent palpitations. He admits to precordial discomfort, weakness, and anxiety. The symptoms started suddenly earlier in the day, and there is no effect on the palpitations with exertion or rest. His past medical history is negative for any cardiac conditions and he is not taking any prescription medications.

On physical examination, his pulse rate is 150/min, the blood pressure is 124/70 mm Hg, and the heart sounds are normal. Carotid sinus pressure gradually changes the rate to 100/min, but when the carotid pressure is released, the pulse rate returns to 150/min. **Which of the following is the most likely diagnosis?**

(A) atrial flutter with 2:1 block

(B) paroxysmal atrial tachycardia with 2:1 block

(C) sinus arrhythmia

(D) atrial fibrillation

(E) nodal tachycardia

47. A 25-year-old man presents to the emergency department complaining of left precordial chest pain that radiates to the left shoulder but not down the left arm. The pain is accentuated by lying supine as well as inspiration and relieved by sitting up. The pain is accompanied by fever and chills.

On physical examination, his blood pressure is 105/75 mm Hg, pulse is 110/min and regular, and temperature 37.5°C. The heart sounds are normal, there is a biphasic rub, and the lungs are clear. The ECG shows ST-segment elevation in all leads except aVR and V1. On the third hospital day, the patient's blood pressure falls, his jugular venous pressure is now elevated, the heart sounds are faint, and his lungs have bibasilar crackles. **Which of the following is the most likely diagnosis?**

(A) a second pulmonary embolus

(B) extension of a myocardial infarct

(C) cardiac tamponade

(D) secondary bacterial infection

(E) rupture of a chordae tendineae

48. An 80-year-old man presents to the emergency department with symptoms of increasing shortness of breath over the previous week. The symptoms are worse on exertion and lately he is waking up at night feeling short on breath. He reports no chest pain or any fever, cough, or sputum production. His past medical history is significant for type 2 diabetes and hypertension.

On physical examination he appears short of breath, the blood pressure is 170/95 mm Hg, pulse is 100/min and regular. The jugular venous pressure is 7 cm above the sternal angle; there is a loud second heart sound and a systolic ejection murmur at the right sternal border which does not radiate. The lungs have bibasilar crakles up to the scapula. The CXR has bilateral infiltrates and vascular redistribution. His echocardiogram reports aortic sclerosis, concentric left ventricular hypertrophy (LVH), and normal ejection fraction. (See Figure 1–11.) **Which of the following is the most likely mechanism for this condition?**

(A) valvular heart disease

(B) diastolic dysfunction

(C) systolic dysfunction

(D) hibernating myocardium

(E) hypertrophic obstructive cardiomyopathy (HOCM)

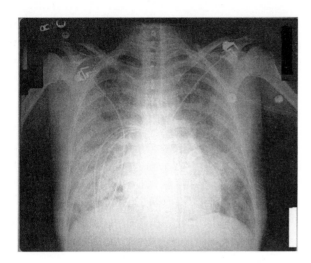

Figure 1–11.

49. A 68-year-woman presents to the emergency department complaining of chest pain for the past 30 minutes. The pain is retrosternal in location and it radiates to her neck. She has no history of cardiac conditions or similar episodes of chest discomfort, and her past medical history includes hypertension and dyslipidemia.

On physical examination, she is diaphoretic and in moderate distress. The blood pressure is 150/90 mm Hg, the heart sounds are normal, and the lungs clear on auscultation. The ECG is shown in Figure 1–12. **Which of the following mechanisms is the most likely cause of her condition?**

(A) coronary plaque rupture
(B) aortic inflammation
(C) pericardial inflammation
(D) vasculitis
(E) myocarditis

RIGHT CORONARY ARTERY

Figure 1–12. (Reproduced, with permission, from Fuster V et al, *Hurst's the Heart*, 11th ed. New York: McGraw-Hill, 2004:1356.)

50. A 62-year-old man presents to the emergency department because of new symptoms of fevers, chills, and malaise. His past medical history is significant for a prosthetic aortic valve replacement 5 years ago because of aortic stenosis from a bicuspid valve.

On physical examination, the blood pressure is 130/85 mm Hg, heart rate is 88/min, and temperature 38.5°C. He has a 2/6 systolic ejection murmur heard best at the aortic region and a mechanical second heart sound, but no other abnormalities on examination. **Blood cultures are most likely to grow which of the following?**

(A) fungi

(B) bartonella

(C) diptheroids

(D) *Staphylococcus epidermidis*

(E) *Streptococcus bovis*

51. A 58-year-old man with no prior cardiac history presents to the emergency department with symptoms of retrosternal chest pain starting at rest and lasting 30 minutes. The pain radiates to the left arm and is associated with diaphoresis and dyspnea.

On physical examination, his blood pressure is 150/90 mm Hg, pulse is 100/min, the heart sounds are normal, and the lungs are clear to auscultation. **Which of the following is the next most appropriate investigation?**

(A) CT scan—chest

(B) CXR

(C) cardiac troponin

(D) ECG

(E) myocardial perfusion imaging

52. A 37-year-old African-American woman is seen in the office for evaluation of an elevated blood pressure of 140/100 mm Hg at rest. She has no associated symptoms and her past medical history is negative. Her family history reveals that her father also has hypertension.

On physical examination the pertinent negatives are a normal funduscopic examination, normal heart sounds, absence of an S4, and no renal bruits. Table 1–1 shows laboratory investigations for this patient. **Which of the following is the most likely diagnosis?**

TABLE 1–1. LABORATORY INVESTIGATIONS

Urinalysis

pH	5.2
Albumin	Negative to trace

Biochemistry

Serum Na	140 mEq/L
K	3.5 mEq/L
Cl	100 mEq/L
CO_2	25 mEq/L
Creatinine	1.0 mg/100 mL
Fasting sugar	90 mg/100 mL
Calcium	9.0 mg/100 mL
Uric acid	5.0 mg/100 mL

(A) Cushing syndrome

(B) primary aldosteronism

(C) essential hypertension

(D) pyelonephritis

(E) bilateral renal artery stenosis

53. An 8-year-old boy is brought to the clinic for evaluation of symptoms of easy fatigability. He reports no chest pressure, shortness of breath, or weakness. The symptoms of the fatigue are more pronounced when he is playing with his friends and his mother notes that he usually cannot keep up with his peers. His past medical history and family history is noncontributory.

On physical examination, the blood pressure is 140/90 mm Hg, heart rate is 80/min, and there is a soft continuous murmur in the upper back. The femoral pulses are diminished in volume as compared to the carotid pulses, and the ECG reveals minimal LVH. The patient's x-ray and MR are shown in Figure 1–13. **What is the most likely diagnosis?**

(A) aortic stenosis

(B) patent ductus arteriosus

(C) coarctation of the aorta

(D) pulmonary valvular stenosis

(E) peripheral pulmonary stenosis

Figure 1–13.

54. A 64-year-old male executive is evaluated in the clinic for routine follow up after a large anterior MI 3 years ago. At the time he developed anterior Q-waves and his course was complicated by heart failure. On his ECG there is anterior Q-waves and persistent ST elevation. Since then he has done well and has no symptoms of chest pain on exertion, shortness of breath, or palpitations. He continues on his medications which are aspirin, metoprolol, enalapril, and atorvastatin. **What is the abnormality seen on the patient's x-ray shown in Figure 1–14?**

(A) calcific pericarditis
(B) left ventricular aneurysm
(C) pericardial effusion
(D) left ventricular hypertrophy
(E) normal

Figure 1–14.

55. A 70-year-old man is evaluated in emergency department for symptoms of dyspnea, orthopnea, and paroxysmal nocturnal dyspnea. His past medical history is significant for hypertension, type 2 diabetes, chronic kidney disease, and hypothyroidism. Medications are furosemide, enalapril, atorvastatin, metformin, and insulin.

On physical examination he has generalized cardiomegaly and pulmonary and systemic venous hypertension. The ECG is shown in Figure 1–15. **What is the cardiac rhythm seen on the ECG?**

(A) ectopic atrial tachycardia

(B) atrial flutter with 2:1 AV conduction

(C) sinus tachycardia

(D) supraventricular tachycardia

(E) atrial fibrillation with rapid ventricular response

56. A 77-year-old woman comes to the emergency department because of feeling "light-headed and dizzy." Except for the irregular pulse, her physical examination is normal. **What is the rhythm in the lead tracing shown in Figure 1–16?**

(A) first-degree heart block

(B) second-degree heart block

(C) third-degree heart block

(D) premature ventricular beats

(E) premature atrial beats

57. A 42-year-old woman is seen in the office for assessment of anterior chest pain of a somewhat atypical nature. The pain is in the anterior chest and occurs intermittently at rest and on exertion but there is no consistency. The pain does not change with respiration and she reports no other symptoms. The patient's pain

Figure 1–15.

Figure 1–16.

has been present for a number of years now and there is no change in the frequency or quality of the pain. Her physical examination is normal. An ECG is done and shown in Figure 1–17. It is not changed from a previous tracing 6 months ago. **What is the interpretation of the ECG?**

(A) inferior wall infarction
(B) anterior wall infarction
(C) ventricular aneurysm
(D) nonspecific changes
(E) pericarditis

Figure 1–17. (Reproduced, with permission, from Fauci AS, Braunwald E, Kasper DL, Harrison's Online, www.accessmedicine.com. New York: McGraw-Hill, 2008. Figure e19-27.)

58. A 67-year-old woman is seen in the emergency department complaining of retrosternal chest pain which started 30 minutes prior to presentation. Her medical history is significant for angina, hypertension, and dyslipidemia. The pain is similar to her usual angina but more severe and nonresponsive to sublingual nitroglycerine.

Her initial ECG reveals ST-elevation in the inferior leads and she is treated with aspirin and thrombolytic therapy. A follow up ECG obtained just after she received the thrombolytic therapy is shown in Figure 1–18. **What is the rhythm seen on the ECG?**

Figure 1–18.

(A) atrial fibrillation

(B) atrial flutter

(C) second-degree heart block

(D) Wenckebach phenomenon

(E) nonsustained ventricular tachycardia

59. A 78-year-old man with chronic kidney disease presents to the emergency department because he is feeling unwell. He can not elaborate any specific symptoms other than generalized malaise. His past medical history also includes heart failure, hypertension, and type 2 diabetes. Medications are ramipril, insulin, furosemide, and metoprolol.

On physical examination, the blood pressure is 155/90 mm Hg, heart rate is 100/min, and respiration 24/min. His heart sounds are normal, there is no edema, and the lungs clear on auscultation. An ECG is performed and shown in Figure 1–19. **What is the most likely diagnosis based on the ECG findings?**

(A) hyperkalemia

(B) hypercalcemia

(C) hypernatremia

(D) pericarditis

(E) ventricular aneurysm

Figure 1–19. (Reproduced, with permission, from Fauci AS, Braunwald E, Kasper DL, Harrison's Online, www.accessmedicine.com. New York: McGraw-Hill, 2008. Figure e19-26.)

60. A 58-year-old man whom you have followed dies suddenly, spurring you into doing some research on sudden death. **Which of the following is the most likely cause for this individual?**

    (A) extensive coronary atherosclerosis
    (B) electrolyte disturbance
    (C) pulmonary embolism
    (D) acute stroke
    (E) CHF

61. A 66-year-old man is evaluated in the clinic for routine follow-up of his essential hypertension. He is doing well with no symptoms and reports adherence to his medications without any medication related side effects. His blood pressure is 130/75 mm Hg after 10 minutes of rest in a quiet room. **Which of the following statements regarding essential hypertension is correct?**

    (A) over 95% of patients are salt-sensitive
    (B) it comprises about 90% of hypertensives in general population
    (C) renin levels are invariably high
    (D) women have a poorer prognosis
    (E) alcohol reduces risk

DIRECTIONS (Questions 62 through 121): The following group of numbered items is preceded by a list of lettered options. For each question, select the one lettered option that is most closely associated with it. Each lettered option may be used once, multiple times, or not at all.

Questions 62 through 64: For each of the following patients, select the characteristic ECG findings.

    (A) shortened PR interval
    (B) lengthened PR interval
    (C) lengthened QU interval
    (D) shortening of the QT interval
    (E) narrow-based (<0.20 second) peaked T wave
    (F) flattened P waves

62. An 80-year-old man presents with nausea, vomiting, and decreased urine output. He has a history of hypertension and chronic kidney disease (Stage 3, GFR [glomerular filtration rate] 50 mL/min). He is taking spironolactone and nifedipine for treatment of hypertension.

63. A 52-year-old woman presents with polyuria, polydypsia, constipation, and fatigue. She has no significant past medical history, and she is not on any medications. She was recently diagnosed with hyperparathyroidism.

64. A 64-year-old man with heart failure is recently started on 80 mg/day of furosemide. He now feels weak and tired, but notes that his heart failure symptoms have improved. There is no change in his urine output and he gets a good diuretic response every time he takes his furosemide. His potassium level is 2.5 mmol/L.

Questions 65 through 68: For the following patients, select the hemodynamic parameters that are most likely to apply.

    (A) decreased right atrial pressure (RAP), low cardiac output (CO), and increased systemic vascular resistance (SVR)
    (B) increased RAP, decreased CO, increased SVR
    (C) increased RAP, decreased CO, decreased SVR
    (D) decreased RAP, increased CO, decreased SVR

65. A 52-year-old man with alcoholic cirrhosis develops a variceal bleed with hypotension. His blood pressure is 85/60 mm Hg, pulse 120/min, and heart sounds are normal. The JVP is not visible, the lungs are clear, and his extremities are pale, cool, and clammy. What would central hemodynamic monitoring reveal?

66. A 73-year-old man has an inferior infarct with ST elevation documented on right-sided precordial leads. He is hypotensive (blood pressure 90/70 mm Hg) and tachycardic. The JVP is 10 cm, the heart sounds are normal, lungs are clear, and his extremities are cool. What would central hemodynamic monitoring reveal?

67. A 20-year-old man is being treated for acute lymphoblastic leukemia. While neutropenic, he becomes severely hypotensive with a temperature of 38.5°C. His blood pressure is 80/60 mm Hg, pulse 120/min, and heart sounds are normal. The JVP is below the sternal angle, lungs are clear, and his extremities are warm and flushed. What would central hemodynamic monitoring reveal?

68. A 78-year-old woman has an acute anterior wall MI with hypotension and pulmonary congestion. Her blood pressure is 90/70 mm Hg, pulse 110/min, JVP at 8 cm, and the heart sounds are normal. The lungs have bibasilar crackles, and her extremities are cool and diaphoretic. What would central hemodynamic monitoring reveal?

Questions 69 and 70: Select the most typical clinical and auscultation findings for the following patients.

   (A) soft S1 and holosystolic murmur radiating from the apex to the axilla
   (B) early and midsystolic murmur, pulmonary edema, and elevated JVP
   (C) diminished S1 only
   (D) clear lungs and elevated JVP

69. An asymptomatic 19-year-old female student presents for routine follow-up. On auscultation there is a murmur which on echocardiogram appears to be due to congenital mitral regurgitation. What might the physical findings include?

70. A 60-year-old man is admitted to the hospital because of an acute myocardial infarct. On the third day post infarct there is, on auscultation, a new murmur. Echocardiogram reveals acute mitral regurgitation. What might the physical findings include?

Questions 71 through 75: For each of the following patients, select the characteristic ECG finding.

   (A) prolonged PR interval
   (B) broad-notched P wave in lead II
   (C) short QT interval
   (D) short PR interval
   (E) LVH

71. A 25-year-old woman develops exertional dyspnea and fatigue. Her past history is significant for rheumatic fever as a child. Auscultation of the heart reveals a loud first heart sound and a low-pitched middiastolic sound.

72. A 70-year-old man with a prior anterior MI comes for his routine evaluation. He feels well and has no symptoms. He is taking metoprolol 100 mg bid, aspirin 81 mg od, enalapril 10 mg bid, and simvastatin 40 mg od for secondary prevention.

73. A 20-year-old woman develops palpitations and dizziness. Her blood pressure is 100/70 mm Hg, pulse 140/min, and heart sounds are normal. She has had symptoms of palpitations for many years.

74. A 64-year-old woman with metastatic breast cancer presents with fatigue and malaise. She recently started noticing polyuria and polydypsia. On examination, her JVP is below the sternal angle, heart sounds are normal, and she has tenderness over her thoracic spine.

75. A 78-year-old man develops recent-onset chest pain and dyspnea on exertion. His blood pressure is 150/90 mm Hg, pulse 90/min, and a systolic ejection murmur at the left sternal border that radiates to the carotids. His carotid pulse is also diminished.

Questions 76 through 79: For each of the following statements, select whether it is applicable to metoprolol and/or captopril.

   (A) true of metoprolol but not captopril
   (B) true of captopril but not metoprolol
   (C) true of both captopril and metoprolol
   (D) true of neither captopril nor metoprolol

76. Useful in heart failure.

77. The effects on the heart result in a prominent negative inotropic effect.

78. The treatment of chronic atrial fibrillation.

79. Mechanism of action is calcium blockade.

Questions 80 through 84: For each of the following statements, select whether it is applicable to one of the following medications.

  (A) losartan
  (B) enalapril
  (C) spironolactone
  (D) metoprolol
  (E) nifedipine
  (F) digoxin
  (G) furosemide

80. Direct action on vascular smooth muscle.

81. Inhibition of angiotensin converting enzyme I (ACE I).

82. Myocardial stimulant.

83. Used for primary pulmonary hypertension.

84. May decrease mortality by direct myocardial protective action against catecholamines.

Questions 85 through 89: For each of the following patients, select the characteristic arterial pulse finding.

  (A) pulsus tardus
  (B) pulsus paradoxus
  (C) hyperkinetic pulse
  (D) bisferiens pulse
  (E) dicrotic pulse
  (F) pulsus alternans
  (G) delayed femoral pulse
  (H) pulsus bigeminus

85. A 75-year-old woman with hypertension develops fatigue and dyspnea on exertion. Her blood pressure is 160/60 mm Hg and pulse 80/min. The second heart sound is diminished and there is an early diastolic murmur that radiates from the right sternal border to the apex. Your clinical diagnosis is aortic regurgitation.

86. A 64-year-old man with two previous MIs develops shortness of breath at rest and has difficulty lying down. His blood pressure is 95/70 mm Hg, pulse 100/min, and JVP is 8 cm. The cardiac apex is dilated and displaced laterally, heart sounds are normal, but there is a soft third heart sound. Your clinical diagnosis is ischemic cardiomyopathy.

87. An 18-year-old man notices occasional lightheadedness when standing up quickly. He also has difficulty playing sports because of easy fatigue and shortness of breath. Examination reveals normal heart sounds, but a loud systolic ejection murmur at the right sternal border. The murmur decreases with elevating the legs and increases in the standing position. Your clinical diagnosis is hypertrophic cardiomyopathy (HOCM).

88. A 76-year-old woman presents with new-onset syncope. She has also noticed early fatigue on exertion for the past year. On examination, there is a systolic ejection murmur at the right sternal border that radiates to the carotids. Your clinical diagnosis is aortic stenosis.

89. A 62-year-old man with a 40-pack/year history of smoking presents with increased sputum production and marked SOB. On examination, he is using accessory muscles of respiration, and breath sounds are diminished with expiratory wheezes. Your clinical diagnosis is chronic obstructive pulmonary disease (COPD) exacerbation.

Questions 90 through 94: For each of the following cardiac abnormalities, select the characteristic JVP finding.

(A) Cannon *a* wave
(B) prominent *x* descent
(C) Kussmaul sign
(D) slow *y* descent
(E) prominent *v* waves
(F) positive abdominojugular reflux

90. Tricuspid regurgitation.

91. Right atrial myxoma.

92. Right ventricular infarction.

93. Right-sided heart failure.

94. Complete heart block.

Questions 95 through 99: For each patient with a systolic murmur, select the most likely diagnosis.

(A) aortic stenosis
(B) hypertrophic obstructive cardiomyopathy (HOCM)
(C) mitral regurgitation (chronic)
(D) tricuspid regurgitation
(E) mitral valve prolapse
(F) pulmonary stenosis

95. A 25-year-old woman is found to have a midsystolic murmur on routine evaluation. The murmur does not radiate but it does increase with standing. She otherwise feels well and the rest of the examination is normal.

96. A 75-year-old man is bought to the hospital because of a syncopal episode. There was no incontinence or post-event confusion. On examination, his blood pressure is 140/80 mm Hg, pulse 72/min with no postural changes. His second heart sound is diminished and there is a systolic ejection murmur that radiates to the carotids. With the Valsalva maneuver, the murmur decreases in length and intensity.

97. A 22-year-old woman with no past medical history is found to have a systolic ejection murmur on routine physical examination. She has no symptoms and feels well. The murmur is heard along the right and left sternal borders and it decreases with handgrip exercises.

98. A 45-year-old woman has developed increasing shortness of breath on exertion and fatigue. She has a loud systolic ejection murmur heard best at the left sternal border, and the murmur increases with standing. A double apical impulse is also felt.

99. A 65-year-old man with a previous history of an anterior MI comes for follow-up. On examination, he has a systolic murmur heard best at the apex and radiating to the axilla. Transient external compression of both arms with blood pressure cuffs 20 mm Hg over peak systolic pressure increases the murmur.

Questions 100 through 105: For each patient with shortness of breath and peripheral edema, select the most likely diagnosis.

(A) cardiac tamponade
(B) constrictive pericarditis
(C) restrictive cardiomyopathy
(D) right ventricle myocardial infarction (RVMI)

100. A 56-year-old man presents with shortness of breath, fatigue, and edema. He has also noticed weight gain, abdominal discomfort, and distension. He has a prior history of lung cancer treated with radiotherapy to the chest. There is no history of liver or cardiac disease in the past. On examination, he has an elevated JVP, prominent y descent of neck veins, and positive Kussmaul sign. The heart sounds are normal. The CXR shows a normal cardiac silhouette and the ECG has low voltages.

101. A 28-year-old woman recently developed symptoms of chest pain that changed with positioning. It was worse when lying down and relieved when sitting up. The pain is better now but she notices increasing dyspnea and edema. On examination, the blood pressure is 85/60 mm Hg with a positive pulsus paradoxus, low volume pulse at 110/min, and the

heart sounds are distant. The JVP is at 7 cm with a negative Kussmaul's sign. There are low voltages on the ECG, and a large cardiac silhouette on the CXR.

102. A 69-year-old woman complains of some atypical chest pain 2 days prior to presentation. On examination, the JVP is at 8 cm, positive Kussmaul sign, and normal heart sounds. The lungs are clear. The ECG is abnormal, and the CXR shows a normal cardiac silhouette.

103. A 55-year-old woman with metastatic lung cancer presents with dyspnea and pedal edema. On examination, the JVP is at 10 cm, with a negative Kussmaul sign. The heart sounds are diminished and the lungs have bibasilar crackles. The ECG shows QRS complexes of variable height.

104. A 64-year-old presents with dyspnea and edema. He had previous coronary bypass surgery 5 years ago, which was uncomplicated. Since then he has had no further chest pain. On examination, his JVP is at 8 cm, with prominent Kussmaul's sign. The heart sounds are easily heard but there is an early diastolic filling sound (pericardial knock).

105. A 55-year-old woman is recently diagnosed with amyloidosis. She is now noticing increasing shortness of breath, fatigue, and edema. On examination, the JVP is at 10 cm with a negative Kussmaul's sign but prominent x and y descent. The blood pressure is 90/70 mm Hg, no pulsus paradoxus, pulse 100/min with low volume, and normal heart sounds.

Questions 106 through 110: For each patient with systemic disease, select the most typical cardiovascular involvement.

(A) focal myocardial necrosis
(B) proximal aortitis
(C) endothelial plaques
(D) systolic scratchy sound
(E) restrictive cardiomyopathy

106. A 45-year-old man develops new symptoms of sudden-onset flushing involving his head and neck lasting a few minutes. He also notices watery diarrhea and abdominal pain when the flushing occurs. Serotonin and its metabolites are elevated in his urine and serum.

107. A 25-year-old man has noticed increasing lower-back and gluteal pain. It is dull and associated with morning stiffness lasting 1 hour, and then it improves after activity. On examination, there are no active inflammatory joints but he has limited forward and lateral flexion of the lumbar spine, as well as decreased chest expansion. X-rays of his pelvis and lumbar spine show changes of sacroiliitis.

108. A 31-year-old woman has new-onset headaches and blood pressure elevation. She also notices that the symptoms come episodically and consist of palpitations, headache, anxiety, and marked blood pressure elevation. She undergoes a workup for secondary causes of hypertension, and is found to have elevated free catecholamines in her urine.

109. A 22-year-old university student notices unintentional weight loss and palpitations for 1 month. She also complains of sweating and feeling hot all the time. On examination, her pulse is regular at 110/min and blood pressure 96/60 mm Hg; she has a diffuse enlargement of the thyroid gland. Her thyroid-stimulating hormone (TSH) is low and free T3 and T4 are elevated.

110. A 60-year-old man presents with shortness of breath, increasing abdominal distention, and lower leg edema. He has no prior history of cardiac, renal, or liver disease. On examination, the JVP is at 8 cm with a negative Kussmaul sign but prominent x and y descent. The blood pressure is 95/75 mm Hg, no pulsus paradoxus, pulse 100/min with low volume, and normal heart sounds. There is shifting dullness of the abdomen and pedal edema. His blood glucose and hemoglobin A1C are elevated.

Questions 111 through 116: For each patient with dyslipidemia, select the most appropriate treatment.

   (A) fibric acid derivatives (clofibrate, gemfibrozil)

   (B) nicotinic acid

   (C) bile acid-binding resins (cholestyramine, colestipol)

   (D) hepatic hydroxymethylglutarylcoenzyme A (HMG-CoA) reductase inhibitors (lovastatin, simvastatin, pravastatin)

   (E) lifestyle modification

   (F) estrogens (Premarin, estradiol)

111. A 63-year-old woman with Type 2 diabetes is seen for follow-up after a fasting lipid profile. She has no other medical conditions and feels well. Her diabetes is well controlled and the last hemoglobin A1C value was 6.5%. Her total cholesterol (T-chol) is 240 mg/dL, HDL 50 mg/dL, low-density lipoprotein (LDL) 160 mg/dL, and triglycerides 150 mg/dL.

112. A 42-year-old woman, who is an executive at a large company, is seen for her annual evaluation. She is concerned about her risk for future cardiac events since a colleague was just diagnosed with angina. She has no other medical illness and is a lifetime nonsmoker. Her fasting lipid profile is T-chol 240 mg/dL, HDL 55 mg/dL, LDL 160 mg/dL, and triglycerides 140 mg/dL.

113. A 57-year-old man comes to see you for follow-up 4 weeks after being discharged from hospital for unstable angina. His coronary angiogram showed moderate nonstenotic disease in two vessels. The cardiologist asks you to follow up on his fasting lipid profile since it was not checked in the hospital. His T-chol is 240 mg/dL, LDL 120 mg/dL, HDL 50 mg/dL, and triglycerides 130 mg/dL.

114. A 58-year-old woman is admitted to hospital with left-sided hemiparesis. She is diagnosed with an ischemic right cortical stroke, and started on aminosalicylic acid (ASA) for secondary prevention. Her carotid ultrasound reveals no arterial stenosis. She has no other significant past medical history but she does smoke half pack a day. Her fasting lipid profile is T-chol 240 mg/dL, HDL 50 mg/dL, LDL 160 mg/dL, and triglycerides 130 mg/dL.

115. A 56-year-old man is diagnosed with the *metabolic syndrome*, which consists of hypertension, insulin resistance, dyslipidemia, and abdominal obesity. He has no prior history of cardiac or vascular disease and is otherwise well. His fasting T-chol is 270 mg/dL, HDL 50 mg/dL, LDL 150 mg/dL, and triglycerides 150 mg/dL. His Framingham risk calculation approximates a 10-year risk for cardiac events of 10%–20%.

116. A 60-year-old woman is concerned about her risk for cardiovascular disease since she is post-menopausal now. She has no symptoms of cardiac or vascular disease and her only cardiac risk factor is hypertension for the past 5 years, which is well controlled. Her fasting T-chol is 240 mg/dL, HDL 55 mg/dL, LDL 160 mg/dL, and triglycerides 140 mg/dL.

Questions 117 through 121: For each patient with high blood pressure, select the most appropriate medication.

   (A) thiazides

   (B) spironolactone

   (C) clonidine

   (D) prazosin

   (E) beta-blockers

   (F) hydralazine

   (G) ACE inhibitors

   (H) calcium channel blockers

117. A 54-year-old man with diabetes has a persistently elevated blood pressure averaging 150/90 mm Hg. He has complications of peripheral neuropathy and a urinalysis is positive for microalbuminuria.

118. A 60-year-old woman with no past medical history has an elevated blood pressure of 165/80 mm Hg on routine evaluation. Repeated measurements over the next month confirm the elevated pressure. Physical examination, routine blood count, and biochemistry are all normal.

119. A 26-year-old woman develops new-onset hypertension. She has no other medical problems and is not taking any medications. She undergoes an evaluation for secondary hypertension and is found to have unilateral renal artery stenosis.

120. A 70-year-old man has isolated systolic hypertension. On examination, his blood pressure is 170/80 mm Hg and heart and lungs are normal. He has no other medical conditions.

121. A 57-year-old man has a blood pressure of 155/90 mm Hg on routine evaluation. He had coronary artery bypass grafting 4 years earlier, after which he has had no further chest pain. The rest of the examination is normal, and the elevated blood pressure is confirmed on 2 repeat visits.

Answers and Explanations

1. **(D)** Wenckebach, or Mobitz type I second-degree AV block, is characterized on ECG by progressive lengthening of the PR interval until there is a nonconducted P wave. The magnitude of PR lengthening declines with each beat, so the RR intervals characteristically shorten prior to the dropped beat. It is almost always caused by abnormal conduction across the AV node, and the QRS complex is usually of normal duration.

   Progressive PR shortening is incorrect as the PR interval increases in Mobitz type I, and this type of arrhythmia results in bradycardia, and not tachycardia. When the AV block is 2:1 it is difficult to distinguish type I from type II block. *(Fauci, Chapter 225)*

2. **(D)** The ventricular inhibited (VVI) pacemaker functions when the heart rate falls below a preset interval. If a QRS is detected, the pacemaker is inhibited. If a QRS is not sensed, the pacing stimulus is not inhibited and the ventricle is stimulated. Pacemaker modes and function are named using a 5-letter code. The first letter indicates the chamber(s) that is paced (O, none; A, atrium; V, ventricle; D, dual; S, single), the second is the chamber(s) in which sensing occurs (O, none; A, atrium; V, ventricle; D, dual; S, single), the third is the response to a sensed event (O, none; I, inhibition; T, triggered; D, inhibition + triggered), the fourth letter refers to the programmability or rate response (R, rate responsive), and the fifth refers to the existence of antitachycardia functions if present (O, none; P, antitachycardia pacing; S, shock; D, pace + shock). Almost all modern pacemakers are multiprogrammable and have the capability for rate responsiveness using one of several rate sensors: activity or motion, minute ventilation, or QT interval. The most commonly programmed modes of implanted single- and dual-chamber pacemakers are VVIR and DDDR, respectively, although multiple modes can be programmed in modern pacemakers. *(Fauci, Chapter 225)*

3. **(D)** Sinus tachycardia is the most common ECG finding in pulmonary embolism. The specific ECG signs of pulmonary embolism such as the S1, Q3, T3 are rarely seen except in cases of massive pulmonary embolism. In submassive pulmonary emboli, the ECG may show nonspecific ST changes and sinus tachycardia.

   On occasion, pulmonary embolism can precipitate atrial flutter or fibrillation. One of the most useful roles of the ECG is to rule out MI when a massive embolism is present. *(Fauci, Chapter 256)*

4. **(C)** The radiation of this patient's systolic ejection murmur, diminished second heart sound, and radiation to the carotids are all suggestive of aortic stenosis. Aortic stenosis is most likely to be associated with angina pectoris, syncope, and exertional dyspnea. Exertional syncope is caused by either systemic vasodilation in the presence of fixed or inadequate cardiac output, an arrhythmia, or both. Syncope at rest is most frequently a result of a transient ventricular tachyarrhythmia.

   While regurgitant valvular lesions (aortic or mitral insufficiency) can also have a systolic ejection murmur as well due to the increased stroke volume, the diminished carotid upstroke and radiation of the murmur to the carotids is more in keeping with this patient having aortic stenosis. *(Fauci, Chapter 230)*

5. **(C)** Common findings in infective endocarditis include petechiae, Roth spots, Osler nodes, Janeway lesions, splinter hemorrhages, stroke, and infarction of viscera, or extremities.

Many of the complications are thought to be embolic but may include vasculitis. Autopsy studies reveal that many systemic emboli go unrecognized. Brain, lung, coronary arteries, spleen, extremities, gut, and eyes are common locations for emboli. *(Fauci, Chapter 118)*

6. **(B)** The slow channel for calcium assumes considerable importance in the region of the sinus node and AV node. For diltiazem, this results in both antiarrhythmic and negative inotropic effects. Different classes of calcium channel blockers have differential effects on these slow channels, explaining the different clinical properties of the various calcium-channel-blocking drugs.

The other medications listed do not have any effect on the slow calcium channel. *(Fauci, Chapter 224)*

7. **(D)** Pericarditis secondary to transmural infarction is very common and most cases appear within 4 days. The most common manifestation of pericarditis is a friction rub along the left sternal border. It is evanescent, lasting only a few days. The pain is usually perceived by the patient to be different than that of the infarct. It is worsened by inspiration, swallowing, coughing, or lying down. It frequently is associated with a low-grade fever. While re-infarction is a possibility, the repeat ECG does not support the diagnosis. The diffuse ST-segment elevation (not in an arterial territory) and PR-segment depression are both characteristic ECG features of pericarditis. The diagnosis of pulmonary embolus and aortic dissection are not supported by the clinical history and ECG changes which are characteristic of pericarditis. *(Fauci, Chapter 232)*

8. **(A)** Calcium plays a role in excitation–contraction coupling, and in drug effects and heart failure. *(Fauci, Chapter 217)*

9. **(C)** This patient has preeclampsia and needs treatment of her hypertension and close follow-up. In the past, there was concern that rigorous drug treatment would harm the fetus. Approximately 5%–7% of all pregnant women develop preeclampsia which is defined as new-onset hypertension with BP> 140/90 mmHg and proteinuria > 300 mg/24h after 20 weeks of gestation.

Studies now show benefit in controlling blood pressure with drugs, but ACE inhibitors and angiotensin receptor blockers (ARB) are contraindicated because they cause renal abnormalities in the fetus. Women who develop hypertension during pregnancy have a higher risk of developing hypertension in later life.

Preeclampsia does not improve during the third trimester, it leads to premature birth or low-birth-weight babies, and injures the placenta. *(Fauci, Chapter 7)*

10. **(E)** There is a possible indication (but not an obligation) to insert a temporary pacemaker if a new LBBB occurs. If LBBB and a Mobitz type II AV block occur, there is general agreement on the usefulness of pacing. Temporary pacemaker is not required for first-degree block.

For second-degree block of the Wenckebach type (usually with an inferior infarction), pacing is only required if symptoms of bradycardia and hypotension cannot be controlled medically. The necessity for temporary pacing during an acute myocardial infarction (AMI) does not necessarily indicate that permanent pacing will be required. *(Fauci, Chapter 225)*

11. **(D)** Pulmonary hypertension is associated with an increased intensity of the second heart sound, which coincides with the end of the T wave on ECG. It is the pulmonic component of the second heart sound that is increased. Pulmonary stenosis or aortic stenosis can cause dyspnea on exertion but auscultation will reveal a systolic murmur and decreased second heart sound (pulmonic component or aortic component). The normal apical impulse and absence of left-sided heart failure make cardiomyopathy less likely as the cause for his dyspnea.

As well, there may be prominent *a* waves in the jugular venous pulse, a right ventricular heave, an ejection click, and a right ventricular fourth heart sound. When signs and symptoms are apparent, the pulmonary hypertension is usually moderate to severe. *(Fauci, Chapter 244)*

12. **(D)** The patient most likely has PSVT, since the tachycardia terminates after carotid sinus massage (CSM). CSM increases vagal tone (parasympathetic) which decreases AV nodal conduction and terminates AV node re-entry arrhythmias. Sinus tachycardia differs from PSVT tachycardia in that it does not start or stop abruptly; it will slow down with CSM but will resume the previous rate once the maneuver is stopped. In PSVT, the QRS is usually narrow without clearly discernible P waves. The ECG does not support the other answers, since ventricular tachycardia is a regular wide complex rhythm, atrial flutter can be a regular narrow complex tachycardia but usually atrial flutter waves are seen, and finally atrial fibrillation is an irregular rhythm with no atrial activity. A wide QRS in PSVT can result from a preexisting bundle branch block, or a functional bundle branch block secondary to the tachycardia. This can make the distinction from a ventricular arrhythmia quite difficult. *(Fauci, Chapter 226)*

13. **(D)** In the absence of critical CAD, angina pectoris occurs most frequently with aortic stenosis. *(Fauci, Chapter 230)*

14. **(B)** In aortic stenosis, the first sound is usually normal; the second sound is characteristically diminished because of the increased ventricular pressure and the stenotic valve is less mobile. There can be a single S2 either because A2 and P2 are superimposed, or A2 is absent or very soft. Severe aortic stenosis may be accompanied by paradoxical splitting of S2. *(Fauci, Chapter 230)*

15. **(B)** AV dissociation is the independent beating of atria and ventricles, and is recognized on the ECG by fixed PP and RR intervals but variable PR intervals. Surgical removal of the atria would result in no atrial activity (absence of p waves) seen on the ECG; re-entry phenomenon can cause retrograde p waves and a fixed PR interval, and finally AV dissociation can

result from a drug side effect but not amlodipine which has no effect on the AV node, unlike metoprolol.

AV block is one cause of AV dissociation. *(Fauci, Chapter 225)*

16. **(E)** Nitroglycerine is usually used in the setting of severe pulmonary congestion with adequate blood pressure. With significant hypotension, inotropic agents are generally administered prior to nitroglycerine. *(Fauci, Chapter 239)*

17. **(A)** A ventricular septal defect is considered a relatively high-risk lesion for infective endocarditis.

Mitral valve prolapse with regurgitation, asymmetric septal hypertrophy, and pure mitral stenosis are considered an intermediate risk. Atrial septal defects of the secundum type are considered low risk. *(Fauci, Chapter 118)*

18. **(A)** The myxoma is a solitary globular or polypoid tumor varying in size from that of a cherry to a peach. About 75% are found in the left atrium, and most of the remainder in the right atrium. The clinical presentation is with one or more of the classical triad of constitution symptoms (fatigue, fever, anemia), embolic events, or obstruction of the valve orifice.

Sarcomas are the most common malignant tumors of the heart but are usually seen on the right side, while rhabdomyomas and fibromas are more commonly seen in children, and usually occur in the ventricles. *(Fauci, Chapter 233)*

19. **(A)** Diltiazem and verapamil may be of help in both acute paroxysms of atrial flutter and chronic management. The other choices have no effect on the AV node to slow down flutter, and atropine accelerates AV conduction. At times, catheter ablation of the flutter pathway is required in chronic atrial flutter. Surgical ablation is reserved for cases where other surgical interventions are required. *(Fauci, Chapter 226)*

20. **(C)** Exercise electrocardiography represents an increasingly popular noninvasive method for early detection of latent ischemic heart disease.

As with other diagnostic tests, the exercise ECG is of most clinical value when the pretest probability of disease is moderate (ie, 30%–70%). In men over 40 and women over 50 who plan to start vigorous exercise and have other cardiovascular risk factors, the use of exercise ECG is possible to screen for latent coronary artery disease. *(Fauci, Chapter 237)*

21. **(D)** Contrast media used in cardiac catheterization may result in renal impairment. The group at highest risk includes diabetics with renal disease and those with preexisting renal failure. Good hydration is essential. Other manifestations of contrast media include nausea and vomiting (common), and anaphylactoid reactions characterized by low-grade fever, hives, itching, angioedema, bronchospasm, and even shock. Side effects are reduced with the use of new low osmolality contrast media. *(Fauci, Chapter 223)*

22. **(E)** Pericarditis in clinical practice is commonly idiopathic and frequently assumed to be of possible viral origin. Coxsackieviruses are a common cause, but herpes viruses are not. Although TB, rheumatic fever, and MI can cause pericarditis, they are unlikely in this case given the prodrome of a viral illness prior to onset of symptoms. *(Fauci, Chapter 232)*

23. **(C)** The "wedge" pressure is an approximation of the pressure in the left atrium. Left-heart catheterization is a more accurate measurement, but involves a slightly increased risk and it is not measured directly. End-expiratory PA diastolic pressure is very close (2–4 mm) to wedge pressure as well. A discordance between wedge pressure and PA diastolic pressure suggests the presence of pulmonary hypertension. *(Fauci, Chapter 246)*

24. **(C)** CT scan of the chest is most efficient and rapid method of establishing the diagnosis of aortic dissection in the emergency room. Aortic dissection is a medical emergency requiring prompt attention. Other cardiac and pulmonary causes of chest pain can be quickly ruled out with ECG and CXR. CT scan of the chest is sensitive (93%–100%) in ruling out

dissection. Transesophageal echocardiography is equally as sensitive but not a transthoracic echo. The ease and rapidity of obtaining a CT scan at any time of the day makes it the imaging modality of choice. *(Fauci, Chapter 242)*

25. **(A)** Increased pulmonary blood flow is characteristic of an atrial septal defect (ASD). Pulmonary blood flow is greater because of increased blood flow from the right atrium, which receives blood from the vena cava and left atrium (left to right shunting). When severe pulmonary hypertension develops (late finding) only then will pulmonary blood flow be equal to or less than systemic blood flow. The left ventricle is usually normal in ASD, but with worsening pulmonary hypertension the right ventricle will enlarge. *(Fauci, Chapter 229)*

26. **(B)** Angina or infarction in young patients should prompt the physician to consider congenital coronary artery anomaly or congenital coronary artery aneurysm. Acquired coronary artery aneurysm can be caused by atherosclerosis, trauma, angioplasty, atherectomy, vasculitis, mycotic emboli, Kawasaki syndrome, or arterial dissection.

   The other valvular lesions such as mitral stenosis, coarctation, and atrial septal defect do not result in typical angina-type symptoms. Despite the patient's young age it should not lead to the diagnosis that this is noncardiac chest pain since the symptoms are so stereotypical of angina. *(Fauci, Chapter 237)*

27. **(D)** This patient has aortic regurgitation based on the diastolic murmur (from the valve incompetence), systolic murmur (from large stroke volume), and carotid pulse findings. This pulse pattern is seen in aortic regurgitation, and is known as a water hammer or Corrigan pulse. A bisferiens pulse (in the bisferiens wave form there are two pressure peaks) may be present as well. The blood pressure in diastole is usually low (because of the aortic insufficiency) and the systolic blood pressure is elevated (because of the large stroke volume) resulting in a large pulse pressure. The other valvular lesions may cause either a systolic (mitral regurgitation or aortic stenosis) or diastolic (mitral stenosis)

murmur, but none of them will result in the carotid pulse physical findings and large pulse pressure as seen in this patient. *(Fauci, Chapter 230)*

28. **(B)** This patient's ECG is characteristic of digoxin toxicity and the digoxin should be discontinued. Digoxin toxicity may cause any dysrhythmia. Classically, dysrhythmias that are associated with increased automaticity and decreased AV conduction occur (ie, paroxysmal atrial tachycardia with 2:1 block, accelerated junctional rhythm, or bidirectional ventricular tachycardia [torsade de pointes]). Sinus bradycardia and other bradyarrhythmias are very common. Slow atrial fibrillation with very little variation in the ventricular rate (regularization of the RR interval) may occur. This arrhythmia is likely slow atrial fibrillation. Symptoms of digitalis toxicity include anorexia, nausea, fatigue, dizziness, and visual disturbances. The presence of hypokalemia increases the likelihood of digitalis toxicity. The addition of a beta-blocker or calcium channel blocker is not appropriate at this time given the patient's slow heart rate. Once the effects of the digoxin have worn off and a rate-controlling drug is required for her atrial fibrillation then one of these two agents may be considered rather than digoxin given her chronic kidney disease. *(Fauci, Chapter 225)*

29. **(A)** This patient has chronic constrictive pericarditis. Rheumatic fever does not cause pericarditis. Usually, no cause is found for constrictive pericarditis. Some patients do give a history of previous acute pericarditis. TB is now an uncommon cause, but metastatic spread of cancer to the pericardium can cause constriction. *(Fauci, Chapter 232)*

30. **(E)** Electrical cardioversion is the method of choice in patients who are hemodynamically unstable. Often, very low amounts of energy during cardioversion will convert atrial flutter. The other maneuvers listed increase AV blockade and are useful for diagnosis, but not for converting the atrial flutter to sinus rhythm *(Fauci, Chapter 226)*

31. **(C)** It is now known that the predominant mechanism for atrial flutter is right atrial macro-reentry with circular activation. Atrial flutter typically originates from the right atrium and most often involves a large circuit that travels around the area of the tricuspid valve. This type of atrial flutter is referred to as typical atrial flutter. Less commonly, atrial flutter can result from circuits in other areas of the right or left atrium. Atrial flutter is characterized by regular atrial activation with an atrial rate of >240 beats/min. The ventricular response depends on the conduction of the AV node; usually there is 2:1 or 3:1 conduction. *(Fauci, Chapter 226)*

32. **(B)** Aldosterone, renin, and vasopressin are generally increased in heart failure. Retention of fluid is complex and not due to any one factor; however, hormones may contribute. Growth hormone does not have fluid-retaining properties. The exact mechanisms that initiate renal conservation of salt and water are not precisely understood, but may include arterial volume receptors sensing a decrease in the *effective* arterial blood volume that occurs in heart failure. *(Fauci, Chapter 227)*

33. **(A)** ST elevation persisting 2 weeks after an infarct, an abnormal pericardial impulse, and a bulge on the left ventricular border on x-ray are characteristic of an aneurysm. Ventricular aneurysms are most often a result of a large anterior infarct. The poor prognosis associated with these aneurysms is due to the associated left ventricular dysfunction, rather than to the aneurysm itself.

Acute infarction is associated with chest pain which this patient did not have, and early repolarization changes are seen in young healthy patients and they usually don't have Q waves on the ECG or physical exam finding of a dilated left ventricle. Finally, hibernating myocardium is usual seen in non-Q-wave MIs where there may be residual myocardium that is still viable. *(Fauci, Chapter 239)*

34. **(D)** This patient has aortic stenosis based on the clinical history and characteristic findings on physical examination such as the systolic

murmur and diminished carotid upstroke. In aortic stenosis, there is normal or increased overall cardiac size, and dilatation of the proximal ascending aorta, not stenosis. *(Fauci, Chapter 230)*

35. **(D)** This combination has the lowest risk, although the total cholesterol is on borderline, the high HDL cholesterol is protective. *(Fauci, Chapter 350)*

36. **(B)** Coarctation is the third most common form of congenital cardiac disease. One-third of the patients will be hypertensive. The femoral pulses are weak, delayed, and even absent. Besides coarctation of the aorta, aortic occlusive disease, dissection of the aorta, and abdominal aneurysm may lead to differential blood pressure in arms and legs. The other answers listed will not result in the clinical findings described in this patient. *(Fauci, Chapter 229)*

37. **(D)** He likely has LVH based on the long history of hypertension, and physical findings.

    ECG changes of LVH include left axis deviation (not right axis), high-voltage QRS complexes in V5 and V6, deep S waves in V1 and V2, and prolonged QRS in the left precordial leads. PR interval prolongation is not a feature of LVH. Age, orientation of the heart in the chest, and noncardiac factors make the ECG an imperfect tool for diagnosing or excluding LVH. *(Fauci, Chapter 221)*

38. **(A)** Low urinary sodium content is usually seen in patients with untreated HF. High urinary specific gravity, nocturia, and daytime oliguria also occur in patients with HF. These changes are the result of the activation of the renin-angiotensin-aldosterone system. Proteinuria or rbc casts are not a usual feature of HF unless there is concomitant renal disease. *(Fauci, Chapter 227)*

39. **(C)** Atrial fibrillation is particularly common in older individuals with hyperthyroidism. Thyroid disease may affect the heart muscle directly or there may be excessive sympathetic stimulation. Common symptoms of thyrotoxic heart disease include palpitations, exertional dyspnea, and worsening angina. Pericardial effusion, and aortic insufficiency are not usual finding in thyrotoxicosis, and the cardiac output is increased in hyperthyroidism, not decreased. *(Fauci, Chapter 335)*

40. **(D)** A discussion about the risks and benefits of anticoagulation is the most appropriate next management step for this patient, in addition to investigating why she has developed atrial fibrillation. Since the duration of atrial fibrillation is not known, it is presumed to be chronic. There is an increased risk of cardioembolic events if restoration of sinus rhythm is attempted before anticoagulating the patient for 3–4 weeks so cardioversion and antiarrhythmic therapy are not appropriate choices. Aspirin is only modestly effective in reducing cardioembolic events and not the first choice. Beta-blockers are not indicated since the rate is controlled (indicating she has underlying AV nodal disease). *(Fauci, Chapter 226)*

41. **(B)** Cotton-wool spots (nerve fiber layer infarcts), flame hemorrhage, and papilledema can occur in patients with accelerated hypertension. Fibrinoid necrosis occurs on the arterioles of many organs. Earlier manifestations of arteriosclerosis include thickening of the retinal vessel wall. This is manifested by obscuring of the venous column at arterial crossings. The other choices are not seen in hypertensive retinopathy. *(Fauci, Chapter 29)*

42. **(A)** Tendon xanthomas, xanthelasma, and arcus senilis are characteristics of familial hypercholesterolemia. The disorder is inherited in an autosomal dominant manner. Tendon xanthomas and xanthelasma are not seen in patients with diabetes, myxedema, or chronic kidney disease unless they have concomitant familial hyperlipidemia. *(Fauci, Chapter 350)*

43. **(C)** Acute pericarditis is most often idiopathic and is typically self-limited (usually within 2–6 weeks). While small effusions are common, tamponade is unusual, as are heart failure and constriction. Other diseases causing pericarditis should be searched for, and may influence the prognosis. *(Fauci, Chapter 232)*

44. (D) Orthostatic hypotension (systolic dropping by 20 mm or more) is particularly common in the elderly and in diabetics because of autonomic neuropathy. Management includes avoidance of precipitating factors, simple adaptive maneuvers, volume expansion, and pharmacologic agents. While thyrotoxicosis, volume depletion from diuretic therapy and venous varicosities can result in a postural drop in blood pressure, the autonomic response will cause an increase in heart rate. *(Fauci, Chapter 370)*

45. (E) In mitral valve prolapse, the first heart sound is usually preserved followed by a systolic click and late systolic murmur. The click is actually the most common finding. General physical examination may reveal scoliosis, pectus excavatum, straightened thoracic spine, or narrow anteroposterior diameter of chest. *(Fauci, Chapter 230)*

46. (A) The symptoms and signs are like any sudden paroxysmal tachycardia, but the ventricular rate is the clue to the diagnosis of atrial flutter with 2:1 block. Paroxysmal tachycardia with a pulse rate close to 150/min is very suggestive of atrial flutter with 2:1 block, and the most likely diagnosis to rule out on the ECG. In this case, a rate change to 100/min with CSM is due to 3:1 block. *(Fauci, Chapter 226)*

47. (C) Careful observation for increasing effusion and tamponade are essential in patients with acute pericarditis. The classic findings of cardiac tamponade include arterial hypotension and pulsus paradoxus. Management of acute viral or idiopathic pericarditis includes analgesia (usually aspirin every 3–4 hours initially) and rest if the pain is severe. Occasionally, nonsteroidal anti-inflammatory drugs (NSAIDs) are required (eg, ibuprofen or indomethacin). The other choices are less likely as the clinical scenario and ECG are characteristic of acute pericarditis, and not of pulmonary embolism, or myocardial infarction. Rupture of a chordae tendineae can lead to acute mitral regurgitation and pulmonary edema, but the absence of a holosystolic murmur makes this unlikely. *(Fauci, Chapter 232)*

48. (B) Diastolic dysfunction is an important cause of heart failure in the elderly. It is commonly associated with a history of hypertension and diabetes. Normal ejection fraction and aortic sclerosis rule out either systolic or valvular heart disease as causes. In HOCM there is nonconcentric hypertrophy. *(Fauci, Chapter 227)*

49. (A) Acute rupture of an atherosclerotic plaque is now recognized as the most common cause of ST-elevation MI. Pericarditis has diffuse ST elevation in multiple leads and aortic stenosis does cause angina but not ST elevation on the ECG. Vasculitis is a very rare and unusual cause of coronary ischemia and therefore unlikely. Myocarditis does not cause ST-segment elevation. *(Fauci, Chapter 238)*

50. (D) *S. epidermidis* is still the most frequent early and late cause of endocarditis in patients with prosthetic heart valves. The other organisms are seen less frequently in late prosthetic valve endocarditis. *(Fauci, Chapter 118)*

51. (D) This man has acute coronary syndrome (ACS) until proven otherwise. The ECG is the most useful initial investigation since it identifies individuals with ST-segment elevation who may be candidates for either thrombolysis or primary angioplasty (PCI). The troponins are important in diagnosing myocardial necrosis. The other investigations may be important in looking for alternate causes of chest pain once ST-elevation MI has been ruled out. *(Fauci, Chapter 238)*

52. (C) Essential hypertension is the most likely diagnosis. A secondary cause for hypertension is found in only 5%–10% of patients, with 90%–95% labeled as essential hypertension. Current recommendations for initial workup of a hypertensive patient include serum chemistry (glucose, potassium, creatinine), urinalysis, and ECG. Her positive family history of hypertension also makes essential hypertension the most likely diagnosis in her.

The normal potassium and bicarbonate (TCO2) level make renal artery stenosis and an endocrine cause of hypertension such as Cushing or primary aldosteronism unlikely.

Stimulation of the rennin-aldosterone system in renal artery stenosis will cause similar biochemical changes in the electrolytes. *(Fauci, Chapter 221)*

53. **(C)** Coarctation of the aorta is the diagnosis.

There is a *reverse 3* deformity of the esophagus, the belly of which represents the dilated aorta after the coarctation. The border of the descending aorta shows a medial indentation called the *3* or *tuck* sign, the belly of the *3* representing the poststenotic dilation and the upper portion by the dilated subclavian artery and small transverse aortic arch. *(Fauci, Chapter 229)*

54. **(B)** Note the abnormal humped contour of the left ventricular border, with a curvilinear calcification following the abnormal cardiac contour. The presence of calcification in the ventricular wall and the abnormal left ventricular contour alerts one to the consideration of a ventricular aneurysm. Calcific pericarditis will not have calcification in the ventricle as seen in this CXR, and while pericardial effusion and LVH can cause an enlarged cardiac silhouette on the CXR, it does not cause an abnormal contour of the left ventricle or calcification. *(Fauci, Chapter 239)*

55. **(B)** The cardiac rhythm is atrial flutter with 2:1 AV conduction. QRS complexes occur with perfect regularity at a rate of about 150/min. Their normal contour and duration indicate that ventricular activation occurs normally via the AV junction–His-Purkinje system. Flutter waves, regular ventricular rate at 150/min make the diagnosis of atrial flutter, rather than atrial fibrillation, sinus tachycardia, or ectopic atrial tachycardia. *(Fauci, Chapter 226)*

56. **(B)** The PR interval of the first two complexes is normal at 0.20 seconds. The QRS duration is 0.16 seconds. The third P wave is nonconducted. This cycle recurs in the remainder of the strip. This is second-degree heart block of the Mobitz type II variety. Note the wide QRS. When this type of heart block develops, either de novo or in the course of an AMI, a cardiac pacemaker is usually recommended, as the incidence of complete heart block is high in this situation.

In first-degree heart block the PR interval is longer than 0.20 s, it does not change, and there are no dropped beats. In third-degree heart block there is no relationship between the atrial and ventricular rate. *(Fauci, Chapter 225)*

57. **(D)** The ST is depressed in leads II, III, aVF, and V4–V6. These nonspecific abnormalities do not indicate significant coronary heart disease, especially in a young patient with no cardiovascular risk factors. Further evaluations should be guided by clinical circumstances. *(Fauci, Chapter 221)*

58. **(E)** The underlying rhythm is a regular sinus rhythm, interrupted by regular wide QRS complex beats that terminate after 3 beats. This is non-sustained ventricular tachycardia that is frequently seen in acute MI when reperfusion of the infarct artery occurs.

The regular wide QRS complex beats and the lack of atrial activity preceding them rule out atrial flutter and atrial fibrillation.

59. **(A)** No atrial activity is detected. The ventricular rate is slightly irregular. Beat number 4 is a ventricular premature contraction. The T waves are tall and markedly peaked. This type of T wave is characteristic of hyperkalemia, as is the absence of visible atrial activity.

Hypercalcemia causes abbreviation of the ST segment and shortening of the QT interval, which are not seen in this ECG. The ECG changes are not that of pericarditis (diffuse ST segment elevation and PR segment depression) or ventricular aneurysm (persistent ST segment elevation in the anterior leads more than 4 weeks after an anterior MI).

The potassium level was 8.2 mmol/L. *(Fauci, Chapter 221)*

60. **(A)** Sudden death, defined as death within 1 hour of onset of symptoms, is usually caused by cardiac disease in middle-aged and elderly patients, but in younger age groups noncardiac causes predominate. There is a bimodal distribution in the population, with the first

peak before 6 months of age (sudden infant death syndrome). The most common coronary artery finding is extensive chronic coronary atherosclerosis, although acute syndromes do occur. *(Fauci, Chapter 267)*

61. **(B)** Over 90% of hypertensives in the general population have essential hypertension. Only about 60% of hypertensives are very sensitive to salt. About 20% of hypertensives have low-renin essential hypertension. This is more common in Blacks. Male sex, Black race, youth, smoking, DM, excess alcohol ingestion, hyper-cholesterolemia, more severe hypertension, and evidence of end-organ damage are among the factors that suggest a poor prognosis. *(Fauci, Chapter 241)*

62. **(E)** In renal impairment, potassium-sparing diuretics can cause life-threatening hyper-kalemia. The characteristic findings of hyper-kalemia are a narrow-based, peaked T wave in conjunction with a widened QRS complex. Other causes of widened QRS complexes do not coexist with a narrow-peak T wave. Also, the PR interval prolongs and the P wave flat-tens with hyperkalemia. *(Fauci, Chapter 221)*

63. **(D)** With severe hypercalcemia, the QT interval is markedly shortened. There is a correlation between the length of QT interval and the degree of hypercalcemia. *(Fauci, Chapter 221)*

64. **(C)** Hypokalemia results in prolongation of the QT interval and terminal U wave. The delayed repolarization in hypokalemia is best expressed at QU rather than QT prolongation since it can be difficult to separate the T wave from the U wave. In severe cases, the ST seg-ments become depressed. A prolonged QT interval can be a risk factor for polymorphic ventricular tachycardia (Torsades des pointes). *(Fauci, Chapter 222)*

65. **(A)** Hypovolemic shock is characterized by low right atrial pressure, a low cardiac output with normal or high systemic vascular resistance. The low right atrial filling pressure and low PA wedge pressure reflect the inadequate venous return. *(Fauci, Chapter 264)*

66. **(B)** This man has a right ventricular MI. Primary right ventricular failure is character-ized by a disproportionately high right atrial pressure with normal or high wedge pressure. The cardiac output is usually low and sys-temic vascular resistance is usually normal or increased. *(Fauci, Chapter 264)*

67. **(D)** In septic shock, right atrial pressure, and systemic vascular resistance are low. Cardiac output can be normal or high in early sepsis. *(Fauci, Chapter 264)*

68. **(B)** Cardiogenic shock is characterized by high right atrial pressure (although it can be normal at times), high PA wedge pressure, high sys-temic vascular resistance, and low cardiac output. *(Fauci, Chapter 264)*

69. **(A)** In chronic, compensated mitral regurgita-tion, there is a holosystolic murmur, which starts with S1 and extends to or past the aortic component of S2. The S1 is diminished, and there is increased splitting of S2. The murmur also radiates from the apex to the axilla. This condition is often tolerated for years before symptoms develop. *(Fauci, Chapter 230)*

70. **(B)** CAD is the most common cause of acute mitral regurgitation in the United States. The murmur is often midsystolic early on, and a thrill may be present. The apex is usually hyperdynamic but actual forward stroke volume is usually diminished. The presenta-tion is usually dominated by acute pulmonary edema and occurs most often 2–7 days post-MI. *(Fauci, Chapter 239)*

71. **(B)** ECG changes in mitral stenosis are due to enlargement and hypertrophy of the left atrium and asynchronous atrial activation.

    The notched P wave is most prominent in lead II. In lead V1, the P wave has a negative terminal deflection. *(Fauci, Chapter 230)*

72. **(A)** A prolonged PR interval is a common find-ing in asymptomatic elderly patients that have age-related degeneration of the AV node. Drugs such as beta-blockers (metoprolol) may exacerbate the condition or even cause PR

prolongation in excessive doses. *(Fauci, Chapter 225)*

73. **(D)** In Wolff–Parkinson–White syndrome, the PR interval is short, the QRS is widened, and there is slurring of the upstroke of the R wave. The shortened PR interval reflects faster than normal conduction through an accessory pathway. The ventricular complex represents a fusion beat. The blurred upstroke of the QRS (delta wave) represents ventricular activation via the accessory pathway. The normal end portion of the QRS represents activation via the normal route through the AV node. *(Fauci, Chapter 226)*

74. **(C)** Hypercalcemia may prolong the QRS and shorten the ST and QT intervals. Serious arrhythmias rarely occur with hypercalcemia. *(Fauci, Chapter 221)*

75. **(E)** The ECG in severe aortic stenosis shows LVH, but is not perfectly sensitive and is not specific. Bundle branch blocks and ST–T changes can occur, but some patients have a normal ECG. *(Fauci, Chapter 230)*

76. **(C)** Beta-blockers and ACE inhibitors are both indicated in the treatment of heart failure patients with systolic dysfunction. *(Fauci, Chapter 227)*

77. **(A)** Beta-blockers have a negative inotropic effect on the heart. Despite this they improve survival in patients with left ventricular dysfunction and heart failure. *(Fauci, Chapter 227)*

78. **(A)** In chronic atrial flutter, control of ventricular rate is the goal of therapy. Beta-blockers, $Ca^{2}+$ calcium channel blockers, and digoxin are drugs commonly used. *(Fauci, Chapter 226)*

79. **(D)** Neither ACE inhibitors or beta-blockers mediate their effects by calcium channel blockade. *(Fauci, Chapter 226)*

80. **(E)** Nifedipine has direct effects on vascular smooth muscle. *(Fauci, Chapter 241)*

81. **(B)** Enalapril exerts its effect by inhibiting formation of angiotensin II. This lowers systemic vascular resistance. In addition, ACE inhibitors have a natriuretic effect by inhibition of aldosterone secretion. *(Fauci, Chapter 241)*

82. **(F)** Digoxin is a direct inotropic agent, but is usually reserved for patients with heart failure who are symptomatic after treatment with ACE inhibitors and diuretics. *(Fauci, Chapter 227)*

83. **(E)** Long-acting nifedipine has been a useful adjunct to the treatment of primary pulmonary hypertension, but great care must be used as even low doses of vasodilators can cause untoward reactions in patients with pulmonary hypertension. Lung transplants have provided a major therapeutic modality for managing severe pulmonary hypertension.

ACE inhibitors and hydralazine have been tried, but are not effective. *(Fauci, Chapter 244)*

84. **(D)** There are numerous potential mechanisms that might explain the beneficial effects of beta-blockers in left ventricular dysfunction, and post-MI. The benefit is additive to that provided by ACE inhibitors. *(Fauci, Chapter 239)*

85. **(C)** A hyperkinetic pulse occurs in the setting of an elevated stroke volume (anemia, fever, anxiety) or an abnormally rapid runoff from the arterial system (aortic regurgitation, patent ductus arteriosus, arteriovenous fistula). *(Fauci, Chapter 230)*

86. **(E)** A dicrotic pulse has a peak in systole and another in diastole. It occurs in patients with very low stroke volume, especially dilated cardiomyopathy. *(Fauci, Chapter 220)*

87. **(D)** The bisferiens pulse, two systolic peaks, occurs in HOCM and aortic regurgitation. In aortic regurgitation, the bisferiens pulse can occur both in the presence or absence of aortic stenosis. *(Fauci, Chapter 231)*

88. **(A)** The pulsus tardus of aortic stenosis is the result of mechanical obstruction to left ventricular ejection and often has an accompanying thrill. The characteristic feel of the pulse is caused by a delayed systolic peak. *(Fauci, Chapter 230)*

89. **(B)** Pulsus paradoxus, a drop of >10 mm Hg in systolic blood pressure during inspiration, is caused by pericardial tamponade, airway obstruction, or superior vena cava obstruction. At times, the peripheral pulse may disappear completely during inspiration. *(Fauci, Chapter 220)*

90. **(E)** Tricuspid regurgitation increases the size of the *v* wave. When tricuspid regurgitation becomes severe, the combination of a prominent *v* wave and obliteration of the *x* descent results in a single, large, positive systolic wave. *(Fauci, Chapter 220)*

91. **(D)** Right atrial myxoma, or tricuspid stenosis, will slow the y descent by obstructing the right ventricular filling. The y descent of the JVP is produced mainly by the tricuspid valve opening and the subsequent rapid inflow of blood into the right ventricle. *(Fauci, Chapter 220)*

92. **(C)** Right ventricular infarction and constrictive pericarditis frequently result in an increase in JVP during inspiration (Kussmaul sign). Severe right-sided failure can also be a cause. *(Fauci, Chapter 220)*

93. **(F)** Right-sided heart failure is the most common cause of a positive abdominojugular reflux (normal JVP at rest, increases during 10 seconds of firm midabdominal compression, and only drops when pressure is released). *(Fauci, Chapter 220)*

94. **(A)** Large *a* waves occur with increased resistance to filling (tricuspid stenosis, pulmonary hypertension) or when the right atrium contracts against a tricuspid valve closed by right ventricular systole (*Cannon a* waves) in complete heart block or other arrhythmias. *(Fauci, Chapter 220)*

95. **(E)** Most murmurs diminish with standing. The two exceptions are HOCM, which becomes louder, and mitral valve prolapse, which becomes longer and louder. *(Fauci, Chapter 230)*

96. **(A)** With the Valsalva maneuver, most murmurs will decrease. The location and radiation of this patient's murmur suggests aortic stenosis. The exceptions are the murmurs of HOCM and mitral valve prolapse, which increase.

    After release of the Valsalva maneuver, right-sided murmurs tend to return to baseline more rapidly. *(Fauci, Chapter 230)*

97. **(B)** The murmur of HOCM often decreases with submaximal isometric exercise (handgrip). Murmurs across normal or obstructed valves will be increased.

    Handgrip can also accentuate an S3 or S4. *(Fauci, Chapter 231)*

98. **(B)** HOCM often has a bisferiens pulse. It can also be found in pure aortic regurgitation or combined aortic regurgitation and aortic stenosis. *(Fauci, Chapter 231)*

99. **(C)** The location and radiation of this murmur suggests mitral insufficiency. The maneuver of inflating bilateral blood pressure cuffs will increase the murmurs of mitral regurgitation, ventricular septal defect, and aortic regurgitation. Other murmurs are not affected. *(Fauci, Chapter 230)*

100. **(B)** Constrictive pericarditis is characterized by a prominent y descent of the neck veins and low voltage on ECG. The presence of a positive Kussmaul sign helps differentiate the syndrome from cor pulmonale and restrictive cardiomyopathies. *(Fauci, Chapter 232)*

101. **(A)** Cardiac tamponade can occur with as little as 200 mL of fluid if the accumulation is rapid. Physical examination reveals a pulsus paradoxus (>10 mm Hg inspiratory decline in systolic arterial pressure), a prominent *x* descent of the jugular veins, but no Kussmaul sign. The ECG may show low voltage. *(Fauci, Chapter 232)*

102. **(D)** RVMI is characterized by high neck veins, ECG abnormalities, and often a right-sided S3. The low cardiac output associated with RVMI can often be treated by volume expansion. Although a third of patients with inferoposterior infarctions have some degree of right ventricular necrosis, extensive RVMI is uncommon. *(Fauci, Chapter 239)*

103. **(A)** Electrical alternans (a beat-to-beat alternation in one or more component of the ECG signal) can occur in pericardial effusion and numerous other conditions. Total electrical alternans (P–QRS–T) and sinus tachycardia is relatively specific for pericardial effusion (often with tamponade). *(Fauci, Chapter 232)*

104. **(B)** A pericardial knock is characteristic of constrictive pericarditis. It is in fact an early S3, occurring 0.06–0.12 seconds after aortic closure. S1 and S2 are frequently distant. *(Fauci, Chapter 232)*

105. **(C)** The combination of absent pulsus and absent Kussmaul sign with prominent *x* descent favors a restrictive cardiomyopathy.

    Unlike constrictive pericarditis, restrictive cardiomyopathies frequently present with an enlarged heart, orthopnea, LVH, and bundle branch blocks. *(Fauci, Chapter 231)*

106. **(C)** The cardiac lesions of gastrointestinal carcinoids are almost exclusively in the right side of the heart and occur only when there are hepatic metastases. Fibrous plaques are found on the endothelium of the cardiac chambers, valves, and great vessels. These plaques can distort cardiac valves; tricuspid regurgitation and pulmonic stenosis are the most common valvular problems. *(Fauci, Chapters 231 and 344)*

107. **(B)** The proximal aortitis of seronegative arthritis (ankylosing spondylitis, Reiter syndrome, psoriatic arthritis, or associated with inflammatory bowel disease) can result in aortic regurgitation and AV block. *(Fauci, Chapter 242)*

108. **(A)** Focal myocardial necrosis and inflammatory cell infiltration caused by high circulating levels of catecholamines are seen in about 50% of patients who die with pheochromocytoma.

    Hypertension can further impair left ventricular function. *(Fauci, Chapter 337)*

109. **(D)** The Means–Lerman scratch, a systolic scratchy sound heard at the left second intercostal space during expiration, is thought to result from the rubbing of the hyperdynamic pericardium against the pleura. Palpitations, atrial fibrillation, hypertension, angina, and heart failure are more common cardiac manifestations of hyperthyroidism. *(Fauci, Chapter 335)*

110. **(E)** DM can result in a restrictive cardiomyopathy in the absence of large-vessel CAD. Histology reveals increased collagen, glycoprotein, triglycerides, and cholesterol in the myocardial interstitium. Abnormalities may be present in small intramural arteries. *(Fauci, Chapter 231)*

111. **(D)** Patients with diabetes have the same rates of coronary heart disease events as patients with established CAD. Therefore, diabetes is now considered a coronary heart disease equivalent when assessing risk even if the patient has not had any previous cardiac symptoms. The current guidelines support risk reduction efforts (both lifestyle and drug therapy) in patients with diabetes similar to those recommended for patients with CAD (secondary prevention). The goal for LDL is <100 mg/dL in patients with diabetes and secondary goals include considering fibrates for those with high triglycerides and nicotinic acid for low HDL cholesterol. Lifestyle modification is recommended for everyone irrespective of risk. *(Fauci, Chapter 338)*

112. **(E)** When assessing patients for cardiovascular risk, it is always important to consider recommendations in light of their risk level. For primary prevention (no known symptomatic CAD), there are risk calculators available to estimate an individual's future risk (see www.nhlbi.nih.gov/guidelines/cholesterol/ for a risk calculator based on the Framingham database). The treatment recommendations and goals should match the patient's risk level.

In this individual, she has no risk factors for CAD and her 10-year risk for cardiovascular events is low. The goals for LDL in her are <160 mg/dL, and drug therapy should be only considered if her LDL >190 mg/dL. For her, the best advice is lifestyle modification such as dietary modification, exercise, and weight loss if indicated, since these changes will lower triglycerides, raise HDL, and lower LDL. Repeat screening is recommended every 5 years. *(Fauci, Chapter 235)*

113. **(D)** For patients with established CAD, their future risk for further cardiovascular events is high (10-year risk >20%). In such individuals, the goals of LDL level are adjusted lower to match the increased risk. For secondary prevention, the LDL level target is <100 mg/dL. For all individuals at increased risk, lifestyle modification is stressed as a key component therapy. In this patient, given the recent diagnosis of CAD and the elevated LDL level, treatment with a "statin" is also indicated. *(Fauci, Chapter 235)*

114. **(D)** Recent evidence has suggested that lipid modification for patients with ischemic stroke (that is not cardioembolic in origin) by lowering LDL level with statins is beneficial in reducing future stroke risk. This evidence comes from the analysis of cardiovascular statin trials that have a lower rate of ischemic strokes in patients taking the medication as compared to the placebo group. In addition, lifestyle modification is important for this individual, especially smoking cessation. *(Fauci, Chapter 364)*

115. **(D)** The metabolic syndrome is frequently identified among individuals given the increasing rates of obesity and diabetes in Western society. This individual has multiple atherogenic risk factors (obesity, hypertension, increased LDL) and his 10-year risk for cardiac events is approximated at 10%–20% by the risk calculator. At this risk level, the LDL goal is <130 mg/dL and treatment threshold for starting drug therapy is >130 mg/dL. Lifestyle modification too is an important component of the overall treatment. *(Fauci, Chapter 236)*

116. **(E)** Many observational studies have verified the increased risk of CAD in women after menopause, and this formed the basis for recommending estrogen therapy to lower cardiovascular risk in postmenopausal women. Recently, two large randomized clinical trials have shown no benefit with estrogen replacement in postmenopausal women as a means of reducing cardiovascular risk. With this evidence, estrogen replacement is not recommended for cardiac risk modification, and is only indicated to treat the symptoms of menopause. For postmenopausal women at increased risk of cardiac disease, statins are considered first-line therapy in modifying risk since there are randomized trial data from multiple trials supporting their effectiveness in women. Since this patient has only one risk factor, her future 10-year risk is low (<10%) and lifestyle modification is the best advice. She will require follow-up lipid risk assessment in 5 years. *(Fauci, Chapter 235)*

117. **(G)** ACE inhibitors have no adverse effects on glucose or lipid metabolism and minimize the development of diabetic nephropathy by reducing renal vascular resistance and renal perfusion pressure. The goal for blood pressure control in diabetics is set at 130/80 mm Hg which is lower than in nondiabetics. This lower pressure is important in preventing progression of renal disease and other end-organ damage. *(Fauci, Chapter 241)*

118. **(A)** Thiazides have been a cornerstone in most trials of antihypertensive therapy. Their adverse metabolic consequences include renal potassium loss leading to hypokalemia, hyperuricemia from uric acid retention, carbohydrate intolerance, and hyperlipidemia. The current U.S. Joint National Committee (JNC-7) guidelines suggest starting with thiazide diuretics because of their proven efficacy in lowering mortality and morbidity in large clinical trials. Other agents are considered if there are comorbidities such as diabetes or CAD. *(Fauci, Chapter 241)*

119. **(G)** Although contraindicated in bilateral stenosis, ACE inhibitors are the drug of choice in unilateral renal artery stenosis.

When ACE inhibitors are used in patients with impaired renal function, renal function should be monitored twice a week for the first 3 weeks. *(Fauci, Chapter 241)*

120. **(A)** Thiazides seem to work particularly well in Blacks and the elderly. Younger individuals and Whites respond well to beta-blockers, ACE inhibitors, and calcium channel antagonists. Isolated systolic hypertension is a common occurrence in the elderly. It is due to arteriosclerosis of the large arteries. Treatment of isolated systolic hypertension with low-dose thiazides results in lower stroke rates and death. The goal for treatment is a blood pressure of 140/90 mm Hg. *(Fauci, Chapter 241)*

121. **(E)** Beta-blockers are the most appropriate choice for the treatment of hypertension in patients with CAD. They lower mortality in patients with CAD as well as hypertension. ACE inhibitors can also be used, especially if there is left ventricular dysfunction, or the patient has multiple cardiovascular risk factors such as diabetes or dyslipidemia. *(Fauci, Chapter 241)*

CHAPTER 2

Dermatology
Questions

DIRECTIONS (Questions 1 through 5): The following group of numbered items is preceded by a list of lettered options. For each question, select the one lettered option that is most closely associated with it. . Each lettered option may be selected once, multiple times, or not at all.

Questions 1 and 2: For each patient with a skin lesion, select the most likely diagnosis.

- (A) psoriasis
- (B) eczema
- (C) hypersensitivity reactions
- (D) lichen planus
- (E) toxic erythemas
- (F) lichen planus
- (G) Kaposi sarcoma
- (H) melanotic nodules
- (I) maculopapular rash
- (J) serum-filled bullae

1. A 19-year-old man develops new lesions at the sites of skin trauma. The lesions appear as sharply marginated erythematous papules with silvery-white scales.

2. A 32-year-old man with human immunodeficiency virus (HIV) infection develops skin tumors and patches on the legs with some on the face. They are palpable, firm, and appear violaceous with some nodules appearing purple brownish.

Questions 3 through 5: For each patient, select the associated skin and clinical findings.

- (A) rarely involves border of scalp
- (B) discoloration of upper eyelids
- (D) never a permanent effect on skin
- (E) potentially aggravated by contact with the skin
- (F) worse on weekends
- (G) high likelihood of malingering
- (H) associated with squamous cell cancer
- (I) extensive large plaques
- (J) lesions at various stages (progression of lesions)

3. A 22-year-old man is diagnosed with psoriasis, and has never received any treatment. What might the findings include?

4. A 63-year-old woman develops skin lesions, and difficulty getting out of a chair. A clinical diagnosis of dermatomyositis is made. What might the findings include?

5. A 43-year-old woman develops a rash on her arms and hands after starting a new job in a factory. The lesions have well-demarcated erythema and edema with superimposed closely spaced vesicles and papules. What might the findings include?

DIRECTIONS (Questions 6 through 21): For each of the questions in this section select the one lettered answer that is the best response in each case.

6. A 19-year-old woman with asthma has a chronic rash with distribution on her hands, neck, and elbow creases. It is very itchy, and the skin appears thickened with increased skin markings. There are some areas of fissures in the skin at the elbow creases and hands. (See Figure 2–1.) **Which of the following is the most appropriate advice?**

Figure 2–1.

(A) psychoanalysis
(B) warm clothing
(C) dry environment
(D) environmental manipulation
(E) vigorous exercise

7. A 74-year-old man develops a new single 1.5-cm lesion on his face. It is firm and nodular with a dome shape and central keratotic plug. Excisional biopsy confirms keratoacanthoma. **Which of the following best characterizes this lesion?**

(A) rapid growth
(B) distinct pathology
(C) usual occurrence on the trunk
(D) a malignant potential
(E) a dark brown color

8. A 85-year-old woman has large blistering lesions on the abdomen and thighs that come and go without therapy (See Figure 2–2.). Nikolsky sign is negative. **Which of the following is the most likely diagnosis?**

Figure 2–2.

(A) pemphigus vulgaris (PV)
(B) dermatitis herpetiformis (DH)
(C) bullous pemphigoid
(D) herpes gestationis
(E) erythema multiforme

9. A 69-year-old woman develops dark, velvety pigmentation in her axillae. She has noticed 10 lb weight loss over the past 3 months with heartburn and early satiety. She notices no other symptoms. (See Figure 2–3.) **Which of the following conditions should she be studied for?**

(A) a visceral carcinoma
(B) lymphoma
(C) diabetes mellitus
(D) sarcoidosis
(E) an allergy

Figure 2–3. (Reproduced, with permission, from Wolff K and Johnson RA, *Fitzpatrick's Color Atlas & Synopsis of Clinical Dermatology*, 5th ed. New York: McGraw-Hill, 2005:87.)

10. A 22-year-old woman develops an acute contact dermatitis to a household-cleaning agent. **Which of the following treatments is most appropriate during the bullous, oozing stage?**

   (A) wet dressings
   (B) systemic corticosteroids
   (C) topical anesthetics
   (D) systemic antibiotics
   (E) antihistamines

11. Which of the following is a characteristic of ringworm of the scalp as compared with other dermatophytoses?

   (A) more frequent occurrence in childhood
   (B) high degree of contagiousness
   (C) ability to invade the dermis

   (D) sensitivity to penicillin
   (E) ability to spread to other organs

12. A 27-year-old man develops warts on his hand. **Which of the following is a correct statement concerning these skin lesions?**

   (A) are viral in etiology
   (B) may be premalignant lesions
   (C) are found mainly in patients with lymphoma
   (D) are contagious in children only
   (E) may be treated with griseofulvin

13. A 27-year-old man develops a painless 1-cm sore on his penis. It appears ulcerated with a raised margin and minimal serous exudates. (See Figure 2–4.) **Which of the following is the most appropriate next step in the diagnosis?**

Figure 2–4. (Reproduced, with permission, from Wolff K and Johnson RA, *Fitzpatrick's Color Atlas & Synopsis of Clinical Dermatology*, 5th ed. New York: McGraw-Hill, 2005:915.)

   (A) biopsy
   (B) Gram stain
   (C) serology
   (D) ultrasound
   (E) skin test

14. A 64-year-old woman notices bullous-type lesions over her thighs and axilla. They are itchy, but not painful, and she has no other symptoms. On examination, there are large tense, serous-filled bullae on the affected areas. A biopsy confirms the diagnosis of bullous pemphigoid. **Which of the following histologic features is typical of this condition?**

(A) nonspecific changes
(B) immunoglobulin A (IgA) deposits
(C) lesions within the epidermis (acantholysis)
(D) basement membrane lesions
(E) immunoglobulin M (IgM) deposits

15. A 27-year-old woman has a 1-year history of loosely formed bowel movements associated with some blood and abdominal pain. She develops multiple painful erythematous nodules on her lower legs. **Which of the following is the most likely diagnosis? (See Figure 2–5.)**

Figure 2–5. (Reproduced, with permission, from Wolff K and Johnson RA, *Fitzpatrick's Color Atlas & Synopsis of Clinical Dermatology*, 5th ed. New York: McGraw-Hill, 2005:149.)

(A) erythema multiforme
(B) erythema migrans
(C) erythema nodosum
(D) cutaneous lymphoma
(E) necrobiosis lipoidica

16. **Which of the following best describes mycosis fungoides?**

(A) fungal infection of the epidermis
(B) benign skin lesion
(C) cutaneous lymphoma
(D) dermatitis
(E) form of eczema

17. A 58-year-old man complains of an enlarged, pitted nose, and a facial rash that "flushes" in response to drinking hot liquids or alcohol. The rash is on both cheeks, and it is red and flushed in appearance, with some telangiectatica and small papules. (See Figure 2–6.) **Which of the following is the most likely diagnosis?**

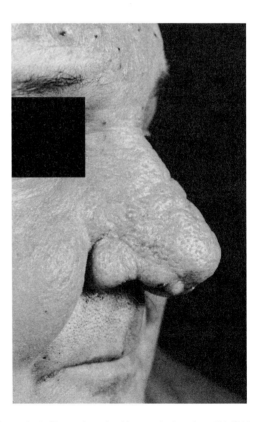

Figure 2–6. (Reproduced, with permission, from Wolff K and Johnson RA, *Fitzpatrick's Color Atlas & Synopsis of Clinical Dermatology*, 5th ed. New York: McGraw-Hill, 2005:11.)

(A) acne vulgaris

(B) pemphigus

(C) rosacea

(D) psoriasis

(E) seborrheic dermatitis

18. An 81-year-old man presents with pallor, glossitis, cheilitis, and vitiligo. **Which of the following is the most likely diagnosis?**

(A) sickle cell anemia

(B) cold agglutinin syndrome

(C) methemoglobinemia

(D) pernicious anemia

(E) polycythemia

19. A 70-year-old man develops multiple pruritic skin lesions and bullae mostly in the axillae and around the medial aspects of his groin and thighs. There are some lesions on his forearms and on his lower legs (first appeared in this location), and moderately painful oral lesions. Nikolsky sign is negative. There is no eye involvement. **Which of the following is the most likely diagnosis?**

(A) dermatitis herpetiformis (DH)

(B) pemphigus vulgaris (PV)

(C) bullous pemphigoid

(D) cicatricial pemphigoid

(E) epidermolysis bullosa (EB)

20. A man presents with bullous lesions on his face, armpit, and chest. He initially had them only in his mouth. They appear round and oval with serous fluid and some are "flabby." When pressure is applied to the lesion, the fluid spreads laterally. A clinical diagnosis of pemphigus vulgaris (PV) is made. (See Figure 2–7.) **Which of the following is the usual age of onset for this condition?**

Figure 2–7. (Reproduced, with permission, from Wolff K and Johnson RA, *Fitzpatrick's Color Atlas & Synopsis of Clinical Dermatology*, 5th ed. New York: McGraw-Hill, 2005:104.)

(A) under 10 years of age

(B) 10–20 years of age

(C) 20–40 years of age

(D) 40–60 years of age

(E) 60–80 years of age

21. **Which of the following is the most likely drug to cause pemphigus vulgaris (PV)?**

(A) captopril

(B) D-penicillamine

(C) sulfonamides

(D) hydralazine

(E) quinidine

DIRECTIONS (Questions 22 through 28): The following group of numbered items is preceded by a list of lettered options. For each question, select the one lettered option that is most closely associated with it. Each lettered option may be selected once, multiple times, or not at all.

Questions 22 and 23: For each patient with a skin lesion, select the most common associated features.

(A) associated with adenocarcinoma

(B) autosomal dominant inheritance

(C) viral etiology

(D) adenocarcinoma

(E) neural tumors most frequently appear during old age

(F) multiple neural tumors

22. A young child is found to have axillary freckling. The lesions appear light brown with sharp margination and are of variable size from small tiny "freckle"-like macules to larger patches. What other characteristics does this disorder include?

23. A 68-year-old woman develops grayish-brown, thickened skin in the axillae. Examination shows increased pigmentation, with accentuated skin lines and the skin appears "dirty." This skin is thickened and has a velvety texture on palpation. What other findings are associated with this disorder?

Questions 24 through 28: Match the following descriptions with the correct diagnosis.

(A) basal cell cancer

(B) basal cell nevus syndrome (BCNS)

(C) melanoma

(D) actinic keratosis

(E) keratoacanthoma

(F) seborrheic keratosis

(G) lipoma

(H) mongolian spot

(I) spider angioma

(J) glomus tumor

(K) squamous cell cancer

24. Malignant, but does not metastasize beyond the skin.

25. Malignant, and may metastasize beyond the skin.

26. More common in women and patients with cirrhosis.

27. More common in Asian children than Caucasian children.

28. May develop in long-standing scars.

DIRECTIONS (Questions 29 through 42): For each of the questions in this section select the one lettered answer that is the best response in each case.

29. A 60-year-old man presents with the skin lesion pictured in Figure 2–8. **Which of the following is the most likely diagnosis?**

Figure 2–8.

(A) erythema nodosum

(B) acanthosis nigricans

(C) herpes zoster

(D) alopecia variegata

(E) bullous pemphigoid

30. An 18-year-old woman has severe acne for many years. She has tried many topical therapies with no lasting benefit. On examination, she has multiple inflammatory papules on her

face, with some even larger nodules and cysts. **Which of the following is the most appropriate next step in management?**

(A) dietary controls
(B) radiotherapy
(C) ultraviolet light
(D) tetracycline
(E) isotretinoin

31. A 70-year-old man comes to the emergency department because of a skin rash and severe itching. He appears ill; there is a generalized skin rash that is scaly, erythematous, and thickened. His palms, soles, and scalp are also involved. **Which of the following is the most likely diagnosis?**

(A) pemphigus vulgaris
(B) rosacea
(C) erythroderma (exfoliative dermatitis)
(D) dermatitis herpetiformis
(E) disseminated varicella

32. A 32-year-old woman comes to the emergency department because of a generalized erythematous skin rash. She was recently started on trimethoprim-sulfamethoxazole (Septra) for a urinary tract infection. Examination shows the diffuse rash involving her whole body including the palms and soles. Except for generalized lymphadenopathy, the rest of the examination is normal. **Which of the following is the most appropriate interpretation of the generalized lymphadenopathy finding?**

(A) a viral infection
(B) pyoderma
(C) lymphoma
(D) leukemia
(E) nothing specific

33. A 62-year-old man develops scaling and non-scaling patches, and plaques over his chest and back. They are itchy, but not painful. The rest of the examination is normal, except for lymphadenopathy. Examinations of the blood film and skin biopsy histology, both, reveal unusu-

ally large monocytoid cells. (See Figure 2–9.) **Which of the following is the most likely diagnosis?**

(A) leukemia

Figure 2–9.

(B) visceral B-cell lymphoma
(C) primary cutaneous T-cell lymphoma
(D) viral infection (usually Epstein-Barr)
(E) paraneoplastic syndrome secondary to lung cancer

34. **Which of the following statements about the prognosis of cutaneous T-cell lymphoma is true?**

(A) rapidly downhill
(B) determined by the type of medical care
(C) rarely fatal
(D) remissions and exacerbations, but with eventual progression to a fatal outcome
(E) eventual complete recovery, regardless of treatment

35. **Which of the following treatments is used for most patients with cutaneous T-cell lymphoma?**

    (A) antibiotics

    (B) antiviral medication

    (C) aggressive systemic chemotherapy to ensure cure

    (D) symptomatic treatment

    (E) early use of high-dose systemic steroids

36. A 72-year-old man is newly diagnosed with bullous pemphigoid. **Which of the following is the most appropriate next step in the management?**

    (A) plasmapheresis

    (B) low-dose prednisone (10–20 mg/day)

    (C) high-dose prednisone (50–100 mg/day)

    (D) azathioprine (150 mg/day)

    (E) dapsone (100–150 mg/day)

37. **Which of the following features indicates a more negative prognosis for patients with malignant melanoma?**

    (A) female sex

    (B) location on the leg

    (C) dark pigmentation of the lesion

    (D) nodularity of the lesion

    (E) level A invasion

38. A 34-year-old man presents with a chronic and progressive skin rash. He has a history of poorly controlled Crohn disease and has lost 20 lb in the past 6 months. On examination, there are dry, scaly patches, and plaques, which are sharply marginated and bright red around his mouth, and anogenital regions. There is also involvement of the flexural regions of the arms. **Which of the following is the most likely diagnosis?**

    (A) ichthyosis

    (B) acquired zinc deficiency

    (C) Paget disease

    (D) candidiasis

    (E) herpes simplex

39. A 26-year-old woman develops discomfort on her lower legs and notices a skin rash. On examination, there are tender nodules on her shins with an erythematous base. **Which of the following conditions is this rash associated with?**

    (A) caused by aspergillosis

    (B) usually occurs in children

    (C) more common in males than females

    (D) only caused by malignant disease

    (E) can occur with streptococcal infection

40. Which of the following differentiates a patch from a macule?

    (A) it is more easily palpable

    (B) a patch is erythematous

    (C) a patch can contain fluid

    (D) the etiology is very different

    (E) it is larger

41. A 19-year-old man develops a rash in the groin area. On examination, it is a large well-demarcated area of tan-brown discoloration around his left inguinal area. There is some scaling of the lesion when brushed with a tongue depressor. (See Figure 2–10.) **Which of the following is the most appropriate initial diagnostic test?**

Figure 2–10. (Reproduced, with permission, from Wolff K and Johnson RA, *Fitzpatrick's Color Atlas & Synopsis of Clinical Dermatology*, 5th ed. New York: McGraw-Hill, 2005:699.)

(A) punch biopsy of skin

(B) Tzanck smear

(C) potassium hydroxide (KOH) preparation of scrapings

(D) blood culture for fungi

(E) diascopy

42. A 7-year-old boy develops a skin rash in the right axillary area. On examination, there are superficial small pustules, with some that have ruptured and formed golden-yellow crusts. The area is itchy, but not painful, and he has no systemic symptoms. Treatment with oral antibiotics is started. **Which of the following statements about this condition is most likely correct?**

(A) caused by fungi of the *Microsporum* species

(B) caused exclusively by staphylococcal infections

(C) characterized by premalignant changes

(D) treated by improved hygiene

(E) characterized by papulosquamous lesions

DIRECTIONS (Questions 43 through 53): Each set of matching questions in this section consists of a list of lettered options followed by several numbered items. For each numbered item, select the most appropriate lettered option(s). Each lettered option may be selected once, multiple times, or not at all.

Questions 43 through 48: For each patient with a skin lesion, select the most likely diagnosis or associated condition.

(A) generalized vitiligo

(B) localized vitiligo

(C) telangiectasia

(D) erythroderma

(E) tuberculoid leprosy

(F) sarcoid

(G) limited scleroderma

(H) dermatomyositis

(I) secondary syphilis

(J) diabetes

(K) eruptive xanthoma

43. A 20-year-old man who recently emigrated from Southeast Asia has chronic skin lesions on his back and chest. On examination, there are multiple well-defined hypopigmented macules with raised edges. They vary in size from 1.0 to 5.0 cm, and some have lost sensation to touch and pinprick.

44. A 47-year-old woman has symptoms of heartburn and skin changes in her hands. She notices pain and discomfort in her hands while washing dishes with cold water, and that the fingers sometimes become pale and colorless when they are painful. The fingers then change color to blue, and red after warming. On examination, there are areas of telangiectasias on her face.

45. A 25-year-old woman presents with a diffuse skin rash, starting a few days after starting antibiotics for a urinary tract infection. On examination, her skin was warm to touch, and red in color.

46. A 32-year-old man notices the sudden eruption of tiny nodules on his lower arms and knees. On examination, he has multiple crops of papules on his lower arms and knees. They are dome shaped, discrete, and have a yellow center with surrounding areas of redness.

47. A 24-year-old man presents with malaise, fever, and a new rash on his abdomen. Eight weeks ago he had a painless 1-cm ulcer on his penis that resolved spontaneously. On examination, there are faint pink brownish-red macules on his abdomen ranging in size from 0.5 to 1.0 cm.

48. A 51-year-old man with obesity (body mass index [BMI] >30) presents with skin changes in his right axilla. On examination, there is increased pigmentation and the skin appears dirty. The area feels velvety and the skin folds are accentuated.

Questions 49 through 53: For the following medications, select the most appropriate skin manifestations.

    (A) dystrophic nail changes

    (B) may mottle teeth

    (C) black pigmentation of face

    (D) erythema nodosum

    (E) morbilliform eruption in patients with acquired immune deficiency syndrome (AIDS)

    (F) gingival hyperplasia

    (G) reactions in patients with nasal polyps

49. Bleomycin.

50. Chloroquine.

51. Birth control pills.

52. Tetracycline.

53. Sulfamethoxazole and trimethoprim.

Answers and Explanations

1. **(A)** Koebner phenomenon is typically seen in psoriasis. The kind of injury eliciting the phenomenon is usually mechanical, but ultraviolet light or allergic damage to the skin may be provocative. Koebner phenomenon can also occur in lichen planus, lichen nitidus, keratosis follicularis, and pemphigoid. The Koebner phenomenon has been used to study early skin changes in these diseases. *(Wolff, p. 53)*

2. **(G)** Kaposi sarcoma often manifests as multiple blue dermal plaques. Lesions have two prominent features: accumulation of spindle cells and presence of vascular elements. Classical Kaposi sarcoma is an indolent disease of later life and is much more common in men than in women. Kaposi sarcoma in association with HIV infection is a much more aggressive disorder. In all types of Kaposi, the deoxyribonucleic acid (DNA) of human herpes virus 8 has been identified. *(Wolff, p. 538)*

3. **(I)** Psoriasis does not present a progression of lesions unless therapy is applied. Lesions vary in size and configuration from patient to patient and in the same patient from time to time and vary from drop-shaped lesions to large plaques. Nail changes are characteristic. *(Wolff, p. 53)*

4. **(B)** In dermatomyositis, the dermatitis may be the most striking feature of the illness or so minor as to be easily overlooked. The classic manifestation is a purplish-red heliotrope erythema of the eyelids, upper cheeks, forehead, and temples, often with edema of the eyelids and of the periorbital tissue. Telangiectasia and skin atrophy can also occur. The typical hand changes involve scaly, bluish-red plaques around the base of the nails and backs of the joints of the fingers. These are most frequently found in elderly patients and are called Gottron papules. There is an association with malignancy in those over 55 years of age. *(Wolff, p. 370)*

5. **(E)** The history should not reveal worsening eruption during the weekend. Allergy, acne, diabetes, psoriasis, xeroderma, or seborrheic dermatitis may all be mistaken for occupational disorders. The list of possible occupational skin hazards is long. At times, a site visit to the workplace is required to confirm the diagnosis. First aid in the workplace often involves sensitizing agents that worsen the situation. Skin problems can be severe and permanent. Relatively few patients are malingerers. *(Wolff, p. 22)*

6. **(D)** A change of environment is among the best treatments for atopic dermatitis. The patient should be kept in as dust-free an environment as possible and should not wear rough garments. Maintenance of adequate humidity is also important. *(Wolff, p. 34)*

7. **(A)** This tumor as a rule occurs on exposed, hairy skin. It grows rapidly but involutes slowly, occasionally up to 1 year. It is more common in white-skinned males. The lesion starts as a small, rounded, flesh-colored or reddish papule. It grows rapidly and may reach 10–20 mm in a few weeks. There are telangiectasias just below the surface and the center contains a horny plug or is covered by a crust concealing a keratin-filled crater. Histology can be difficult to differentiate from squamous cell cancer. *(Wolff, p. 286)*

8. **(C)** Bullous pemphigoid is most common in the elderly, and the disease often starts with urticaria-like and pruritic erythematous lesions, before classic blisters occur. The blisters arise from inflamed and normal skin, unlike in pemphigus where they arise from normal skin. As well, unlike pemphigus, mucosal lesions are minimal or absent. There are antibodies to skin basement membrane, but unlike pemphigus, antibody levels do not correlate with disease activity. *(Wolff, p. 112)*

9. **(A)** Patients with acanthosis nigricans should be studied for a visceral carcinoma. There are hereditary, drug-induced, and benign forms of acanthosis nigricans as well. Given this patient's symptoms, a gastric malignancy should be ruled out. Diabetics get a benign form of the disorder. Other dermatoses associated with malignancy include dermatomyositis, flushing, acquired ichthyosis, and thrombophlebitis migrans. *(Wolff, p. 88)*

10. **(A)** Ointments are not used, but wet dressings are applied several times a day, using Burow solution or boric acid, and baths are also included in the treatment. The key aspect of care is prevention. When contamination does occur, washing the affected area is the first mode of treatment. Oral corticosteroids are only used in severe cases. In less severe cases, topical class I glucocorticoid preparations can be helpful. *(Wolff, p. 32)*

11. **(A)** Ringworm of the skin is most common in children because of their intimacy with animals and other children. The lesions are round or oval scaly patches. Secondary bacterial infection is common with certain fungi. *(Wolff, p. 709)*

12. **(A)** Verrucae are viral in etiology. The human papillomavirus is a DNA-containing virus of the papovavirus group that includes animal tumor viruses. Although most warts are not felt to be premalignant, there is evidence to show that genital warts are correlated with malignancy. *(Wolff, p. 787)*

13. **(C)** This is likely a case of primary syphilis. Serology is the most appropriate test; it can remain negative for a period up to 1 month after the infection is contracted. The serologic test for syphilis usually is positive within 1 week after the chancre appears. With therapy, the chancre heals rapidly, but will heal in 4–6 weeks even without treatment. Genital chancres are usually painless, unless superinfected, but extragenital chancres (eg, fingers) can be quite painful. Biopsy is usually not necessary for diagnosis, and the spirochetes are seen with dark-field examination, not with Gram stain. *(Wolff, p. 919)*

14. **(D)** In bullous pemphigoid, biopsy reveals immunoglobulin G (IgG) deposits in the basement membrane area. In pemphigus vulgaris, the immune deposition and damage is within the lower zone of the epidermis. IgA deposits are seen in dermatitis herpetiformis. *(Wolff, p. 112)*

15. **(C)** About 15% of patients with ulcerative colitis will develop skin manifestations. Typical lesions include erythema nodosum, pyoderma gangrenosum (painless, but can heal with scarring), aphthous ulcers, and ocular inflammation (episcleritis, iritis, uveitis). The activity of the skin manifestations typically parallels the severity of the colonic disease. *(Wolff, p. 152)*

16. **(C)** Mycosis fungoides is best described as a cutaneous T-cell lymphoma. Lesions may remain confined to the skin for years, and internal organ involvement occurs when the disease advances into late stages. It is a disorder involving T lymphocytes. Treatment is usually palliative rather than curative. *(Wolff, p. 526)*

17. **(C)** Rhinophyma is a complication of rosacea. It can be treated surgically by shaving off the excessive tissue with a scalpel, but regrowth occurs in time. There is very little evidence to support the association between alcoholism and rhinophyma. The other conditions do not cause flushing or blushing-type appearance. Psoriasis and seborrheic dermatitis have lesions that have white dry scales. *(Wolff, p. 9)*

18. **(D)** Glossitis and cheilitis result from the vitamin deficiency affecting rapidly turning over tissues. Patients may complain of a "burning" tongue, and examination reveals atrophy of papillae, a deep red mucosa, and a "cobblestone" appearance. Vitamin B_{12} administration rapidly relieves these symptoms. The vitiligo is caused by an associated autoimmune disorder. *(Fauci, Chapter 100)*

19. **(C)** The description and age range (60–80) is typical of bullous pemphigoid. PV is usually associated with a positive Nikolsky sign (pressure on blister leads to lateral extension), and very severe oral lesions. Cicatricial pemphigoid is also a disease of the elderly, but is rare and usually involves the eyes as well. EB is an inherited disorder that usually presents in earlier life. DH does not usually affect mucous membranes, and the lesions are grouped in clusters. However, it can mimic early bullous pemphigoid, and biopsy is needed for confirmation. Permanent remission is frequent, and continued therapy would not be required. *(Wolff, p. 112)*

20. **(D)** PV is most common from 40 to 60 years of age, whereas bullous pemphigoid is seen most frequently after the age of 80. Dermatitis herpetiformis is most common in the age group from 30 to 40, but has a wide age range. *(Wolff, p. 106)*

21. **(B)** Captopril and other drugs can cause PV, but D-penicillamine is the most likely to cause the disease. Drug-induced PV usually, but not invariably, remits when the offending agent is withdrawn. *(Wolff, p. 108)*

22. **(B)** Neurofibromatosis is inherited in an autosomal manner. Incomplete forms are frequent. The skin manifestations include café au lait spots (more than 6 required for diagnosis), axillary freckles, cutaneous neurofibromas, and pigmented iris hamartomas (Lisch nodules). There are numerous other manifestations as well, including neural tumors. *(Wolff, p. 453)*

23. **(A)** Early recognition of acanthosis nigricans warrants a thorough search for underlying pathology such as malignancy or insulin resistance. The earliest changes are usually pigmentation, dryness, and roughness of the skin. The skin is gray brown or black, palpably thickened, and covered by small papillomatous elevations, which give it a velvety texture. The most common sites are axillae, back, neck, anogenital region, and the groin. *(Wolff, p. 88)*

24. **(A)** Basal cell tumors have a substantial capacity for local destruction but metastasize very rarely. *(Wolff, p. 287)*

25. **(C)** Melanoma can spread beyond the skin. Only about 3%–4% of squamous cell cancers metastasize, but metastasis is quite common in melanoma. Melanoma is the most dangerous primary skin cancer. *(Wolff, pp. 280, 308)*

26. **(I)** Spider angiomas are seen in both women and patients with cirrhosis. Spider angiomas are small A-V malformations that are seen on the skin, particularly on the anterior chest. *(Wolff, pp. 280, 287)*

27. **(H)** Mongolian spots are congenital gray-blue macular lesions, characteristically located on the lumbosacral area, although they can occur anywhere on the skin. They are almost always (99%–100%) in infants of Asiatic or Amerindian origin, although reports in Black, and rarely, White infants have occurred. They usually disappear in early childhood, and generally the lesions are solitary. *(Wolff, p. 189)*

28. **(K)** Squamous cell carcinoma of the skin can arise in areas of inflammation such as burn scars, chronic ulcers, radiation dermatitis, and chronic cutaneous lupus erythematosis. Other early lesions include solar keratoses, cutaneous horns, arsenical keratoses, and Bowen disease. *(Wolff, p. 280)*

29. **(E)** Bullous pemphigoid is most common in older adults. It is not as severe as pemphigus vulgaris, and histology reveals an absence of acantholysis, and immunofluorescence reveals specific antibodies in the basement membrane area. *(Wolff, p. 112)*

30. (E) Tetracyclines are commonly used in the treatment of moderate acne, but may be associated with risk of dental discoloration or photosensitivity. Isotretinoin is the most effective drug for severe acne, but is teratogenic, and may cause lipid abnormalities, hepatoxicity, and night blindness. It cannot be combined with tetracycline because of the risk of pseudotumor cerebri. *(Wolff, p. 6)*

31. (C) Exfoliative dermatitis is a rare skin condition, but because of its severity, patients with this syndrome are often admitted to a hospital. The syndrome can be primary, appearing in otherwise healthy individuals, or secondary to malignancy, contact dermatitis, drugs, or other dermatologic diseases (eg, psoriasis). Even mild cases require systemic treatment for the severe itching. Antihistamines are usually the first choice. *(Wolff, p. 164)*

32. (E) Most cases of exfoliative dermatitis will have widespread lymphadenopathy, whether they are primary or secondary forms. Biopsy will usually reveal nonspecific changes and is only warranted if there is a suspicion of lymphoma. *(Wolff, p. 166)*

33. (C) These large cells are typical of Sézary syndrome, a leukemic form of cutaneus T-cell lymphoma (CTCL). This is frequently an early presentation of mycosis fungoides or CTCL. There may be a relationship to human T-cell lymphotropic virus (HTLV) I and II, but it is not universal. CTCL is a malignancy of helper T cells (CD^{4+}). *(Wolff, p. 524)*

34. (D) The typical course of mycosis fungoides is an initial erythematous stage (which might become diffuse and cause an exfoliative dermatitis as in this case), a plaque stage, and a tumor stage. The course is usually progressive through these stages, but all stages can be bypassed. The early stages may progress slowly with remissions or exacerbations. The disease can be rapidly progressive, particularly when the tumor stage is reached. The disease is invariably fatal. *(Wolff, p. 534)*

35. (D) There is no curative therapy, and most experts provide treatment only when symptoms occur. Therapy includes topical treatments such as tar cream plus ultraviolet light or local nitrogen mustard, and systemic treatment with steroids and radiation therapy.

Chemotherapy regimens are used but not with great success. *(Wolff, p. 534)*

36. (C) Severe cases require systemic steroids, often with the addition of azathioprine. Dapsone is useful in mild cases, and occasionally in very mild cases (or for local recurrences) topical glucocorticoid therapy will suffice. *(Wolff, p. 112)*

37. (D) Nodular melanoma is invasive from the start. Women do better than men; trunk lesions and depigmented lesions carry a worse prognosis. Prognosis is directly related to depth of the lesion. *(Wolff, p. 308)*

38. (B) Zinc deficiency can present as a persistent dermatitis around the mouth, with acral involvement that begins as vesicles but is soon crusted. Later it goes on to involve the scalp, hands and trunk, and feet. Treatment is zinc replacement in the diet. It has been described after prolonged parenteral alimentation, malabsorption states, intestinal bypass surgery, and chronic alcoholism. There is an inherited form (autosomal recessive) of the syndrome called acrodermatitis enteropathica. The inherited form occurs in infants and is also treated with zinc. *(Wolff, p. 442)*

39. (E) Erythema nodosum is a hypersensitivity vasculitis associated with many infections, drugs, malignancies, and inflammatory conditions (sarcoidosis). The peak age is 20–30 and it occurs more commonly in females. The lesions are rare in children. It is a nodular erythematous eruption, usually on the extensor aspects of the legs, less commonly on the thighs and forearms. It regresses by bruise-like color changes in 3–6 weeks without scarring. *(Wolff, p. 152)*

40. **(E)** A macule is a flat, colored lesion not raised above the surface of the surrounding skin. It is less than 1 cm in diameter. A patch differs from a macule only in size, being greater than 1 cm in diameter. *(Wolff, p. xxvii)*

41. **(C)** A KOH preparation is useful when performed on scaling skin lesions, when a fungal etiology is suspected. The scraped scales are placed on a microscope slide, treated with one or two drops of KOH solution, and examined for hyphae, pseudohyphae, or budding yeast. A Tzanck smear is a cytologic technique for the diagnosis of herpes virus infection from vesicles, and diascopy is to assess whether a skin lesion will blanch with pressure. *(Wolff, p. 695)*

42. **(D)** Impetigo is a superficial bacterial infection of skin caused by group A beta-hemolytic streptococci or *Staphylococcus aureus.*

It is characterized by superficial pustules that rupture, resulting in a honey-colored crust. The bullous variant is more likely staphylococcal in origin. Treatment requires improving hygiene and soaking the crust, as well as oral antibiotics. *(Wolff, p. 597)*

43. **(E)** Localized areas of vitiligo can be seen in numerous primary skin disorders. It can also be caused by systemic disorders such as sarcoidosis and tuberculoid leprosy. In the latter disorder, there is associated anesthesia, anhidrosis, and alopecia of the lesions. Biopsy of the palpable border will reveal granulomas. *(Wolff, p. 665)*

44. **(G)** Scleroderma is characterized by typical fibrotic and vascular lesions. These lesions may be periungual telangiectasias that are found in lupus erythematosus and dermatomyositis. Another form of telangiectasia, mat telangiectasia, is seen only in scleroderma. These lesions are broad macules 2–7 mm in diameter. They are found on the face, oral mucosa, and hands. The nail beds of scleroderma patients often reveal loss of capillary loops, with dilatation of the remaining loops when examined under magnification. *(Wolff, p. 389)*

45. **(D)** Drug reactions most frequently result in papulosquamous reactions or diffuse erythroderma. Sulfa drugs frequently cause erythroderma. Other drugs commonly implicated include penicillins, gold, allopurinol, captopril, phenytoin, and carbamazepine. Fever, eosinophilia, and interstitial nephritis frequently accompany the erythroderma. *(Fauci, Chapter 56)*

46. **(K)** Hyperlipoproteinemia is frequently associated with xanthomas, yellow-colored cutaneous papules or plaques. Xanthomas associated with hypertriglyceridemia are frequently eruptive; these yellow papules have an erythematous halo and are most frequently found on extensor surfaces of the extremities and buttocks. *(Wolff, p. 434)*

47. **(I)** The first exanthem of secondary syphilis is always macular and faint. Later eruptions may be papulosquamous and often involve the palms and soles. Associated findings that help make the diagnosis include annular plaques on the face, nonscarring alopecia, condylomata lata, mucous patches, lymphadenopathy, malaise, fever, headache, and myalgia. *(Wolff, p. 919)*

48. **(J)** Obesity is the most common cause of acanthosis nigricans—a velvety, localized hyperpigmentation. Other causes include gastrointestinal malignancy and endocrinopathy such as acromegaly, Cushing syndrome, Stein–Leventhal syndrome, or insulin-resistant diabetes. *(Wolff, p. 88)*

49. **(A)** Cancer chemotherapy most frequently involves rapidly proliferating elements of the skin, resulting in stomatitis and alopecia. Bleomycin, hydroxyurea, and 5-fluorouracil can cause dystrophic nail changes. Other skin manifestations of cancer drugs include sterile cellulitis, phlebitis, ulceration of pressure areas, urticaria, angioedema, and exfoliative dermatitis. The underlying malignancy often makes diagnosis of skin disease more difficult. *(Wolff, p. 1027)*

50. (C) Chloroquine is used for certain skin diseases such as lupus and polymorphous light eruption, but can also cause skin reactions and exacerbate porphyria cutanea tarda. Black pigmentation can involve the face, mucous membrane, and pretibial and subungual areas. *(Wolff, p. 346)*

51. (D) Birth control pills, sulfonamides, and penicillins are common drugs that can cause erythema nodosum. This is a panniculitis characterized by tender, subcutaneous, erythematous nodules characteristically found on the anterior portion of the legs. *(Wolff, p. 152)*

52. (B) The only common skin reaction with tetracyclines is photosensitivity. However, the drug is contraindicated in children under 8 years of age because of the risk of discoloring permanent teeth. *(Wolff, p. 244)*

53. (E) The combination of sulfamethoxazole and trimethoprim causes two distinct cutaneous reactions: an urticarial eruption in the first few days of therapy and a morbilliform eruption occurring a week or more after therapy has begun. This latter reaction is particularly common in patients with AIDS. Sulfonamides cause numerous skin lesions, including Stevens–Johnson syndrome. *(Wolff, p. 568)*

CHAPTER 3

Endocrinology
Questions

DIRECTIONS (Questions 1 through 32): For each of the questions in this section select the one lettered answer that is the best response in each case.

1. A 42-year-old woman presents to the clinic complaining of dry skin, fatigue, and weight gain over the past 3 months. She is not on any medications and there is no significant medical history.

    On physical examination, her blood pressure is 110/70 mm Hg, pulse 52/min, and heart and lungs are normal. Her skin feels rough and dry, but the rest of the examination is normal. Her biochemistry is normal but the thyroid-stimulating hormone (TSH) level is 39 mU/L (0.5–5 mU/L). **Which of the following is the most likely cause for her elevated TSH?**

    (A) trauma
    (B) radioactive iodine ingestion
    (C) autoimmune hypothyroidism
    (D) parathyroid surgery
    (E) medication side-effect

2. A 53-year-old man with gout for many years usually experiences 4–5 attacks a year. He treats each flare with an over-the-counter nonsteroidal anti-inflammatory drug (NSAID), but is not taking any medications for gout prophylaxis.

    On physical examination, there are no active joints presently, but he does have some tophaceous deposits on his left hand. As part of his complete evaluation, screening for renal complications of gout is performed. **Which of the following findings is most likely compatible with chronic gouty nephropathy?**

    (A) nephrotic syndrome
    (B) decreased urinary concentrating ability and proteinuria
    (C) acute kidney injury
    (D) acute tubular necrosis (ATN)
    (E) malignant hypertension

3. A 26-year-old woman presents to the clinic for assessment of various symptoms. She reports feeling fatigue, having poor concentration, and recent weight gain. She was involved in a motor vehicle accident (MVA) 4 months ago, and sustained a concussion from head injury. Her medical history is otherwise negative and she in not taking any medications. A screen for clinical depression is negative and she has no constitutional symptoms.

    On physical examination, the blood pressure is 104/68mm Hg, and heart rate is 56/min. The remaining exam is entirely normal. You suspect hypopituitarism, as a complication of the head injury from the MVA, as a possible diagnosis. **Which of the following is the most common presentation of anterior pituitary hyposecretion?**

    (A) occurrence of myxedema
    (B) decreased melanin pigmentation
    (C) emaciation and cachexia
    (D) loss of axillary and pubic hairs
    (E) amenorrhea

4. A 19-year-old woman presents to the clinic for evaluation of primary amenorrhea. Her physical examination is normal, and she has female sex characteristics and breast development. The only abnormality is the absence of body hair. Among other investigations she also has genetic testing that reveals an XY chromosome pattern. **Which of the following mechanisms is most likely to explain her phenotypic pattern and amenorrhea?**

(A) estrogen receptor defect

(B) excess hormone production

(C) androgen receptor defect

(D) decreased hormone production

(E) abnormal hormone production

5. A 17-year-old woman has skin photosensitivity since childhood but has gotten worse recently. Her skin appears fine indoors, but within a short period of sun exposure, she develops burning, redness, and itching. A diagnosis of erythropoietic protoporphyria is made by a dermatologist. (See Figure 3–1.) **Which of the following treatments is most likely to be helpful?**

(A) phenobarbital

(B) corticosteroids

(C) high carbohydrate diet

(D) beta-carotene

(E) chlorpromazine

6. A 23-year-old woman presents to the clinic for evaluation of irregular periods and infertility. Her clinical examination is entirely normal. Biochemical tests show a reduced estradiol and follicle-stimulating hormone (FSH) levels. She is diagnosed with central hypogonadism. **Which of the following is the most important function of FSH?**

(A) causes ovulation

(B) encourages progesterone secretion

(C) causes the secretory phase of the uterine mucosa

(D) inhibits estrogen secretion

(E) encourages maturation of the follicle

7. A healthy 42-year-old woman is found on routine blood testing to have a calcium level of 12 mg/dL. She feels well and reports no symptoms associated with hyperkalemia. Her past medical history includes a previous cesarean section, and she is not on any medications.

Her physical examination is normal. Further investigations reveal a parathormone

Figure 3–1. (Reproduced, with permission, from Wolff K and Johnson RA, *Fitzpatrick's Color Atlas & Synopsis of Clinical Dermatology,* 5th ed. New York: McGraw-Hill, 2005:257.)

(PTH) level of 750 pg/mL (230–630 pg/mL). **Which of the following findings is also associated with this disorder?**

(A) osteoblastic lesions of bone

(B) polycythemia

(C) prolonged QT interval on electrocardiogram (ECG)

(D) orthostatic hypotension

(E) cystic bone lesions

8. A 32-year-old woman presents to the emergency room because she is feeling unwell and experiencing muscle cramps and generalized fatigue. She had a previous thyroidectomy for a goiter 3 years ago and is taking thyroid supplements.

On physical examination, her blood pressure is 120/70 mm Hg, heart rate 100/min, and the heart and lungs are normal. Muscle strength and bulk are normal but the reflexes are increased symmetrically.

Her serum calcium level is 6.5 mg/dL (8.4–10.2 mg/dL), PTH 130 pg/ml (230–630 pg/ml), TSH 3 mU/L (0.5–5 mU/L), and albumin 4 g/dL (3.5–5.5 g/dL). **Which of the following is the most likely explanation for her low calcium?**

(A) idiopathic

(B) hereditary hypoparathyroidism

(C) postradiation

(D) end-organ resistance due to chronic kidney disease

(E) surgical removal

9. A 27-year-old woman presents to the clinic for evaluation of weight loss, fatigue, and weakness. She is also experiencing nausea and vomiting but no dysphagia.

On physical examination her blood pressure is 98/66mm Hg, and the heart rate is 96/min. The remaining physical examination is normal except for increased generalized skin pigmentation. Laboratory investigations reveal an impaired ACTH stimulation test, and a low serum sodium, and high potassium concentration. (See Figure 3–2.) **Which of the following features is also most likely to be present?**

(A) the skin is shiny and pale

(B) a diabetic glucose tolerance is characteristic

(C) water diuresis is impaired

(D) the urinary steroids are high

(E) the serum calcium is elevated

Figure 3–2. (Reproduced, with permission, from Wolff K and Johnson RA, *Fitzpatrick's Color Atlas & Synopsis of Clinical Dermatology,* 5th ed. New York: McGraw-Hill, 2005:445.)

10. A 32-year-old woman is evaluated in the clinic for symptoms of polyuria and polydipsia. She has no significant past medical history and her only medication is the oral contraceptive pill.

Her physical examination is entirely normal. Urine and serum biochemistry investigations are suggestive of central diabetes insipidus (DI). **Which of the following is the most likely finding on magnetic resonance imaging (MRI) of the brain?**

(A) hypothalamic tumor
(B) hyperintense signals in the cerebral cortex
(C) agenesis of the corpus callosum
(D) lack of hyperintense signals from the posterior pituitary
(E) communicating hydrocephalus

11. A 17-year-old man is seen in the clinic for evaluation of obesity. He has no significant past medical history and reports always being over weight even as a child. His review of symptoms is negative except for dyspnea on exertion, but no other cardiopulmonary symptoms.

On physical examination, the blood pressure is 130/80 mm Hg (with a large cuff), heart rate 84/min, respirations 12/min, and O_2 saturation 99%. His height is 5'7", weight 280 lbs, and BMI 44 kg/m^2. No medical cause for this "essential obesity" is found. **Which of the following abnormalities can he also be expected to have?**

(A) normal mortality risk
(B) hypothyroidism
(C) low PCO_2 values
(D) hypertriglyceridemia
(E) hyperadrenocorticalism

12. A 56-year-old man presents to the emergency department complaining of a change in skin color, fatigue, discomfort in his hand joints, and abdominal pain. He has also noticed increased urine output and thirst.

On examination, his skin appears bronze in color, his liver span is 16 cm, and there is loss of body hair, and testicular atrophy. His ferritin is 600 ng/mL (15–200 ng/mL), aspartate amino transferase (AST) 130 U/L (8–20 U/L), alanine amino transferase (ALT) 150 U/L (8–20 U/L), and total bilirubin 0.5 mg/dL (0.1–1 mg/dL). Coagulation tests and albumin level are normal but the random glucose is elevated at 250 mg/dL. **Which of the following is the most likely diagnosis?**

(A) diabetes mellitus (DM)
(B) amyloidosis
(C) Wilson disease
(D) hemochromatosis
(E) Addison disease

13. A 35-year-old man has had recurrent attacks of abdominal pain and proximal motor neuropathy since puberty. The episodes are precipitated by infections and certain medications. During one of the attacks, the plasma porphobilinogen levels were increased. **Which of the following medications is not considered safe in patients with this condition?**

(A) chlorpromazine
(B) sulfonamide antibiotics
(C) penicillin and derivatives
(D) narcotics
(E) glucocorticoids

14. A 43-year-old man is seen in the clinic for an annual health assessment. He feels well and physical examination including the blood pressure is normal. He weighs 85 kg and is 1.8 m tall. His calculated body mass index (BMI) is 23 kg/m^2. **Which of the following conditions is he most likely at risk for?**

(A) DM
(B) hyperlipoproteinemia
(C) abnormal growth hormone response
(D) atherosclerosis
(E) no increased risk for mortality

15. A 47-year-old woman with bipolar disorder presents to the clinic for assessment of symptoms of polyuria and polydipsia. The symptoms

started gradually but are getting worse over the past 3 months. Her review of symptoms is negative, and there is no family history of type 2 diabetes. Her only medication is lithium used to control her bipolar disorder.

On physical examination, the blood pressure is 124/78 mm Hg, heart rate is 88/min, and the jugular venous pressure is normal. The heart sounds are normal and the lungs clear. The remaining exam is normal. **Which of the following is the most likely explanation for this complication of lithium treatment?**

(A) impaired glucose absorption at the cellular level

(B) decreased production of antidiuretic hormone (ADH)

(C) increased production of ADH

(D) a solute diuresis

(E) impaired ADH action at the distal renal tubular level

16. The 2-year-old daughter of a Jewish couple, whose parents emigrated from Russia, develops progressive loss of motor skills. There is macular pallor on ophthalmic examination, and she has a short stature, thin limbs, but full cheeks. She is also prone to developing hypoglycemia and lactic acidosis. **Which of the following metabolic abnormalities is most likely associated with this disorder?**

(A) glycogen storage

(B) ganglioside accumulation

(C) amyloid accumulation

(D) corneal deposits

(E) cholesterol accumulation

17. A 63-year-old man comes to the clinic for evaluation of edema, and dyspnea on exertion. He has no prior history of cardiac or renal conditions, and on physical examination the pertinent findings are macroglossia, elevated jugular venous pressure (JVP), hepatomegaly, and 3+ pedal edema. (See Figure 3–3.) **Which of the following is the most characteristic neurologic finding associated with this condition?**

Figure 3–3.

His laboratory investigations:

24 hour urine protein excretion:	3.5 g/d
Hemoglobin:	11 g/dL
Fasting glucose:	80 mg/dL
Creatinine:	1.6 mg/dL
Serum immunoelectrophoresis:	positive for a monoclonal immunoglobulin.

(A) peripheral motor and sensory neuropathy

(B) spinal cord compression in the lumbar region

(C) spinal cord compression in the thoracic region

(D) a peripheral neuropathy associated with cerebral manifestations

(E) a Guillain–Barré-type syndrome

18. A 30-year-old man presents to the clinic with recurrent symptoms of flushing, diarrhea, and weight loss. He cannot associate the symptoms with any particular activity, time of day or food ingestion. His past medical history is negative and he is not taking any prescription or recreational medications.

   On physical examination, his blood pressure is 126/74 mm Hg, and the heart rate is 72/min and regular. His remaining physical examination is completely normal. Lab investigations reveal an elevated urinary 5-hydroxyindoleacetic acid (5-HIAA). **Which of the following is the most likely diagnosis?**

   (A) phenylketonuria
   (B) alkaptonuria
   (C) malignant melanoma
   (D) carcinoid syndrome
   (E) disseminated carcinomatosis

19. A 25-year-old woman presents to the clinic with symptoms of polyuria and polydipsia. The symptoms started 1 month ago and she notes that the urine output does change with oral fluid intake. Her past medical history is significant for a prior appendectomy as a child and endometriosis. She is currently on an oral contraceptive pill. So far, investigations have ruled out psychogenic polydipsia and diabetes as causes.

   A fluid deprivation test is performed. At the end of the test, the urine osmolality is 240 mOsm/kg and the serum antidiuretic hormone (ADH) level is elevated. **Which of the following is the most likely diagnosis?**

   (A) adrenal cortex defect
   (B) nephrogenic diabetes insipidus
   (C) central (posterior pituitary) diabetes insipidus
   (D) acute tubular necrosis (ATN)
   (E) Addison disease

20. A 40-year-old woman has lipid investigations suggesting familial hypercholesterolemia (increased cholesterol, increased low-density lipoprotein [LDL], and normal triglycerides). This condition is characterized by increased risk for premature atherosclerosis and by the occurrence of tuberous and tendon xanthomas.

Before making the assumption of familial hypercholesterolemia, secondary causes need to be considered. **Which of the following conditions is most likely to cause secondary hyperlipidemia?**

   (A) cholestatic liver disease
   (B) alcoholism
   (C) estrogen replacement
   (D) malabsorption syndromes
   (E) chronic lung disease

21. A 61-year-old woman with poorly controlled type 2 diabetes is seen in follow-up. Her blood sugars are persistently elevated to levels greater than 200 mg/dL, and her hemoglobin A1C value is 9.5%.

   On examination, she is obese, the blood pressure is 165/90 mm Hg, heart rate is 80/min, and the cardiac and respiratory exams are normal. Sensory testing with a tuning fork reveals that she has sensory loss to her mid-shins in both legs. **Which of the following fasting lipid profiles is most likely to be consistent with her values?**

   (A) high total cholesterol, low LDL, and normal triglycerides
   (B) high total cholesterol, high LDL, low triglycerides
   (C) high total cholesterol, normal LDL, high triglycerides
   (D) high total cholesterol, low LDL, and low triglycerides
   (E) high total cholesterol, high LDL, and high triglycerides

22. A 26-year-old man is evaluated in the clinic for persistent symptoms of back pain and fatigue. There is no history of any mechanical injury and he was previously healthy.

   On examination, he is pale, there is lumber spine tenderness on palpation, and the liver is enlarged with a span of 18 cm. The complete blood count reveals that he is pancytopenic, and there is a vertebral fracture on lumbar x-rays. A bone-marrow biopsy reveals infiltration with lipid-laden macrophages (Gaucher cells). **Which of the following is the most likely diagnosis?**

(A) metachromatic leukodystrophy
(B) inherited Gaucher disease
(C) acquired Gaucher disease
(D) glycogen storage disease
(E) familial hyperchylomicronemia

23. A 19-year-old man presents to the clinic complaining of early fatigue and muscle cramps while playing sports. He is fine when walking or doing less intense levels of work. On physical examination, he appears well and the vital signs are normal. Muscle bulk, tone and strength in the proximal muscles are normal. There is no muscle fatigue with repetitive arm-grip exercises. After an exercise stress test, his serum creatine kinase (CK) is elevated and lactate level is normal. **Which of the following is the most likely diagnosis?**

(A) Gaucher disease
(B) Tay–Sachs disease
(C) McArdle disease (glycogen storage disease)
(D) hemochromatosis
(E) myasthenia gravis

24. A 33-year-old man presents to the emergency department complaining of severe left flank pain that radiates to the front inguinal region. The pain started abruptly and was so intense that he almost felt like "passing out." Nothing seems to relieve the pain.

His physical examination is entirely normal, and in particular there is no fever or costovertebral angle tenderness. Eventually the pain subsides after the passage of "sand-like" urine. A urinalysis reveals flat hexagonal plate like crystals (cystine). **Which of the following statements about this condition is most likely true?**

(A) commonest cause of renal stones
(B) stones are radiolucent on x-ray
(C) increased cystine concentration in the urine
(D) decreased cystine concentration in the urine
(E) acquired disorder of cystine metabolism

25. A 50-year-old man presents to the clinic with symptoms of feeling tired and unsteady on his feet. His history is vague and the details are poor. He does volunteer a decreased appetite and weight loss of 15 lb over the past 6 months.

On physical examination, he appears cachectic, the heart and lungs are normal, but his liver span is 18 cm. His lab tests show a very low magnesium level (0.7 mEq/L). On further questioning, he reports drinking heavily since losing his job. **Which of the following is the most likely explanation for his low magnesium level?**

(A) alcoholism
(B) chronic malabsorption
(C) DM
(D) kwashiorkor
(E) hypervitaminosis E

26. A 27-year-old woman presents to the clinic with symptoms of feeling unwell ever since going on a high vitamin diet. She is also experiencing dry skin, vomiting, headaches, and amenorrhea.

Her physical examination and lab data are positive for hepatomegaly, splenomegaly, leukopenia, anemia, periosteal changes, sparse and coarse hair, and increased serum lipids. **Which of the following is the most likely diagnosis?**

(A) vitamin D intoxication
(B) vitamin D deficiency
(C) vitamin A deficiency
(D) vitamin A intoxication
(E) carotenemia

27. A 25-year-old man requests cholesterol screening because of a family history of premature coronary artery disease (CAD). His lipid levels reveal an elevated total and LDL cholesterol. The high-density lipoprotein (HDL) and triglyceride values are normal. His physical examination is completely normal. **Which of the following is the most common cause of genetic dyslipidemia?**

(A) familial combined hyperlipidemia
(B) familial hypercholesterolemia
(C) familial defective Apo B
(D) Apo C-II deficiency
(E) lipoprotein lipase deficiency

28. A 28-year-old woman with type 1 diabetes presents to the clinic for evaluation of skin lesions on her leg. They are not painful or itchy and have developed gradually over time. There is no history of previous trauma to the site either.

On physical examination the skin changes have a central depression and raised irregular margin. The surrounding area is not red, tender, or indurated. They are shown in Figure 3–4. **Which of the following is the most likely diagnosis?**

(A) eruptive xanthomas
(B) necrobiosis lipoidica diabeticorum
(C) gangrene
(D) staphylococcal infection
(E) erythema nodosum

29. A 54-year-old man comes to the emergency room complaining of severe pain in his right toe. The pain is interfering with his ability to walk and he reports no prior trauma to the toe. He has had multiple less severe episodes in the past, which he always treats with pain medications.

On physical examination, the toe is red, inflamed, and exquisitely sensitive to movement. An x-ray of the toe is normal and needle aspiration of the joint confirms uric acid crystals. He is treated with oral indomethacin (NSAID) for 7 days, and 1 month later he remains symptom free. Allopurinol is recommended for prevention of this condition. **Which of the following is the most likely mechanism of action of allopurinol?**

(A) inhibition of xanthine oxidase
(B) solubilization of uric acid
(C) reactivity with hypoxanthine
(D) anti-inflammatory effect on joint tissue
(E) increased renal tubular secretion of uric acid

Figure 3–4. (Reproduced, with permission, from Wolff K and Johnson RA, *Fitzpatrick's Color Atlas & Synopsis of Clinical Dermatology, 6th ed.* New York: McGraw-Hill, 2009:429.)

30. A 53-year-old woman with a past medical history of chronic kidney disease due to diabetic nephropathy is noted to have hyperphosphatemia and hypocalcemia on routine electrolyte measurement. The disturbance is likely a result of metabolic bone disease seen in patients with chronic kidney disease. **Which of the following findings is most likely associated with this electrolyte disturbance?**

    (A) lethargy
    (B) neuromuscular irritability
    (C) anorexia
    (D) tachyarrhythmias
    (E) nausea and vomiting

31. A 22-year-old man presents to the clinic for routine annual exam. He reports no specific symptoms and feels well. His past medical history is significant for vision difficulty that an ophthalmologist has diagnosed as subluxation of his lens and flattened corneas. He also states that one of his heart valves "leaks" because of an enlargement of the aorta.

    On physical examination, the blood pressure is 122/62mm Hg, heart rate is 72/min regular, and there is a soft S2 and early diastolic murmur heard best at the aortic region radiating to the left sternal border. His lungs are clear and on inspection he is tall in stature with the span of his arms being greater than his height. **Which of the following is the most likely diagnosis?**

    (A) Ehlers–Danlos syndrome
    (B) Marfan syndrome
    (C) Werner syndrome
    (D) Laurence–Moon–Biedl syndrome
    (E) Hunter syndrome

32. A 33-year-old man is complaining of feeling thirsty all the time and passing more urine than usual. His physical examination is normal, except for a JVP below the sternal angle. **Which of the following drugs is most likely to cause this disorder?**

Investigations:

SERUM
sodium: 150 mEq/L
glucose: 120 mg/dL
osmolality: 315 mOsm/kg
URINE
sodium: 10 mE/L
osmolality: 260 mOsm/kg

    (A) lithium
    (B) cyclophosphamide
    (C) barbiturates
    (D) nicotine
    (E) morphine

DIRECTIONS (Questions 33 through 37): The following group of numbered items is preceded by a list of lettered options. For each question, select the one lettered option that is most closely associated with it. Each lettered option may be used once, multiple times, or not at all.

Questions 33 through 37: For each of the following dyslipidemias, select the most characteristic finding.

    (A) palmar plane xanthomas
    (B) triglycerides >1000
    (C) subcutaneous extensor tendon xanthomas
    (D) low serum cholesterol
    (E) normal cholesterol levels
    (F) xanthelasma after age 50 only

33. Hyperchylomicronemia.

34. Hyperbetalipoproteinemia.

35. Type III hyperlipoproteinemia.

36. Hyperprebetalipoproteinemia.

37. Hypertriglyceridemia.

DIRECTIONS (Questions 38 through 68): For each of the questions in this section select the one lettered answer that is the best response in each case.

38. A 20-year-old woman is complaining of passing large amounts of urine. She is otherwise well and her physical examination is normal. The serum sodium is 140 mEq/L and the urinalysis is negative for protein and glucose. The urine sodium is <20 mEq/L, and urine osmolality is 268 mOsm/kg. She weighs 60 kg, and her 24-hour urine output is over 4 L. **Which of the following is the most likely diagnosis?**

    (A) diabetes mellitus (DM)
    (B) psychogenic polydipsia
    (C) diabetes insipidus (DI)
    (D) contracted bladder
    (E) solute diureses

39. A 62-year-old man is seen in the office. He feels well and reports no new symptoms. His past medical history is pertinent for essential hypertension which is treated with ramipril. As part of routine screening, fasting blood work is performed and his glucose is normal, but the lipid profile reveals elevated LDL cholesterol. **Which of the following is the most likely cause for the elevated LDL?**

    (A) an autosomal dominant disease
    (B) an X-linked recessive disease
    (C) a polygenic disease
    (D) a poor diet
    (E) DM

40. A 54-year-old woman is seen in the clinic for routine followup. She has no past medical history and is otherwise healthy with no active symptoms. Her physical examination is normal including her blood pressure and heart rate. Routine fasting blood work reveals normal electrolytes, renal function, and glucose. Her total cholesterol is elevated and you decide to council her on lifestyle intervention. **Which of the following dietary abnormalities is most commonly associated with elevated cholesterol levels?**

    (A) inadequate fiber
    (B) excess calories resulting in obesity
    (C) excess dietary cholesterol
    (D) excess total fat intake
    (E) excess trans-fatty acid intake

41. A 63-year-old asymptomatic woman is seen in the clinic for investigation of a persistently elevated alkaline phosphatase (ALP) level. The elevated ALP is an isolated finding and the remaining liver enzymes are normal. She reports no abdominal symptoms suggestive of biliary colic or hepatitis.

    On physical examination, the vital signs are normal, she is not icteric, the heart sounds are normal and the lungs are clear. The abdomen is soft and the liver span is 12 cm in the mid-clavicular line.

    X-rays of the pelvis show multiple porotic and sclerotic lesions with characteristic whorls of trabeculation. Her excretion of urinary hydroxyproline is also elevated. **Which of the following is the most likely diagnosis?**

    (A) rickets and osteomalacia
    (B) osteogenic sarcoma
    (C) vitamin D deficiency
    (D) Paget disease of bone
    (E) metastatic cancer

42. A 20-year-old man presents to the emergency department complaining of symptoms of generalized weakness with numbness and tingling in his hands. His past medical history is significant for a previous humerus fracture at the age of 12 after falling off his bike. He currently is not on any medication.

    The physical examination is normal, but laboratory investigations reveal that his calcium is 7.4 mg/dL (8.4–10.2 mg/dL). **Which of the following additional serum values is most consistent with the diagnosis of vitamin D deficiency?**

    (A) low vitamin D, low phosphate, high PTH
    (B) low vitamin D, low phosphate, low PTH
    (C) low vitamin D, high phosphate, low PTH

(D) normal vitamin D, low phosphate, high PTH

(E) normal vitamin D, high phosphate, high PTH

43. A 19-year-old woman presents to the clinic for evaluation of symptoms of weight loss, tremor, and heat intolerance. Her past medical history is negative and her only medication is the oral contraceptive pill.

On physical examination, the blood pressure is 96/64 mm Hg, heart rate 110/min, and the thyroid exam reveals an enlarged non-tender gland with no nodules. The heart and lungs are normal but the skin feels warm to touch, and she has a fine tremor of her hands.

Laboratory investigations reveal a low TSH and elevated free T4 and T3 levels. **Which of the following cardiac findings is most likely to occur in her?**

(A) atrial fibrillation
(B) sinus tachycardia
(C) bradycardia
(D) increase in heart size
(E) pericardial effusion

44. A thyroid nodule is found on a 40-year-old woman on routine evaluation. She has no prior history of thyroid disease and clinically feels well with no symptoms suggestive of hyper or hypothyroidism. There is a 20-mm non-tender nodule on the right lobe of the thyroid with no associated lymphadenopathy. Thyroid function tests are normal. **Which of the following is the most appropriate next step in management?**

(A) thyroid scan
(B) fine needle aspiration (FNA) biopsy
(C) repeat assessment in 6 months
(D) partial thyroidectomy
(E) complete thyroidectomy

45. A 40-year-old woman presents to the clinic for evaluation of symptoms of light-headedness associated with sweating, palpitations, and hunger. The symptoms are most pronounced whenever she misses a meal.

On physical examination, her vital signs are normal, as is the heart, lungs, and abdominal examination. Her past medical history is negative and she is not taking any medications. During one such episode, while in hospital, her blood glucose level was 30 mg/dL and the symptoms resolved with drinking some juice. **Which of the following is the most likely diagnosis?**

(A) excess growth hormone
(B) Cushing disease
(C) thyrotoxicosis
(D) tumor of the pancreatic beta-cells
(E) gastrin deficiency

46. A 63-year-old man is newly diagnosed with light-chain amyloidosis (AL). **In which of the following organs, is deposition of amyloid protein most likely to cause symptoms?**

(A) heart
(B) red cells
(C) thyroid
(D) pancreas
(E) liver

47. A 25-year-old woman presents with intermittent symptoms of sweating, palpitations, and hunger. Her past medical history is non-contributory and she is not taking any medications. On physical examination, the blood pressure is 110/70 mm Hg and the heart rate is 80/min. The thyroid exam in normal and there are no signs of hyperthyroidism.

During one such episode, investigations reveal a glucose level of less than 40 mg/dL, with corresponding low serum insulin and high serum glucagon levels. **Which of the following best describes the hormone function of glucagon?**

(A) promotes glycogenolysis and gluconeogenesis
(B) a carbohydrate in structure
(C) effective in lowering blood sugar levels
(D) antigenically similar to insulin
(E) effective in decreasing cyclic adenosine monophosphate (cAMP) in target cells

48. A 34-year-old woman notices lumps on her elbows and yellow patches below her eyelids. She presents to the clinic because the skin changes are cosmetically bothersome. Her past medical history is negative and she is not on any medications.

On examination, she has tendon xanthomas on her elbows and xanthelasma under the eyelids. Her lipid profile is consistent with a diagnosis of familial hypercholesterolemia (increased LDL). **Which of the following statements regarding the treatment of this condition is correct?**

(A) dietary therapy is usually sufficient

(B) cholestyramine is as effective as hepatic hydroxymethylglutaryl-coenzyme A (HMG-CoA) reductase inhibitors (statins)

(C) ninety percent of patients can be controlled with a statin

(D) a statin is the only type of medication suitable for monotherapy

(E) combined therapy is frequently required

49. Which of the following is the most common manifestation of multiple endocrine neoplasia, type I (MEN I)?

(A) Zollinger–Ellison syndrome

(B) an adrenal adenoma

(C) primary hyperparathyroidism

(D) acromegaly

(E) testicular cancer

50. A 51-year-old woman presents to the clinic because she is experiencing irregular periods for the past 6 months, as well as symptoms of hot flashes and night sweats. Her physical examination is normal. Hormone replacement therapy (HRT) is prescribed for her symptoms and she notices a marked improvement in her symptoms. **Which of the following is the most likely additional benefit of HRT?**

(A) decreased CAD

(B) a decreased risk of Alzheimer disease

(C) reduced venothromboembolism

(D) decreased breast cancer risk

(E) decreased osteoporosis-related fractures

51. A 37-year-old woman presents to the emergency room after falling down some stairs at work. She reports no pre-monitory symptoms prior to the fall or any loss of consciousness. Recently she has noticed persistent symptoms of fatigue, muscle weakness, and unexpected weight gain. She has no past medical history and is not taking any medications.

On examination, the blood pressure is 164/92 mm Hg and heart rate is 84/min. There are multiple skin bruises, facial fullness, and truncal obesity with red "stretch marks." Muscle strength in the proximal muscles is 4/5 and the reflexes are normal. **Which of the following is the most appropriate initial diagnostic test?**

(A) computerized tomography (CT) scan of the abdomen

(B) fasting glucose

(C) overnight dexamethasone suppression test

(D) electromyogram (EMG) studies

(E) MR of the brain

52. A 43-year-old woman presents to the clinic for evaluation because she is concerned about increased hand and foot size. Her past health history is only significant for a live birth by cesarean section at the age of 30, and a pregnancy complicated by gestational diabetes.

On examination, she has spade-like hands, coarsened facial features, and a gap between her incisors. Her blood pressure is 155/85 mm Hg and pulse 80/min, cardiac apical beat is sustained with normal heart sounds. **Which of the following is the most likely effect of this syndrome on the muscles?**

(A) enlargement

(B) spasm

(C) increased strength

(D) myositis

(E) rhythmic contraction

53. A 7-year-old boy has demineralized bones with pseudofractures seen on x-rays. Physiologic doses of vitamin D do not result in improvement. **Which of the following is most likely to be associated with this syndrome?**

    (A) hyperphosphatemia
    (B) low 1,25(OH)2 vitamin D levels
    (C) alopecia
    (D) osteoporosis
    (E) mental retardation

54. An 18-year-old girl is brought to hospital because of weakness. She feels well, but is under a lot of stress at school. Most of her time is spent studying, dieting, and exercising. On physical examination she is 5'8" weighs 85lbs, and appears unwell. The blood pressure is 85/70 mm Hg, heart rate is 50/min, and there is prominent muscle wasting. **Which of the following is this patient most likely at risk for?**

    (A) renal failure
    (B) ventricular tachyarrhythmias
    (C) DM
    (D) hyperthermia
    (E) pernicious anemia

55. A 53-year-old man presents to the clinic complaining of sudden onset and severe pain in his left big toe starting the previous evening. He reports no prior episodes of similar symptoms and no recent trauma. On examination there is redness, and swelling in his left big toe, with severe pain on passive range of motion. **Which of the following conditions is most likely associated with this condition?**

    (A) pernicious anemia
    (B) DI
    (C) Alzheimer disease
    (D) anorexia
    (E) renal disease

56. A 27-year-old woman presents to the emergency department complaining of pain in her left shin. The pain started gradually over the past week and she does not recall any fall or injury to the leg. The pain increases when she is walking and is relieved with rest. The physical examination is entirely normal except for point tenderness on palpation over the mid-tibia.

    X-rays of the leg reveal a stress fracture of the tibia, decreased cortical bone density, and increased radiolucency. She is suspected of having osteomalacia (impaired mineralization of bone matrix). **Which of the following is the most common biochemical manifestation of osteomalacia?**

    (A) hyperphosphatemia
    (B) hypoparathyroidism
    (C) decreased vitamin D
    (D) hypercalcemia
    (E) low alkaline phosphatase (ALP)

57. A 44-year-old man presents to the emergency department with symptoms of worsening abdominal distension, edema, and jaundice. He has a past medical history of chronic viral hepatitis B and cirrhosis. Recently he has noticed decreased urine output despite adequate fluid intake.

    On physical examination, he is icteric, the blood pressure is 110/70 mm Hg, heart rate 74/min, JVP is 4 cm, and heart sounds are normal. The abdomen is non-tender but there is tense ascites and pitting edema up to the thigh. **Which of the following is an early manifestation of hepatorenal syndrome?**

    (A) intrarenal vasodilatation
    (B) sodium retention
    (C) potassium retention
    (D) severe jaundice
    (E) polyuria

58. A 21-year-old woman presents to the clinic for assessment of new symptoms of tremor, and incoordination. The symptoms were first noted 3 months ago, and have progressively gotten worse to the point that she fell 1 week ago. Her past medical history is significant for unexplained hepatitis 2 years ago and depression 1 year ago. She is currently not taking any medications.

Her physical examination is pertinent for increased tone and rigidity but normal muscle strength of the upper and lower limbs. She has a coarse tremor of the hands, and coordination tests are normal. An ophthalmologic examination reveals a brownish-pigmented ring at the corneal margin. (See Figure 3–5.) **Which of the following findings is most likely to be present in this patient?**

Figure 3–5.

(A) renal failure
(B) cirrhosis of the liver
(C) elevated ceruloplasmin
(D) sensory loss
(E) increased plasma copper

59. A 57-year-old man presents to the clinic with complaints of increased thirst and urination. Medical history is significant for hypertension which is well controlled on diltiazem. On physical examination, the blood pressure is 135/84 mm Hg, heart rate is 72/min, BMI>30, and the remaining exam is normal. **Which of**

the following is the most appropriate initial diagnostic test?

(A) a urine osmolality
(B) hemoglobin A1C level
(C) a fasting blood sugar (FBS)
(D) a glucose tolerance test (GTT)
(E) random glucose

60. Which of the following is the most likely effect of insulin at the cellular receptor level?

(A) stimulating tyrosine kinase
(B) binding to ion channels
(C) binding to intracellular erb A receptors
(D) stimulating guanylate cyclase
(E) activating G-proteins

61. Which of the following is the most likely metabolic effect of insulin on adipose tissue?

(A) decrease of glucose transport
(B) decrease in glucose phosphorylation
(C) decrease in lipolysis
(D) decrease in lipoprotein lipase
(E) enhancement of glucagon effect

62. A 32-year-old woman presents to the clinic for evaluation of symptoms of heat intolerance, palpitations, diarrhea, weakness, and 10 lb weight loss. The symptoms started gradually but are worse over the past 1 week. She has no other medical history and is not taking any medications. Her family history is negative for thyroid diseases.

On physical examination, her blood pressure is 90/60 mm Hg, heart rate is 110/min, and she has a fine tremor in her hands. The TSH level is suppressed and T3 and T4 are elevated. **Which of the following is most likely to precipitate this condition?**

(A) propylthiouracil administration (PTU)
(B) high-dose prednisone therapy
(C) beta-adrenergic blockade
(D) pneumonia
(E) salicylate administration

63. A 15-year-old youth has not gone through puberty. **Which of the following is the most likely diagnosis?**

    (A) inadequate diet
    (B) normal variation
    (C) pituitary tumor
    (D) Leydig cell dysfunction
    (E) drug side effects

64. A 44-year-old woman was recently diagnosed with breast cancer and undergoes a mastectomy. She now presents to the clinic for follow-up, and states that she is doing well after the surgery. **Which of the following features is most likely to be important in determining response to tamoxifen therapy?**

    (A) metastases confined to liver
    (B) patient more than 5 years premenopausal
    (C) androgen receptors on the tumor cell membrane
    (D) tumor has progesterone receptors (PR)
    (E) metastases confined to brain

65. **Which of the following increases a woman's risk of breast cancer?**

    (A) bilateral oophorectomy before age 40 years
    (B) late first pregnancy
    (C) long-term nursing
    (D) history of breast cancer in an aunt
    (E) multiparity

66. A 65-year-old woman with type 2 diabetes is on hemodialysis for chronic kidney disease. She now presents to the clinic with symptoms of pain in the hands. The symptoms started many months age and are now getting worse. She does not recall any injury to the hands and has not noticed any swelling or redness in the joints.

On examination, the joints are normal with no inflammation or tenderness on palpation. There is full range of motion of the fingers and wrists.

Lab investigations: calcium (7.2 mg/dL), phosphate (5.5 mg/dL), and PTH level (710 ng/L). (See Figure 3–6.) **What is the most likely diagnosis?**

Figure 3–6.

    (A) scleroderma
    (B) gout
    (C) secondary hyperparathyroidism
    (D) pseudogout
    (E) Paget disease

67. A 35-year-old woman presents to the clinic for evaluation of symptoms of fatigue, weakness, and weight gain. The symptoms started gradually and seem to be getting worse. She has no prior medical history and her only medication is the oral contraceptive pill.

On physical examination the blood pressure is 164/90 mm Hg, heart rate is 80/min, heart sounds are normal, and the lungs are clear. Her face is full, and there is central obesity around her abdomen with skin striae that have a deep red color. Investigations are shown in Table 3–1. **Which of the following is the most likely diagnosis?**

TABLE 3–1. CASE WORK-UP

	Normal	Patient
Plasma ACTH pg/mL	<150	<50
Plasma cortisol u/dL	17	35
Urine 17-OH mg/24 h	2 to 10	25
Urine 17-Ks mg/24 h	5 to 15	10
Urine 17-OH response to:		
ACTH IV	Increase × 5	No response
Dexamethasone 0.5 mg	<3.0	No response
2.0 mg	<3.0	No response
Metyrapone 750 mg	Increase × 2	No response

Abbreviation: ACTH–adrenocorticotropic hormone

(A) adrenal hyperplasia secondary to hypothalamic dysfunction
(B) adrenal adenoma with complete autonomy
(C) exogenous steroids, iatrogenic
(D) pituitary tumor
(E) carcinoma of the adrenal

68. A 55-year-old obese woman presents to the clinic for evaluation of multiple symptoms. She notes frequent episodes of vaginal yeast infections in the past 2 months, recent weight loss in spite of a large appetite, and waking up frequently at night to urinate. There is no history of fever or chills, and her only past medical illness is hypertension that is treated with ramipril. **Which of the following is the most likely diagnosis?**

(A) diabetes mellitus (DM)
(B) diabetes incipidus (DI)

(C) vaginitis and cystitis
(D) myxedema
(E) pheochromocytoma

DIRECTIONS (Questions 69 through 79): The following group of numbered items is preceded by a list of lettered options. For each question, select the one lettered option that is most closely associated with it. Each lettered option may be used once, multiple times, or not at all.

Questions 69 through 71: For each patient with a complication of diabetes, select the most likely diagnosis or findings.

(A) microaneurysms and hemorrhage (dot and blot)
(B) vitreal hemorrhage
(C) dilated veins
(D) open-angle glaucoma
(E) erythema multiforme
(F) pyoderma gangrenosum
(G) necrobiosis lipoidica
(H) candidiasis

69. A 72-year-old man with type 2 diabetes notices painless skin lesions on his legs. They have an irregular raised border with a flat depressed center that is hyperpigmented brown in color.

70. A 59-year-old man with type 2 diabetes goes for a screening eye examination. The ophthalmologist reports that the patient has developed nonproliferative retinopathy. (List the findings.)

71. A 35-year-old woman with type 1 diabetes develops progressive vision loss in her left eye. The ophthalmologist reports the development of proliferative retinopathy. (List the findings.)

Questions 72 through 75: For each of the following causes of sexual dysfunction, select the most likely clinical feature.

(A) loss of sexual desire

(B) failure of erection with absent nocturnal penile tumescence (NPT)

(C) absence of emission

(D) absence of orgasm with normal libido and erectile function

(E) failure of detumescence

72. Can be caused by high prolactin level.

73. Rarely indicates organic disease.

74. Can be caused by hematologic disease.

75. Can be caused by vascular disease.

Questions 76 through 79: For each of the following explanations for hirsutism, select the most likely cause.

(A) drugs

(B) adrenal tumor

(C) polycystic ovarian disease (PCOD)

(D) adrenal hyperplasia

(E) idiopathic hirsutism

(F) ovarian tumor

76. Slight elevation of plasma testosterone and androstenedione.

77. Can be associated with anovulation, obesity, and amenorrhea.

78. May stimulate surrounding tissue to secrete androgens.

79. Often associated with elevated 17-hydroxyprogesterone levels.

DIRECTIONS (Questions 80 through 83): For each of the questions in this section select the one lettered answer that is the best response in each case.

80. A 15-year-old girl has been losing weight and exercising vigorously. She feels overweight and wants to lose more weight. On examination, she is thin with muscle wasting. **Which of the following physical signs is also suggestive of the diagnosis?**

(A) salivary gland enlargement

(B) coarse body hair

(C) diarrhea

(D) tachycardia

(E) hypertension

81. A 17-year-old man is brought to the emergency room because of weakness and weight loss. He is diagnosed with an eating disorder and admitted to the hospital. **Which of the following lab values is not consistent with this diagnosis?**

(A) hypokalemia

(B) hypochloremia

(C) metabolic alkalosis

(D) hyperglycemia

(E) low blood urea nitrogen (BUN)

82. A 22-year-old woman is brought to hospital because of syncope. There were no warning symptoms, and she was fine after the event. Recently she has lost 40 lb because of an eating disorder. She weighs 70 lb, looks unwell, and has little muscle bulk. The blood pressure is 80/60 mm Hg and pulse 50/min. **Which of the following is the most likely abnormality on her ECG?**

(A) resting sinus tachycardia

(B) increased QRS voltages

(C) short QT interval

(D) increased T waves

(E) prolonged QT interval

83. A 64-year-old woman with type 2 diabetes for 10 years now develops increasing fatigue, dyspnea, and pedal edema. On examination, her blood pressure is 165/90 mm Hg, pulse 90/min, JVP is 4 cm, heart sounds are normal, lungs are clear, and there is 3+ pedal edema.

Her urinalysis is positive for 3 gm/L of protein and no casts or red blood cells. An abdominal ultrasound reveals normal size kidneys and no hydronephrosis. **Which of the following renal diseases is the most likely diagnosis in this patient?**

(A) acute glomerulonephritis (GN)

(B) obstructive uropathy

(C) glomerulosclerosis with mesangial thickening

(D) renal infarction

(E) polycystic kidneys

DIRECTIONS (Questions 84 through 89): The following group of numbered items is preceded by a list of lettered options. For each question, select the one lettered option that is most closely associated with it. Each lettered option may be used once, multiple times, or not at all.

Questions 84 through 89: For each patient placed on a dietary restriction, select the most likely diagnosis.

(A) diabetes

(B) obesity

(C) hypertension

(D) anorexia nervosa (AN)

(E) gastroesophageal reflux (GERD)

(F) postgastrectomy

(G) Parkinson disease

(H) cirrhosis

(I) Crohn disease

(J) osteoporosis

(K) celiac disease

(L) irritable bowel syndrome

(M) hyperlipidemia

84. A 24-year-old female is placed on a low residue and low fiber diet. She has a long history of right lower quadrant pain, cramps, and diarrhea.

85. A 56-year-old man is started on a low caloric and weight loss diet. He recently started feeling unwell, had vision changes, and noticed numbness in his feet.

86. A 52-year-old woman is started on a low sodium diet. She feels well and is experiencing no symptoms. Her physical examination is normal except for a sustained cardiac apical impulse.

87. A 64-year-old man is placed on a low simple sugar diet. He is experiencing symptoms of crampy abdominal discomfort, nausea, diarrhea, and diaphoresis 15–30 minutes after eating.

88. A 45-year-old woman is placed on a protein restriction diet and a daily laxative regimen. She recently had a hospital admission for confusion related to a chronic illness.

89. A 38-year-old woman is told to limit chocolate and caffeine intake for worsening symptoms. She is also told that weight loss is helpful in improving the symptoms for her condition.

Questions 90 through 94: For each patient with vitamin deficiency or excess, select the most likely diagnosis.

(A) niacin

(B) thiamine

(C) pyridoxine

(D) vitamin C

(E) vitamin A

(F) vitamin E

(G) vitamin K

90. An 83-year-old man with poor nutrition notices easy bruising and bleeding gums. On examination, he has inflamed bleeding gums, multiple areas of ecchymoses, and perifollicular hemorrhages. His coagulation profile and liver function is normal.

91. A 26-year-old woman started developing frequent headaches, dizziness, and double vision after starting a "megavitamin" program. Her examination is normal except for papilledema.

92. A 57-year-old man has dyslipidemia with a low HDL and high triglyceride pattern. Recently the dose of one of his medications was increased and he started experiencing flushing and pruritus secondary to histamine release.

93. A 43-year-old woman with chronic alcoholism presents with shortness of breath and edema. On examination, her blood pressure is 100/60 mm Hg, pulse 110/min, JVP is 8 cm, the cardiac apex is displaced and enlarged, there are bilateral inspiratory crackles, and there is pedal edema.

94. A 52-year-old alcoholic notices a skin rash on his chest, and also has symptoms of diarrhea and abdominal pain. On examination, he has a scaly and pigmented rash on the sun-exposed areas of his skin, the abdomen is soft, and his short-term memory is impaired. He has dermatitis, diarrhea, and dementia syndrome.

Answers and Explanations

1. **(C)** Autoimmune hypothyroidism is the most common cause of hypothyroidism in adults. It is several times more common in women than in men and occurs most often between the ages of 40 and 60. Postablative hypothyroidism (radiation or surgery induced) can also occur if the patient has a history of thyroid surgery or neck radiotherapy. Medications such as amiodarone or lithium can also cause hypothyroidism as a side effect of their use if there is a history of such medication use. *(Fauci, Chapter 335)*

2. **(B)** Diminished concentrating ability and proteinuria occur even when the glomerular filtration rate is near normal in gouty nephropathy. The severity of renal involvement correlates with the duration and magnitude of serum uric acid elevation. Uric acid and monosodium urate deposit in the renal parenchyma. These deposits can cause intrarenal obstruction and elicit an inflammatory response as well. Hypertension, nephrolithiasis, and pyelonephritis can also contribute to the nephropathy of gout. Nephrotic syndrome, acute kidney injury, and ATN are not characteristics of chronic gouty nephropathy, though patients with gout may be at risk for these disorders for other reasons. *(Fauci, Chapter 279)*

3. **(E)** With pituitary hypofunctioning, gonadotropin deficiency is the most common early manifestation in both men and women. In women, this usually presents as a change in the menstrual cycle or amenorrhea, and in men as decreased sexual function, loss of secondary sexual characteristics, or infertility. Growth hormone secretion is also impaired early on, but is less clinically apparent in adults, but in children can present as growth disorders. TSH (secondary hypothyroidism) and ACTH (hypocortisolism) deficiency usually develops later in the course of pituitary failure. *(Fauci, Chapter 333)*

4. **(C)** Androgen receptor defect such as androgen insensitivity will result in the phenotypic characteristics seen in this patient. Other disease states due to abnormal intracellular receptors include cortisol resistance; vitamin D-dependent rickets, type II; thyroid hormone resistance; and pseudohypoaldosteronism. Androgen insensitivity syndrome is caused by a mutation in the androgen receptor, and it affects 1 in 100,000 chromosomal males. Because the androgen receptor is X-linked, it only affects males. The phenotypic presentation can vary from complete androgen insensitivity (female external features) to partial insensitivity causing ambiguous or normal male features and infertility. There are several different types of cell membrane receptors. *(Fauci, Chapter 343)*

5. **(D)** Beta-carotene increases the patient's tolerance for sunlight, apparently by quenching active intermediates. Beta-carotene is an effective scavenger of free radicals. Although many affected individuals can tolerate sun exposure while taking beta-carotene, it has no effect on the basic metabolic defect in porphyrin–heme synthesis. The other answers listed have no effect on this type of porphyria. *(Fauci, Chapter 352)*

6. **(E)** FSH is said to encourage maturation of a follicle in the human menstrual cycle. The cardinal hormonal change in phase I is a rise in

FSH caused by a decrease in the level of estrogens and a waning activity of the corpus luteum. In men, FSH stimulates Sertoli cells, which have an important role in spermatogenesis. *(Fauci, Chapter 333)*

7. **(E)** In hyperparathyroidism, bony lesions are lytic and can cause pain. The cortical surfaces are thinned and much of the bone is demineralized. The fibrotic bulging lesions within bone are termed *brown tumors*. Fluid-filled cysts can also occur (osteitis fibrosa cystica). Anemia is common not polycythemia, and the QT interval can be shortened if the calcium is high enough (not prolonged). Hypertension is common. Most patients with hyperparathyroidism have a simple adenoma that functions autonomously, so that hormone is secreted with high calcium. In about 10%–15% of cases, hyperplasia of all the parathyroid glands (chief cell hyperplasia) is the cause. Differentiation from adenoma is important to determine the correct surgical approach. *(Fauci, Chapter 347)*

8. **(E)** Surgical removal is the most common cause of hypoparathyroidism. When the glands, or their blood vessels, have merely been damaged and not removed, tissue often regenerates. Hypoparathyroidism can frequently follow thyroid surgery. The incidence varies and depends on the extent of resection, the skill of the surgeon, and the degree of diligence in diagnosing hypocalcemia. Hereditary hypoparathyroidism is a rare disorder and less likely in this patient given her history of thyroid surgery. Hypocalcemia due to end-organ resistance (PTH ineffective) to PTH occurs in chronic kidney disease or vitamin D deficiency of any cause. In this patient's case, the PTH level would be elevated if her hypocalcemia was due to end-organ resistance. *(Fauci, Chapter 347)*

9. **(C)** Water diuresis is impaired in primary adrenocortical insufficiency (Addison). Lack of aldosterone also favors the development of hyperkalemia and mild acidosis. The decreased circulating volume, secondary to aldosterone deficiency, is one of the factors resulting in elevated basal antidiuretic hormone (ADH) levels, and thus hyponatremia. Patients with Addison do not have impaired glucose handling or elevated serum calcium values. Lack of endogenous steroid production leads to decreased urinary steroid excretion in Addison. *(Fauci, Chapter 336)*

10. **(D)** Because DI is usually caused by destruction, or agenesis, of the posterior pituitary, its normal signaling is lost. Pituitary DI can also result from trauma, tumors (both primary and secondary), granulomas, infections, inflammatory diseases, chemical toxins, congenital malformations, and genetic disorders.

    Depending on the cause, the MRI may demonstrate other associated findings. *(Fauci, Chapter 334)*

11. **(D)** Hypertriglyceridemia may result in part from hyperinsulinism, because insulin is one of the factors involved in lipoprotein secretion by the liver. With massive obesity, there is an increased prevalence of cardiovascular disease, hypertension, diabetes, pulmonary disorders, and gallstones. Young men with morbid obesity have a 12-fold higher mortality risk than the general population. Even in old age (65–74 years), the mortality is doubled in obese men. Cardiovascular disease is the most important factor. Increased cortisol production in not a feature of obesity and suggests a diagnosis of Cushing disease. Patients with obesity also have normal thyroid function and PCO_2 values. Occasionally, the POC_2 may be elevated in the "obesity hypoventilation" syndrome. *(Fauci, Chapter 75)*

12. **(D)** High ferritin, hepatomegaly, skin changes, and <u>diabetes</u> suggest hemochromatosis. The arthritis is characterized by chondrocalcinosis, but, unlike idiopathic chondrocalcinosis, the hands are usually involved first. The arthropathy often progresses despite phlebotomy. Liver disease is usually the presenting feature. Skin pigmentation is predominantly by melanin. Heart failure is the most common cardiac problem. Addison disease does not involve the liver, and Wilson usually presents at an earlier age and does not cause diabetes. In amyloidosis, skin pigmentation is not a feature. *(Fauci, Chapter 351)*

13. **(B)** In patients with acute intermittent porphyria, oral phenothiazines may be used for abdominal or muscle pains, and narcotics may also be used, but barbiturates should be avoided. Sulfonamides are unsafe, but penicillin and its derivatives are safe. Other unsafe medications include alcohol, carbamazepine, valproic acid, and synthetic estrogens and progestogens. Most heterozygotes remain asymptomatic unless a precipitating factor such as a drug or weight loss is present. Poorly localized abdominal pain is the most common symptom. *(Fauci, Chapter 352)*

14. **(E)** One of the most efficient ways to define obesity is by BMI, which is calculated by weight/height^2, calculated using kilograms for weight and meters for height. This man's BMI is between 23 and 24 kg/m^2 and confers no special risk. (The acceptable range is 20–25.) *(Fauci, Chapter 75)*

15. **(E)** Nephrogenic diabetes insipidus (DI) is caused by a defect in the action of ADH on the distal renal tubules. This can be genetic, and variants include X-linked recessive, autosomal dominant, and autosomal recessive. Numerous drugs can cause the syndrome, as can many forms of renal disease. Prolonged lithium use is a frequent cause of nephrogenic DI. Hypercalcemia and hypokalemia can also cause the syndrome. In nephrogenic DI induced by lithium the production of ADH by the posterior pituitary is normal. *(Fauci, Chapter 334)*

16. **(B)** Glycogen storage is not characteristic of Tay–Sachs disease. Ganglioside accumulation can now be diagnosed by decreased hexosaminidase in peripheral leukocytes. Tay–Sachs is characterized as a lysosomal storage disease. Mental retardation, seizures, blindness, and a retinal cherry-red spot are characteristic.

It is most common in Ashkenazi Jews and is inherited in an autosomal recessive manner. *(Fauci, Chapter 355)*

17. **(A)** In addition to peripheral motor and sensory neuropathy, cardiac involvement, tongue enlargement, gastrointestinal (GI) manifestations, and carpal tunnel syndrome are also seen in amyloidosis. The specific diagnosis requires tissue biopsy with presence of amyloid with specific stains. In primary amyloidosis and myeloma, the amyloid protein is of the AL type. In reactive amyloidosis, the protein is of the amyloid A protein (AA) type. *(Fauci, Chapter 324)*

18. **(D)** Carcinoid syndrome is characterized by increased levels of 5-hydroxyindolacetic acid. The syndrome occurs in relation to malignant tumors that have metastasized, usually with hepatic implants. Gastrointestinal carcinoids are most commonly found in the appendix. These are very slow growing, thus the 5-year survival rate is 99%. Many carcinoids are discovered as incidental findings on autopsy. *(Fauci, Chapter 344)*

19. **(B)** Nephrogenic diabetes insipidus is the failure of the kidney to respond to ADH. It can be acquired, genetic, or medication related. Central diabetes insipidus is most commonly caused by a primary deficit in the secretion of vasopressin by the posterior pituitary. It is usually caused by agenesis or destruction of vasopressin-producing neurons by either a developmental, acquired, genetic, or idiopathic disorder. Addison disease or adrenal cortex defects do not cause symptoms of polyuria or polydipsia, and ATN usually causes oligouria. *(Fauci, Chapter 334)*

20. **(A)** Important secondary causes include DM, obesity/dietary intake, hypothyroidism, renal disease (nephritic syndrome), and cholestatic liver disease. Alcohol in small amount improves lipid profiles and in excess causes increase in triglycerides. Estrogen too improves lipid profiles. The other choices are not important in affecting lipid levels.

In familial hypercholesterolemia, there is an increased incidence of CAD, and hypercholesterolemia occurs along with tuberous xanthomas, arcus senilis, and atheromas. Most affected individuals are heterozygous for the mutant gene. *(Fauci, Chapter 350)*

21. **(E)** In type 2 diabetes, high levels of insulin and insulin resistance have multiple effects on lipid metabolism. These include increases in triglycerides, low HDL, and normal to high LDL. The high triglycerides respond to insulin therapy and to weight loss, while the low HDL responds to exercise. *(Fauci, Chapter 350)*

22. **(B)** The diagnosis is inherited Gaucher disease since it is an autosomal recessive disorder. There is no acquired form of the disease. The glucocerebrosides are derived from lipid catabolites, from the membranes of senescent leukocytes and erythrocytes. Although the juvenile form may have severe neurologic symptoms (mental retardation, spasticity, ataxia), the adult form usually has no neuro-logic symptoms. Like Tay–Sachs, it is a lysoso-mal storage disease with a predilection for Ashkenazi Jews. *(Fauci, Chapter 355)*

23. **(C)** There are many types of glycogen storage diseases, each caused by a different enzymatic abnormality. The best-known types of glycogen storage disease are those that have hepatic hypo-glycemic pathophysiology (eg, von Gierke disease) or those that have muscle energy patho-physiology (McArdle disease). In McArdle' symptoms usually develop in adulthood, and it is marked by cramps and muscle injury with strenuous exercise, but not with usual activities. Gaucher and Tay–Sachs disease are lysosomal storage diseases. *(Fauci, Chapter 357)*

24. **(C)** Cystinuria is commonly associated with hexagonal crystals in the urine. Cystine, lysine, arginine, and ornithine are excreted in great excess by patients homozygous for the disease. The tissues manifesting the transport defect of cystinuria are the proximal renal tubule and the jejunal mucosa. It is inherited as an autoso-mal recessive trait. Cystine kidney stones (1% of all renal stones) are the major clinical manifestation, and they are radiopaque. *(Fauci, Chapter 359)*

25. **(A)** Magnesium deficiency is most commonly due to alcoholism. Renal loss and malabsorp-tion are also common causes. Magnesium defi-ciency is not seen in hypervitaminosis E.

Causes of magnesium deficiency also include milk diets in infants, the diuretic phase of acute tubular necrosis, chronic diuretic therapy, acute pancreatitis, and inappropriate antidiuretic hormone. The symptoms of hypomagnesemia include anorexia, nausea, tremor, and mood alteration. Symptoms can also be caused by the associated hypocalcemia or hypokalemia. *(Fauci, Chapter 387)*

26. **(D)** Symptoms of vitamin A intoxication occur in infants or adults ingesting over 50,000 IU of vitamin A daily. The prognosis is good when vitamin A intake ceases. Rare occurrences of hypercalcemia with vitamin A intoxication have been reported. *(Fauci, Chapter 71)*

27. **(A)** Familial combined hyperlipidemia has an incidence of 1/100. It is an autosomal-dominant disorder and different affected family members may display different dyslipidemic phenotypes. Familial hypercholesterolemia (1/500) and familial defective Apo B (1/1000) are also common. The other two disorders (Apo C-II deficiency and lipoprotein lipase defi-ciency) are extremely rare. *(Fauci, Chapter 350)*

28. **(B)** Necrobiosis lipoidica diabeticorum is more frequent in females and may antedate other clin-ical signs and symptoms of diabetes. The plaques are round, firm, and reddish-brown to yellow in color. They most commonly involve the legs but can also involve the hands, arms, abdomen, and head. This in not a staphylococcal skin infection since it is not tender, indurated or warm to touch, and erythema nodosum is characterized by round, tender elevated lesions usually on the anterior shin. *(Fauci, Chapter 338)*

29. **(A)** Allopurinol inhibits the enzyme xanthine oxidase, resulting in decreased uric acid pro-duction. Allopurinol is particularly useful in the treatment of uric acid nephrolithiasis in gouty individuals. Even if the gouty individual has calcium oxalate stones, allopurinol may be helpful. *(Fauci, Chapter 327)*

30. **(B)** Neuromuscular irritability is a clinical fea-ture of hypocalcemia if it is severe enough. Hyperphosphatemia rarely causes any symptoms

directly. Its secondary effects on calcium can result in hypocalcemic tetany or metastatic calcification. The usual cause of hyperphosphatemia is uremia. Anorexia, nausea, and vomiting are not usual clinical features of hypocalcemia or hyperphosphatemia. They may occur if the patient has advanced chronic kidney disease and associated uremia. Hypocalcemia prolongs the QT interval, and in severe cases predispose to polymorphic VT (Torsades) but this is a rare occurrence. For the majority of patients with hypocalcemia there are no associated tachyarrhythmias. *(Fauci, Chapter 347)*

31. **(B)** The severe form of Marfan syndrome is caused by a mutation in a single allele of the fibrillin gene (FBN1). The gene product is a major component of elastin-associated microfibrils. Long, thin extremities; ectopia lentis; and aortic aneurysms are the classical triad. Milder forms of the disease probably also occur but are hard to classify. Mutations in the FBN2 gene can also cause Marfan syndrome, but without aneurysms. *(Fauci, Chapter 357)*

32. **(A)** Nephrogenic DI can be caused by drugs such as lithium, amphotericin, cisplatin, and rifampin. Metabolic factors, vascular disease, ureteral obstruction, and genetic factors can also cause nephrogenic DI. *(Fauci, Chapter 334)*

33. **(B)** Very elevated triglycerides are a prominent feature of this disorder. In the familial type 1 form, the defect is believed to be a deficiency of lipoprotein lipase activity. It is a rare autosomal recessive syndrome, and usually presents in childhood with typical eruptive xanthoma and abdominal pain secondary to acute pancreatitis. Secondary hyperchylomicronemia (diabetes, hypothyroidism, uremia) is a much more common syndrome. *(Fauci, Chapter 350)*

34. **(C)** Subcutaneous xanthomas begin to appear at about age 20 and may involve Achillis tendons, elbows, and tibial tuberosities. Familial hypercholesterolemia may be monogenic or polygenic in its inheritance. The disorder is common, and heterozygous familial hypercholesterolemia is felt to affect 1 in 500 individuals.

It can be secondary to other diseases such as hypothyroidism, nephrotic syndrome, or even porphyria. Xanthelasmas after the age of 50 are often not related to any dyslipidemia at all. *(Fauci, Chapter 350)*

35. **(A)** In the rare familial form, raised yellow plaques appear on palms and fingers, and reddish-yellow xanthomas occur on the elbows. This disorder is felt to be secondary to accumulation of abnormal chylomicron and very low-density lipoprotein (VLDL) remnants. It is probably due to inherited homozygous defects in Apo E-II structure. *(Fauci, Chapter 350)*

36. **(E)** Triglycerides are over 150 and are raised by alcohol intake, estrogens, stress, insulin, and physical activity. Cholesterol levels are average or mildly elevated. HDL is usually low. Dietary therapy and the maintenance of ideal weight is the cornerstone of therapy. *(Fauci, Chapter 350)*

37. **(B)** Hypertriglyceridemia is usually secondary to DM or drugs, rather than a genetic disorder. It can be a normal response to caloric excess or alcohol ingestion and is common in the third trimester of pregnancy. *(Fauci, Chapter 350)*

38. **(C)** She has diabetes insipidus either nephrogenic or central. In DM, there is an obligatory osmotic diuresis due to the elevated glucose level, but in DI there is lack of water resorption in the tubules. Both result in polyuria, but in DM, there will be substantial glucosuria as well. The large amount of urine output (usually >50 mL/ kg/day) is characteristic of polyuric states, such as DI, not a bladder problem. Psychogenic polydipsia is commonly seen in patients with psychiatric problems on medications. *(Fauci, Chapter 334)*

39. **(D)** In Western societies, most dyslipidemias are secondary. The most common predisposing cause is diet, and the second common is DM. His normal fasting glucose rules out DM. Hypothyroidism, renal disease, alcoholism, and anorexia nervosa are also associated with secondary dyslipidemias. Many drugs

(eg, estrogen, glucocorticoids) can also cause secondary dyslipidemias. *(Fauci, Chapter 350)*

40. **(D)** The most important factors in diet-induced cholesterol elevation are the amount of total fat and saturated fat consumed. Cholesterol intake is next in importance. Obesity and caloric excess usually result in high triglyceride levels. *(Fauci, Chapter 350)*

41. **(D)** The elevated ALP and hydroxyproline are diagnostic for Paget disease. The bony lesions are osteoblastic, and the sacrum and pelvis are most frequently involved, followed closely by the tibia and femur. Hypercalcemia is not usually a feature of Paget, though can occur as a complication of immobilization. The etiology is unknown. Symptoms may be absent or severe (pain, deformity). In metastatic cancers of most types the lesion are lytic, and the other metabolic abnormalities listed do not have an elevation in hydroxyproline. *(Fauci, Chapter 349)*

42. **(A)** Many affected persons with vitamin D deficiency have no demonstrable abnormality except for hypocalcemia, hypophosphatemia, and increased PTH levels. Decreased calcium absorption, which is vitamin D dependent, results in mild hypocalcemia that leads to the secondary hyperparathyroidism. This in turn results in increased renal phosphate excretion and hypophosphatemia. *(Fauci, Chapter 347)*

43. **(B)** Sinus tachycardia is the most common cardiac manifestation in a young individual with hyperthyroidism. Atrial fibrillation and cardiomegaly are common cardiac manifestations, but are more common in the elderly. Other symptoms include palpitations, tachycardia, nervousness, sweating, and dyspnea. Pericardial effusions are not typical findings in hyperthyroidism, and cardiac dilation may occur but only in severe prolonged hyperthyroidism that is untreated resulting in a cardiomyopathy. *(Fauci, Chapter 335)*

44. **(B)** Needle biopsy can be used in numerous diseases, but the main rationale is to differentiate benign from malignant nodules. A thyroid scan is appropriate if the TSH is suppressed suggesting a possible "hot" nodule (hyperfunctioning nodules are very rarely malignant). The specimen must be read by an experienced cytologist. It is difficult to diagnose differentiated follicular carcinoma or to differentiate lymphoma from Hashimoto thyroiditis. Papillary carcinoma is the easiest diagnosis to make by needle biopsy. Thyroid surgery (either complete removal or partial resection) is only indicated if the nodule is malignant, or there is local pressure symptoms related to the size of the nodule. A repeat assessment is not appropriate without confirming first that the nodule is not malignant. *(Fauci, Chapter 335)*

45. **(D)** Tumor of the pancreatic beta cells, such as an insulinoma, is the cause of her symptoms. Classification of hypoglycemia includes spontaneous causes such as reactive or fasting hypoglycemia and pharmacologic or toxic causes. The diagnosis of insulinoma is most certain when Whipple triad is fulfilled: symptoms consistent with hypoglycemia, low plasma glucose, and relief of symptoms with elevation of plasma glucose to normal. Cushing disease and excess growth hormone will result in elevated blood glucose levels and diabetes (not decreased glucose values). Thyrotoxicosis and gastrin deficiency do not cause hypoglycemia. *(Fauci, Chapter 344)*

46. **(A)** Cardiac failure and arrhythmias frequently occur in cardiac amyloid. The ECG reveals low-voltage QRS complexes and conduction disturbances. Red cells are not involved, and involvement of the thyroid, liver, and pancreas is usually asymptomatic. The precursors of the AL, amyloid protein found in primary AL and myeloma, are kappa and lambda light chains. Serum amyloid A protein (SAA) is the precursor for the AA amyloid found in secondary AL. *(Fauci, Chapter 324)*

47. **(A)** Glucagon promotes glycogenolysis and gluconeogenesis to protect the blood glucose value when hypoglycemia develops. This person has either fasting or reactive hypoglycemia. Glucagon exerts a marked effect on carbohydrate, fat, and lipid metabolism, and

increases cAMP in many tissues. It is the first counterregulatory hormone to respond to hypoglycemia, and it does this by increasing glycogenolysis and gluconeogenesis. Glucagonomas of the pancreas present with features such as mild DM, psychiatric disturbances, diarrhea, venous thromboses, and skin findings (necrolytic migratory erythema). *(Fauci, Chapter 338)*

48. **(E)** Combined therapy is frequently required for most patients. In mild cases, dietary therapy may suffice, but the vast majority of patients require drug therapy. Statins are clearly the most effective medications available, but the majority of patients will not have optimal cholesterol control, even with maximum doses of a statin. Homozygous patients always require combination therapy. *(Fauci, Chapter 350)*

49. **(C)** Primary hyperparathyroidism develops in over 87% of those with MEN I. Polyendocrine adenomatosis, type I, frequently includes islet cell tumors of the pancreas, leading to the Zollinger–Ellison syndrome, insulinomas, and glucagonomas. Inheritance is via an autosomal dominant pattern. Hypercalcemia does not usually occur until after the first decade. *(Fauci, Chapter 345)*

50. **(E)** HRT can reduce osteoporosis-related fractures. Estrogens cause thickening of vaginal mucosa and can improve urogenital and postmenopausal symptoms. The evidence for protection against CAD and dementia is epidemiologic. Randomized trials have failed to show a reduction in CAD risk with HRT. The risk of venothromboembolism and breast cancer is increased, not decreased. *(Fauci, Chapter 342)*

51. **(C)** This patient has Cushing syndrome. The diagnosis is established by demonstrating increased cortisol secretion (24-hour urine cortisol collection) or by failure to suppress AM cortisol levels after overnight dexamethasone administration. Investigations for either adrenal tumor or pituitary adenoma (with CT or MR) are only considered once the diagnosis of Cushing syndrome is established. *(Fauci, Chapter 336)*

52. **(A)** Growth hormone excess in acromegaly produces hypertrophy of muscle. Initially, strength may be increased, but this is transient, and a third of patients will experience weakness, likely secondary to myopathy. Muscle spasm and rhythmic contraction (fasciculation) are not clinical features of growth hormone excess. *(Fauci, Chapter 333)*

53. **(C)** Half the affected individuals with vitamin D-resistant rickets have alopecia, and this tends to correlate with severity. Vitamin D-resistant rickets is a familial disorder, with an X-linked recessive pattern, treated with pharmacologic doses of vitamin D. Serum vitamin D levels are normal in this condition.

Rickets and osteomalacia are characterized by impaired mineralization of bone. Osteoporosis is a disorder with a diminished amount of normally mineralized bone. *(Fauci, Chapter 346)*

54. **(B)** Patients with severe eating disorders are at risk of ventricular tachyarrhythmias. Risk of death in anorexia nervosa is also associated with hypothermia, suicide, or pneumonia with emaciation. Because of the danger of ventricular tachyarrhythmias, patients should be followed with ECGs. A prolonged QT interval is a sign of danger. In addition, severe weight loss can lead to both systolic and diastolic dysfunction of the ventricles. Diabetes is not a feature of eating disorders and acute kidney injury can sometimes develop in severe volume depletion states, but not typically seen. *(Fauci, Chapter 76)*

55. **(E)** In gouty patients, nephrolithiasis and uric acid nephropathy may occur. More commonly impaired uric acid excretion is an important risk factor for developing gout in patients with chronic kidney disease. The association of cardiovascular disease, hypertension, pyelonephritis, and hyperlipoproteinemia with gout contributes to the high prevalence of renal disease in these individuals. *(Fauci, Chapter 327)*

56. **(C)** Vitamin D levels are decreased in osteomalacia. In severe osteomalacia, there is bowing of the long bones, inward deformity of the long

bones, and wide osteoid borders on bone surfaces. Hypocalcemia is characteristic of osteomalacia; however, secondary hyperparathyroidism often raises the serum calcium to low normal levels. The PTH-mediated increase in phosphate clearance often produces hypophosphatemia. *(Fauci, Chapter 346)*

57. **(B)** Sodium retention is an important mechanism in the fluid retention leading to ascites formation in patients with cirrhosis. Hepatorenal syndrome frequently complicates hepatic failure. Although it can develop gradually, acute renal failure can also be precipitated by hemodynamic stresses (bleeding, diuresis). The earliest manifestations are intrarenal vasoconstriction and avid sodium retention. Potassium retention is not a feature of the hepatorenal syndrome and oligoria occurs, not polyuria. *(Fauci, Chapter 302)*

58. **(B)** Wilson disease includes cirrhosis of the liver, signs of basal ganglia disease, and a brownish pigmented ring at the corneal margin (Kayser–Fleischer ring). Ceruloplasmin levels are low. The gene for Wilson disease is located on the long arm of chromosome 13. In some cases, it is possible to identify carrier states and make prenatal diagnoses. The relationship between the abnormal gene and the metabolic defect (inability to regulate copper balance) is unclear. Renal failure and sensory loss are not typical findings in Wilson disease. *(Fauci, Chapter 304)*

59. **(C)** This patient may have diabetes and a FBS is the most appropriate test. The gold standard for the diagnosis of DM is still a fasting plasma glucose > 7 mmol/L (126 mg/dL) on two separate occasions. GTTs are rarely required. With typical symptoms, even a markedly elevated random sugar is diagnostic. *(Fauci, Chapter 338)*

60. **(A)** Insulin binding to its receptor stimulates tyrosine kinase activity. Other stimulators of protein kinases include platelet-derived growth factor and epidermal growth factor. Tyrosine phosphorylation results from this interaction. Insulin-resistant states can be caused by prereceptor resistance (mutated insulin, anti-insulin

antibodies) or receptor and postreceptor resistance. *(Fauci, Chapter 338)*

61. **(C)** Insulin's effect on adipose cells results in decreased lipolysis. The action of insulin involves all three major metabolic fuels (carbohydrate, protein, fat). It is active in liver, muscle, and adipose tissue. In each there are anticatabolic as well as anabolic effects. These tend to reinforce each other. *(Fauci, Chapter 338)*

62. **(D)** Infection or other acute medical condition is the usual precipitant for thyroid storm. Radioactive iodine treatment or abrupt withdrawal of antithyroid medications is also implicated. The key diagnostic features are fever, tachycardia, and central nervous system dysfunction. PTU and beta-blocker administration are used in the treatment of hyperthyroidism and not associated with precipitating thyroid storm. Salicylate administration has no effect on thyroid function. *(Fauci, Chapter 335)*

63. **(B)** All the causes listed may delay puberty, but the most common cause by far is normal variation in growth pattern. There is often a family history of delayed puberty in parents or siblings. In these individuals, bone age often correlates better with the onset and progression of puberty than does chronologic age. *(Fauci, Chapter 341)*

64. **(D)** Presence of estrogen receptors (ER) or PR improves the likelihood of response to tamoxifen. If the tumor is both ER and PR positive, the response rate is 70%. Approximately, one-third of unselected women with metastatic breast cancer will respond to tamoxifen. Androgen receptors on the tumor cells and premenopausal status do not affect response to tamoxifen therapy. *(Fauci, Chapter 86)*

65. **(B)** A generally increased risk of breast cancer is associated with late first pregnancy and nulliparity. A history of maternal breast cancer is also a risk factor for developing breast cancer. Prior history of breast cancer is of course a powerful risk factor. Multiparity and oophorectomy do not increase the risk of breast cancer. *(Fauci, Chapter 86)*

66. **(C)** The diagnosis is secondary hyperparathyroidism as a consequence of the chronic renal disease. Calcium deposits are seen in the periarticular areas of the fourth and fifth metacarpophalangeal, third proximal interphalangeal, and fourth distal interphalangeal joints. There is slight soft tissue swelling, especially of the fourth and fifth metacarpophalangeal joints. Calcification in scleroderma is subcutaneous in location. In gout, if monosodium urate is deposited it could appear as a soft tissue mass. *(Fauci, Chapter 346)*

67. **(B)** Adrenal adenoma with complete autonomy (Cushing) is the most likely diagnosis. Autonomous adrenal tumors are adrenocorticotropic hormone (ACTH) insensitive and fail to demonstrate a brisk rise in urinary 17-hydroxycorticoids. Androgenic effects, such as hirsutism, are usually absent. In Cushing syndrome, secondary to an autonomous adrenal tumor, onset is usually gradual, and hirsutism, other androgenic effects, and hyperpigmentation are absent. In a pituitary tumor causing elevated cortisol the ACTH level would be increased, and exogenous steroid use would result in low cortisol and ACTH levels. *(Fauci, Chapter 336)*

68. **(A)** DM is a syndrome consisting of hyperglycemia, large vessel disease, microvascular disease, and neuropathy. The classic presenting symptoms are increased thirst, polyuria, polyphagia, and weight loss. In type 2 diabetes, the presentation can be more subtle and is often made when the patient is asymptomatic. While DI can result in increased urinary volume, the other clinical features seen in this patient are not characteristic of it. Hypothyroidism can cause some of the symptoms experienced by this patient but not the weight loss, frequent yeast infections, or nocturia. *(Fauci, Chapter 338)*

69. **(G)** Necrobiosis lipoidica is a plaque-like lesion with a brown border and yellow center usually found on the anterior leg surface. Pyoderma gangrenosum is not a cutaneous manifestation of diabetes. Perineal pruritus in a diabetic is almost always associated with *Candida albicans*. A severe external otitis can occur in older patients. It is caused by *Pseudomonas aeruginosa* and is characterized by ear pain, drainage, fever, and leukocytosis. Facial nerve paralysis can occur and is a poor prognostic sign. *(Fauci, Chapter 338)*

70. **(A)** Background retinopathy is present in about 90% of diabetes after 25–30 years of disease. Microaneurysms, dilated veins, dot and blot hemorrhages, cotton-wool spots, and hard exudates are common findings. *(Fauci, Chapter 338)*

71. **(B)** Proliferative retinopathy carries a high risk of vitreous hemorrhage, scarring, retinal detachment, and blindness. Proliferative retinopathy is associated with nephropathy and CAD, and is associated with a poor prognosis, for life as well as for vision. *(Fauci, Chapter 338)*

72. **(B)** High prolactin level suppresses luteinizing hormone-releasing hormone (LH-RH), and can result in low plasma gonadotropin and testosterone levels. It may not be obvious on physical examination. Therapy with a dopamine agonist may lower prolactin levels and reverse impotence. *(Fauci, Chapter 333)*

73. **(D)** An absent orgasm, when libido and erectile function are normal, invariably indicates that organic disease is absent. Loss of desire can also be caused by psychologic disturbance, but may indicate androgen deficiency or drug effect. *(Fauci, Chapter 49)*

74. **(E)** Failure of detumescence—priapism—can be caused by sickle cell anemia or chronic granulocytic leukemia. Priapism must be treated promptly to preserve future erectile functioning. *(Fauci, Chapter 49)*

75. **(B)** Vascular disease, by itself or in conjunction with peripheral neuropathy in DM, is a common cause of erectile dysfunction. The lesions can be in large vessels (aortic occlusion, Leriche syndrome), small arteries, or even in the sinusoidal spaces. *(Fauci, Chapter 49)*

76. **(E)** Idiopathic hirsutism may simply represent an extreme of normal androgen production. It is

diagnosed by demonstrating minimal elevation of androgens and exclusion of other causes. Management is primarily by cosmetic therapy, although drugs to suppress androgen production and/or androgen effects on the hair follicle can be used. (*Fauci, Chapter 50*)

77. **(C)** The most severe form of PCOD, Stein–Leventhal syndrome, is associated with chronic anovulation, hirsutism, enlarged cystic ovaries, obesity, and amenorrhea. The spectrum of disease, however, is quite wide, and some patients have only mild hirsutism. (*Fauci, Chapter 50*)

78. **(F)** Krukenberg tumors of the ovary stimulate surrounding ovarian stromal tissue to produce excess androgen. When onset of hair growth (with or without frank virilization) is very rapid, a neoplastic source of androgen is suggested. In addition to ovarian tumors, the potential neoplasms include adenomas and carcinomas of the adrenal gland. (*Fauci, Chapter 50*)

79. **(D)** Attenuated forms of adrenal hyperplasia can present with hirsutism at puberty or in adulthood. Elevated levels of a precursor of cortisol biosynthesis such as 17-hydroxyprogesterone, 17-hydroxypregnenolone, or 11-deoxycortisol can present. ACTH infusion will increase the precursor level, and dexamethasone will suppress it. (*Fauci, Chapter 50*)

80. **(A)** Salivary gland enlargement occurs both in anorexia nervosa (AN) and bulimia (BN). Other common findings in AN include constipation, bradycardia, hypotension, hypercarotenemia, and soft downy hair growth (lanugo). Menses are usually absent. (*Fauci, Chapter 73*)

81. **(D)** Hyperglycemia is not seen in eating disorders, and would suggest an alternate diagnosis for the weight loss such as diabetes. Hypoglycemia and low estrogens and gonadotropins are frequently seen in anorexia nervosa (AN). BUN and creatinine may be elevated. Hypochloremia, hypokalemia, and alkalosis are frequently seen in BN. (*Fauci, Chapter 73*)

82. **(E)** The presence of a prolonged QT interval is most suggestive of serious cardiac arrhythmias in patients with eating disorders. Other ECG features include low QRS voltages, sinus bradycardia, and ST-T changes. (*Fauci, Chapter 73*)

83. **(C)** The patient is most likely to develop glomerulosclerosis. This can be diffuse or nodular (Kimmelstiel–Wilson nodules). Poor metabolic control is probably a major factor in the progression of diabetic nephropathy. Acute GN is unlikely given the lack of casts or red cells in the urine, and patients with renal infarction usually provide a history of flank pain and/or hematuria. The ultrasound results argue against obstructive uropathy and PCKD. (*Fauci, Chapter 338*)

84. **(I)** Low fiber diets are frequently prescribed during flares of inflammatory bowel disease to reduce diarrhea and pain. There is no level 1 evidence to support this practice. Similar diets are often prescribed for diverticulitis or other conditions associated with a narrowed or stenosed colon. It may be prescribed for patients with a new ostomy. When acute symptoms subside, however, restrictions concerning dietary fiber should be stopped. (*Fauci, Chapter 289*)

85. **(A)** Restricting caloric intake and weight reduction are important components of the medical nutrition therapy for patients with diabetes. Most patients should be referred to a dietician to help construct a diet appropriate in caloric intake. (*Fauci, Chapter 338*)

86. **(C)** Some patients with hypertension are salt sensitive, and will lower their blood pressure with salt restriction. Low sodium diets are also recommended in patients with congestive heart failure (CHF), ascites, or chronic renal failure. (*Fauci, Chapter 241*)

87. **(F)** After gastrectomy, avoiding simple sugars and limiting liquids can ameliorate symptoms of dumping. Early dumping occurs within 30 minutes of eating and is characterized by vasomotor symptoms such as palpitations,

tachycardia, lightheadedness, and diaphoresis. Late dumping includes similar symptoms plus dizziness, confusion, and even syncope. It occurs 1.2–3 hours after eating. *(Fauci, Chapter 287)*

88. **(H)** The symptoms of hepatic encephalopathy are improved with protein restriction and a bowel elimination routine with lactulose. It is presumed that this results in lower levels of serum ammonia, but other substances in the serum may be implicated. These include mercaptans, short-chain fatty acids, and phenol. Gamma-aminobutyric acid (GABA) levels in the brain are also increased. Chronic encephalopathy can be controlled with restricting protein intake and taking lactulose (osmotic laxative). Restricting daytime protein intake in patients with Parkinson disease may improve the efficacy of levodopa therapy. *(Fauci, Chapter 302)*

89. **(E)** Chocolate, ethanol, caffeine, and tobacco decrease lower esophageal sphincter pressure. Other effective treatments for GERD include low fat diet, weight loss, avoiding bedtime snacks, and elevating the head of the bed while sleeping. *(Fauci, Chapter 286)*

90. **(D)** Vitamin C deficiency (scurvy) is characterized by a tendency to hemorrhage and perifollicular hyperkeratotic papules in which hair become fragmented and buried. Gums are involved only if teeth are present. It can occur in infants 6–12 months of age who are on processed milk formulas, without citrus fruit or vegetable supplementation. The peak incidence in the United States is in poor and elderly people and alcoholics. It is frequently associated with other nutritional deficiencies (eg, folic acid). *(Fauci, Chapter 71)*

91. **(E)** Excessive vitamin A ingestion can cause abdominal pain, nausea, vomiting, headache,

dizziness, and papilledema. Deficiency of vitamin A can cause night blindness and progress to visual loss. It is common in children in developing countries and is a major cause of blindness. *(Fauci, Chapter 71)*

92. **(A)** Pharmacologic doses of niacin for hypercholesterolemia may cause histamine release, which results in flushing, pruritus, and GI disturbance. Asthma may be aggravated, acanthosis nigricans can occur, and in high doses, elevation of uric acid and fasting blood sugar can occur. Hepatic toxicity, including cholestatic jaundice, has been described with large doses. *(Fauci, Chapter 71)*

93. **(B)** Thiamine deficiency can cause high-output cardiac failure (wet beriberi) or neurologic symptoms (dry beriberi). In North America, thiamine deficiency occurs in alcoholics or those with chronic disease. In alcoholics, deficiency is secondary to low intake, impaired absorption and storage, and accelerated destruction. Genetic factors are important as clinical manifestations occur only in a small proportion of chronically malnourished individuals. Beriberi heart disease is characterized by peripheral vasodilatation, sodium and water retention, and high-output CHF. *(Fauci, Chapter 71)*

94. **(A)** Diarrhea, dementia, and dermatitis are the classic triad for pellagra (niacin deficiency). The diagnosis is based on clinical suspicion and response to therapy, and can be confirmed by demonstrating low levels of the urinary metabolites 2-methylnicotinamide and 2-pyridone. Small doses of niacin (10 mg/day) with adequate dietary tryptophan will cure pellagra secondary to nutritional deficiency. *(Fauci, Chapter 71)*

CHAPTER 4

Gastroenterology
Questions

DIRECTIONS (Questions 1 through 10): The following group of numbered items is preceded by a list of lettered options. For each question, select the one lettered option that is most closely associated with it. Each lettered option may be used once, multiple times, or not at all.

Questions 1 through 6: For each patient with a small bowel tumor, select the most likely diagnosis.

- (A) polypoid adenoma
- (B) leiomyoma
- (C) adenocarcinoma
- (D) primary gastrointestinal (GI) lymphoma
- (E) carcinoid tumor

1. A 56-year-old woman presents with weight loss and watery diarrhea. She also notices periumbilical pain and bloating after eating. A small bowel x-ray reveals an area of narrowing and the lesion is surgically resected. The pathology report shows this to be the most common endocrine tumor of the GI tract.

2. A 72-year-old man is investigated for iron deficiency anemia. There is no clinical history of upper or lower GI bleeding, but his stools are fecal occult blood positive. His colonoscopy is negative for any obvious sources of bleeding, but upper endoscopy reveals ulceration in the distal duodenum that is biopsied. The pathology report shows this to be the most common primary malignancy of the small bowel.

3. A 23-year-old man of Middle-Eastern decent is investigated for symptoms of chronic diarrhea, vomiting, and abdominal cramps. He has lost 20 lb and appears unwell. A small bowel x-ray shows diffuse nonspecific mucosal abnormality. Upper endoscopy is performed to visualize the small bowel and obtain biopsies. The pathology report identifies the mucosal abnormality as "immunoproliferative small intestinal disease" (IPSID). This form of small bowel tumor can be treated with antibiotics in its early stages.

4. A 21-year-old woman develops acute periumbilical pain that localizes to the right lower quadrant. She appears unwell, and on examination, there is tenderness and guarding in the right lower quadrant. A pregnancy test is negative and a pelvic examination rules out pelvic inflammatory disease. A clinical diagnosis of acute appendicitis is made and she has an uncomplicated laparoscopic appendectomy. The pathology report notes acute inflammation and a tumor for which the appendix is a very common site of involvement.

5. A 57-year-old woman with a 20-year history of celiac disease now presents with weight loss, cramps, and abdominal discomfort. She is adherent to her gluten-free diet, and is not taking any new medications. On examination, her abdomen is soft and there is fullness in the right lower quadrant. A small bowel x-ray reveals an area of narrowing in the distal ileum, and there is thickening and nodularity of the mucosal folds. She undergoes surgical resection of the lesion, and the pathology report confirms a tumor that is more common in patients with celiac disease, Crohn disease, or depressed immune function such as human immunodeficiency virus (HIV).

6. A 48-year-old man presents with periumbilical pain made worse by eating and weight loss. A small bowel x-ray reveals an area of narrowing in the distal ileum. The differential diagnosis includes tumors that most commonly involve the distal part of the small bowel.

Questions 7 through 10: For each patient with GI symptoms, select the possible diagnoses and associated findings.

(A) celiac disease
(B) gastrinoma
(C) hyperthyroidism
(D) associated with skin pigmentation
(E) increase in pancreatic enzymes
(F) hypersensitivity reaction
(G) Whipple's disease

7. A 29-year-old woman has recently developed milk intolerance.

8. A 19-year-old man has a long history of weight loss, abdominal distention, bloating, and diarrhea. Investigation reveals steatorrhea, and a small bowel biopsy reveals blunting and flattening of villi.

9. A 53-year-old man presents with weight loss, low-grade fever, and peripheral lymphadenopathy. Steatorrhea is documented, and small bowel biopsy reveals para-aminosalicylic acid (PAS) positive macrophages.

10. A 43-year-old woman has had a 10-year history of severe and recurrent peptic ulcer disease (PUD) that is refractory to medical therapy. She has had ulcers at multiple sites of the small bowel including the distal duodenum and jejunum. She also has chronic diarrhea, but not enough fat to make the diagnosis of steatorrhea. Evaluation for *Helicobacter pylori* infection is negative.

DIRECTIONS (Questions 11 through 35): For each of the questions in this section select the one lettered answer that is the best response in each case.

11. A 79-year-old woman presents to the clinic with symptoms of severe constipation. She reports no weight loss, but does notice occasional bright red bleeding with bowel movements. Her family history is negative for colon cancer and she has never had screening colonoscopy. The medical history includes well-controlled hypertension and osteoporosis. Her physical examination is entirely normal. She is referred for colonoscopy and the only abnormal finding is multiple diverticuli. **Which of the following is the most appropriate next step in management?**

(A) stool softeners
(B) prophylactic surgery
(C) phenolphthalein laxatives
(D) increasing dietary fiber
(E) psychotherapy

12. A 77-year-old woman is brought to the emergency room because of symptoms of nonspecific abdominal discomfort. She has no anorexia, fever, chills, or weight loss. On physical examination, the vital signs are normal, the abdomen is soft and nontender with no masses or organomegaly palpated. Abdominal x-rays show lots of stool in the colon, but no free air or air-fluid levels. Laboratory investigations reveal an amylase of 150 U/L (25–125 U/L), and the rest of her biochemistry and complete blood count are normal. **Which of the following conditions can cause a false-positive elevation in the serum amylase?**

(A) maturity-onset diabetes mellitus (DM)
(B) gastric ulcer
(C) renal failure
(D) sulfonamide therapy
(E) gastric carcinoma

13. A 71-year-old man presents to the clinic for evaluation of progressive weight loss and dysphagia over a 3-month period. The symptoms of dysphagia are getting worse and seem to be more pronounced with solid foods than liquids. His past medical history includes coronary artery disease, hypertension, and dyslipidemia. His physical examination is only pertinent for muscle wasting.

An upper endoscopy reveals a lesion in the esophagus which is confirmed on biopsy to be esophageal cancer. **Which of the following statements regarding this cancer is most likely correct?**

(A) is very responsive to chemotherapy
(B) is more common in females
(C) has a 5-year cure rate of 20%
(D) may be either adenocarcinoma or squamous cell carcinoma
(E) is characterized by significant complications from hemorrhage

14. A 23-year-old woman presents to the clinic complaining of symptoms of weight loss and chronic diarrhea. She has no past health issues and is not taking any medications. On physical examination, she appears unwell and cachectic. Routine laboratory tests reveal a low hemoglobin level and an increased international normalized ratio (INR) even though she is not taking any anticoagulants. The liver enzymes are normal, but the albumin and calcium levels are low, suggesting generalized malnutrition. **Which of the following is the most appropriate initial diagnostic test for malabsorption?**

(A) xylose absorption
(B) Schilling test
(C) x-ray studies
(D) stool fat quantitation
(E) small intestinal biopsy

15. A 33-year-old man presents to the clinic concerned that he might have hepatitis C. His partner was just diagnosed with hepatitis C and now he is inquiring if he might have it as well. He has not had vaccination for either hepatitis A or B in the past. Serologic tests reveal negative hepatitis C antibody, negative hepatitis B surface antigen (HBsAg), and positive antibody to hepatitis B surface antigen. **Which of the following conditions does this serologic pattern best fit with?**

(A) previous hepatitis B infection
(B) chronic active hepatitis
(C) acute hepatitis B infection
(D) poor prognosis
(E) need for vaccine to hepatitis B

16. A 29-year-old woman is found, on routine annual blood testing, to have a small increase in unconjugated bilirubin. There is no evidence of hemolysis and her liver enzymes and function tests are otherwise normal. She has no prior history of liver disease and is not taking any medications. Her physical examination is completely normal with no signs of chronic liver disease. **Which of the following is the most likely diagnosis?**

(A) Crigler–Najjar syndrome
(B) Dubin–Johnson syndrome
(C) Rotor syndrome
(D) Gilbert syndrome
(E) pregnanediol therapy

17. An 18-year-old woman was diagnosed 7 years earlier with precocious pseudopuberty secondary to ovarian tumor. Physical examination reveals oral and lingual dark pigmentation. (See Figure 4–1.) **Which of the following is the most likely diagnosis?**

Figure 4–1.

(A) Peutz–Jeghers syndrome
(B) Gardner syndrome
(C) Lynch syndrome
(D) juvenile polyposis
(E) Turcot syndrome

18. A 63-year-old man presents to the clinic for an annual clinical exam. He is otherwise well and has no new symptoms. His physical examination is normal except digital rectal exam is positive for occult blood on fecal testing. He reports no overt rectal bleeding with bowel movements, and there is no change in his bowel patterns. **Which of the following is the most likely location of bowel cancer?**

    (A) cecum
    (B) sigmoid
    (C) transverse colon
    (D) appendix
    (E) ascending colon

19. A 74-year-old man underwent surgery for peptic ulcer surgery 35 years ago. He now presents with symptoms that include abdominal pain and bloating about 30–40 minutes after eating, accompanied by nausea. If he vomits, the symptoms are relieved.

    On physical examination, the vital signs are normal, there is an old mid-line scar on the abdomen, but no focal tenderness, guarding, masses or organomegaly that is palpated. **Which of the following is the most likely cause for his symptoms?**

    (A) early dumping syndrome
    (B) late dumping syndrome
    (C) bile reflux gastropathy
    (D) retained gastric antrum
    (E) afferent loop syndrome

20. A 29-year-old man with acquired immune deficiency syndrome (AIDS) comes to the emergency department because of progressively increasing abdominal discomfort. The pain started 2 days ago, and is associated with some nausea but no vomiting. He also notes that the pain gets worse with eating, is dull in nature, and seems to radiate through to his back. He has never experienced this type of pain before.

    Physical examination is relevant for voluntary guarding in the mid upper abdomen. His biochemistry is normal except for an elevated amylase at 370 U/L (25–125 U/L). **Which of the following infections can trigger this disorder in AIDS patients?**

    (A) toxoplasmosis
    (B) *Mycobacterium avium* complex
    (C) *Mycobacterium tuberculosis*
    (D) *Pneumocystis carinii*
    (E) herpes virus

21. A 55-year-old man from China is known to have chronic liver disease, secondary to hepatitis B infection. He presents to the clinic because of feeling unwell recently with new symptoms of intermittent right upper quadrant pain, poor appetite, and weight loss.

    On physical examination, he appears unwell, the vital signs are normal, and he is not jaundiced. The abdomen is soft, there are no clinical signs of ascites, but the liver edge is hard and tender. Laboratory investigations show that his hemoglobin level has increased from 130 g/L, 1 year ago, to 165 g/L. **Which of the following is the most appropriate initial diagnostic test?**

    (A) alkaline phosphatase (ALP)
    (B) alpha-fetoprotein (AFP)
    (C) aspartate transaminase (AST)
    (D) alanine transaminase (ALT)
    (E) unconjugated bilirubin

22. A 63-year-old man with a long history of alcohol abuse presents to the clinic complaining of abdominal distension. He is experiencing mild abdominal discomfort and associated nausea and poor appetite.

    On physical examination, there is tense ascites and generalized tenderness of the abdomen but no rigidity. A diagnostic paracentesis of the fluid is performed. **Which of the following ascitic fluid results is most likely to suggest uncomplicated ascites due to portal hypertension from cirrhosis?**

    (A) hemorrhage
    (B) protein >25 g/L
    (C) bilirubin level twice that of serum
    (D) serum to ascites albumin gradient >1.1 g/dL
    (E) more than 1000 white cells/mm^3

23. A 64-year-old woman presents to the emergency department with symptoms of sudden-onset abdominal discomfort after eating a large meal. The pain is constant, localizes to the epigastric area with radiation to her right scapula. She also has symptoms of nausea and vomiting. The pain eventually subsides after 1 hour. She recalls similar episodes of pain in the past but never to this extent in severity or duration of symptoms.

On examination, the vital signs are normal and there is some tenderness in the right upper quadrant on deep palpation. An ultrasound of the abdomen reveals a dilated common bile duct secondary to stones. **Which of the following statements regarding common bile duct stones is most likely true?**

(A) all originate in the gallbladder
(B) always produce jaundice
(C) produce constant level of jaundice
(D) can be painless
(E) indicate anomalies of the bile duct

24. A 53-year-old man presents to the clinic for evaluation of persistent diarrhea lasting more than 1 month. He has also noticed symptoms of facial flushing lasting minutes at a time with no clear precipitant.

On physical examination, his blood pressure is 124/74 mm Hg, heart rate is 84 and regular, and there are facial telangiectasias on head and neck examination. He also has a systolic heart murmur that was not present 2 years before. This murmur is accentuated by deep breathing. **Which of the following is the most appropriate initial diagnostic test?**

(A) urinary vanillylmandelic acid (VMA)
(B) serum noradrenaline levels
(C) barium enema
(D) serum serotonin levels
(E) urinary 5-hydroxyindolacetic acid (5-HIAA)

25. A 29-year-old woman presents to the clinic complaining of symptoms of dysphagia with solids and liquids. The symptoms are worse when she is eating quickly or is anxious. Her physical examination is normal. Esophageal manometry reveals normal basal esophageal sphincter pressure, with no relaxation of the sphincter on swallowing. **Which of the following is the most appropriate next step in management?**

(A) beta-blocker therapy
(B) partial esophagectomy
(C) anticholinergic drugs
(D) balloon dilatation
(E) dietary modification

26. A 34-year-old woman presents to the clinic complaining of severe heartburn, ulcers on her finger tips, and discomfort in her hands in cold weather or while washing with cold water. She describes the hands becoming pale and painful with cold exposure and then becoming red on rewarming.

On physical examination, the pertinent findings are healing lesions of the fingertips that she says were small ulcers, and there are small areas of telangiectasias on her face. Esophageal manometry reveals a decrease in the expected amplitude of smooth muscle contraction. Lower esophageal sphincter tone is subnormal, but relaxes normally with swallowing. **Which of the following statements regarding this condition is most likely correct?**

(A) characterized by systemic signs of inflammation
(B) predominantly treated symptomatically
(C) characterized by a poor prognosis
(D) usually more frequent in men
(E) characterized by death secondary to a renal crisis

27. A 35-year-old man presents to the clinic for assessment of worsening bowel symptoms. He has a prior diagnosis of ulcerative colitis which presented with symptoms of diarrhea, rectal bleeding, crampy abdominal pain, and the passage of mucus. He is taking his medications regularly but the symptoms are getting worse.

   On physical examination, the abdomen is soft, there is no guarding, and the rectal exam is normal. A barium enema is performed and is shown in Figure 4–2. **Which of the following is the most likely diagnosis of this new complication?**

Figure 4–2.

(A) toxic megacolon
(B) amoebic colitis
(C) appendicitis
(D) ischemic colitis
(E) annular carcinoma

28. A 45-year-old man is brought to the emergency department after vomiting up frank blood. This has never occurred before and he reports no prior symptoms of nausea, vomiting, or ASA/NSAID use. His past health history is significant for chronic alcoholism.

   On physical examination, his blood pressure is 94/73 mm Hg, heart rate 110/min, and there are signs of chronic liver disease. He is resuscitated with IV fluids (normal saline) and undergoes urgent endoscopy which reveals the findings shown in Figure 4–3. **Which of the following is the most likely diagnosis?**

Figure 4–3.

(A) esophageal varices
(B) esophageal carcinoma
(C) foreign body
(D) tertiary waves
(E) Barrett esophagus

29. A 33-year-old woman presents to the emergency department with new symptoms of epigastric abdominal pain and associated nausea and vomiting of 2 days duration. The symptoms are persistent and radiate to her back. Eating does not change the character of the pain.

   On physical examination, her abdomen is tender on palpation in the epigastric region, and the remaining examination is normal. Her white count is 13,000/mL, and amylase is 475 U/L (25–125 U/L). **Which of the following is the most common predisposing factor for this disorder?**

(A) drugs
(B) gallstones
(C) malignancy
(D) alcohol
(E) hypertriglyceridemia

30. A 40-year-old taxicab driver presents to the clinic for evaluation of worsening abdominal pain. The symptoms seem to get worse after meals and the pain is described as a dull burning sensation with no radiation. Antacids previously alleviated the pain but do not seem to be effective now and his only medication is prn use of naproxen for lower back pain.

On physical examination, there is epigastric tenderness but no rigidity or masses. Diagnostic upper endoscopy is performed with the findings seen in Figure 4–4. **Which of the following is the most likely diagnosis?**

Figure 4–4.

(A) gastric ulcer
(B) achalasia
(C) esophageal varices
(D) normal
(E) hiatus hernia

31. A 54-year-old man complains of burning epigastric pain that usually improves after a meal, and is occasionally relieved with antacids. On examination, he appears well and besides some epigastric tenderness on palpation, the rest of the examination is normal. Upper endoscopy confirms a duodenal ulcer. **Which of the following statements concerning PUD is most likely correct?**

(A) duodenal ulcer is seen more often in older people than is gastric ulcer
(B) clinically, gastric ulcers are more common than duodenal ulcers
(C) duodenal ulcers can frequently be malignant
(D) infection can cause both types of peptic ulcer
(E) peptic gastric ulcers are usually quite proximal in the stomach

32. A 30-year-old man complains of chronic diarrhea for the past 6 months. There is no weight loss, fever, or abdominal pain. He takes no medications and feels fine. His physical examination is completely normal.

Further history reveals that this man does not take laxatives; however, in an effort to stay slim he eats a lot of sugar-free gum and sugarless candy. **Which of the following explanations is the most likely cause of his diarrhea?**

(A) direct stimulant effect of chemicals in the candies
(B) lack of fiber in his diet
(C) pancreatic insufficiency secondary to chronic protein-calorie malnutrition
(D) secondary intestinal mucosal atrophy
(E) nonabsorbed carbohydrates

33. **Which of the following is a risk factor for** *Helicobacter pylori* **infection?**

(A) excess exposure to antibiotics
(B) female sex
(C) alpha1-antitrypsin deficiency
(D) low socioeconomic indicators
(E) proton pump inhibitor therapy

34. A 73-year-old woman presents to the emergency room complaining of black tarry stools for the previous 2 days and now symptoms of lightheadedness when standing up.

    On physical examination, she has a postural drop in her blood pressure and increase in heart rate. The abdomen is soft and nontender, but digital rectal examination confirms the presence of melena. She recently started using ibuprofen for hip discomfort. She is admitted to the hospital for treatment and upper endoscopy confirms the diagnosis of a gastric ulcer. **Which of the following is the most likely explanation for the gastric ulcer?**

    (A) increasing acid production
    (B) causing direct epithelial cell death
    (C) promoting replication of *Helicobacter pylori*
    (D) an antiplatelet effect
    (E) inhibiting mucosal repair

35. A 52-year-old woman is experiencing abdominal discomfort after meals as well as early in the morning. There is no weight loss or constitutional symptoms, and she has tried antacids but experiences minimal relief. Upper endoscopy reveals a duodenal ulcer and the biopsy is negative for malignancy. **Which of the following is the most appropriate next step in management?**

    (A) 6–8 weeks of omeprazole or ranitidine
    (B) long-term acid suppression with omeprazole
    (C) antibiotic therapy
    (D) antibiotic therapy and omeprazole
    (E) bismuth citrate therapy

DIRECTIONS (Questions 36 through 43): The following group of numbered items is preceded by a list of lettered options. For each question, select the one lettered option that is most closely associated with it. Each lettered option may be used once, multiple times, or not at all.

Questions 36 through 43: For each patient with viral hepatitis, select the most likely viral agents.

(A) hepatitis A virus
(B) hepatitis B virus
(C) hepatitis C virus
(D) hepatitis D virus
(E) hepatitis E virus

36. A 24-year-old man develops acute onset of anorexia, nausea, and vomiting. This is followed by clinical jaundice and right upper quadrant discomfort 1 week later. Four weeks ago, he was traveling in South America, where he ate food from street vendors. On examination, he is icteric with right upper quadrant tenderness but the rest of the examination is normal. His hepatitis serology is positive for an agent that could have been prevented with vaccination.

37. A couple returns from a trip to Central America and develops nonspecific abdominal symptoms followed by clinical jaundice. They stayed at a resort, and ate fresh fruits and salads. Serology for hepatitis virus spread by the fecal–oral route is positive.

38. A 23-year-old sex-trade worker develops acute-onset jaundice and seeks medical attention. There is no history of intravenous drug use or travel. On examination, she is icteric, there is no lymphadenopathy, and the heart and lungs are normal. Her liver span is 14 cm and the liver edge is smooth but tender. Her pelvic examination is normal. Serology for viral hepatitis transmitted via the sexual route is positive.

39. A 34-year-old man is seen for asymptomatic elevations in his AST and ALT. He appears well and the physical examination is normal. There is no prior history of intravenous drug use, blood transfusions, or multiple sex partners. His hepatitis serology is positive for the virus, most likely to lead to chronic infection.

40. A 45-year-old woman is evaluated for chronic elevations in her liver enzymes (AST and ALT). She feels well and her physical examination is normal. Nonviral etiologies, such as medications and autoimmune conditions,

are ruled out. Her serology is positive for the hepatitis virus that can respond to specific antiviral therapy.

41. A 24-year-old woman is pregnant at 14 weeks with her first baby. She feels well and the pregnancy is uncomplicated. Routine screening is positive for chronic viral hepatitis for which perinatal transmission is of major epidemiologic significance.

42. A 38-year-old woman is worried about a recent potential exposure to an individual with active viral hepatitis. She is seeking treatment for viral hepatitis for which passive immunotherapy can provide some protection.

43. A 28-year-old man, who emigrated from North Africa, is evaluated for chronic elevations in liver enzymes (AST and ALT). He has no symptoms of acute hepatitis, and his physical examination is normal with no characteristics of chronic liver disease. His hepatitis serology is positive for a virus that requires the presence of another infectious agent before becoming clinically apparent.

DIRECTIONS (Questions 44 through 66): For each of the questions in this section select the one lettered answer that is the best response in each case.

44. A 53-year-old man presents to the emergency department with severe epigastric abdominal pain. On physical examination, his temperature is 37.2°C, the blood pressure is 110/70 mm Hg, heart rate 110/min, and respirations 20/min. Examination of the heart and lungs is normal, and his abdomen is tender in the epigastric region. His white count is 15,000/mL and amylase is 450 U/L (25–125 U/L). **Which of the following laboratory abnormalities is also most likely to be present?**

(A) hypoglycemia
(B) hypercholesterolemia
(C) hyperglycemia
(D) hypercalcemia
(E) hypercarbia

45. A 43-year-old man presents to the clinic for evaluation of feeling unwell. His symptoms are vague and nonspecific. Physical examination is unremarkable except for evidence of scleral icterus, but no hepatomegaly or ascites. The skin appears normal. **Which of the following is the most likely explanation for why early jaundice is visible in the eyes but not the skin?**

(A) the high type II collagen content of scleral tissue
(B) the high elastin content of scleral tissue
(C) the high blood flow to the head with consequent increased bilirubin delivery
(D) secretion via the lacrimal glands
(E) the lighter color of the sclera

46. A 25-year-old previously healthy man experiences fatigue and malaise. One week ago he had a "viral"-type illness consisting of a sore throat, fever, and myalgias. He now appears jaundiced, but the rest of the physical examination is normal. His investigations reveal a total bilirubin of 4 mg/dL (0.1–1.0 mg/dL) and a direct bilirubin of 0.3 mg/dL (0.0–0.3 mg/dL). **Which of the following is the most likely diagnosis?**

(A) hemolysis
(B) gallstones
(C) alcoholic liver disease
(D) pancreatic carcinoma
(E) Dubin–Johnson syndrome

47. A 28-year-old man presents to the clinic for assessment of frequent bowel movements, crampy abdominal pain, and the passage of mucus. He also notes weight loss of 10 lbs over the past 2 months, despite having a good appetite. There is no history of bloody diarrhea, recent antibiotic use, or foreign travel. He is also complaining of joint discomfort in his hands, knees, and back.

On examination, he is thin, there is muscle wasting, and his abdomen is soft with voluntary guarding in the left lower quadrant. His joints are not actively inflamed and there is an asymmetric distribution of joint involvement. **Which of the following is the most likely diagnosis?**

(A) lymphoma of the bowel
(B) amyloid infiltration
(C) chronic pancreatitis
(D) ulcerative colitis
(E) tropical sprue

48. A 57-year-old man presents to the emergency department complaining of severe diarrhea and abdominal pain. He reports no prior history of diarrhea or bowel disorders, and his past medical history is significant for stable angina, hypertension, and dyslipidemia. Two weeks ago he received antibiotics for the treatment of community-acquired pneumonia. He is evaluated with sigmoidoscopy which reveals a granular friable mucosa. **Which of the following is the most common cause of this syndrome?**

(A) ischemic colitis
(B) rotavirus
(C) *Clostridium perfringens* infection
(D) prior antibiotic therapy
(E) bacterial invasion of the bowel wall

49. A 42-year-old previously well woman presents with pruritus. She is not taking any medications, and only drinks alcohol on a social basis. Her physical examination is entirely normal with no signs of chronic liver disease or jaundice. Laboratory evaluation reveals an alkaline phosphatase level 3 times the upper limit of normal, and an ultrasound of the liver and gallbladder is normal. **Which of the following is the most appropriate next step in diagnosis?**

(A) INR or prothrombin time
(B) antinuclear antibodies
(C) protein immunoelectrophoresis
(D) CT scan of the abdomen
(E) antimitochondrial antibodies

50. A 22-year-old man with Crohn disease presents to the clinic for evaluation of increased symptoms of bloating, abdominal pain, cramping, and non-blood diarrhea. There is no fever or chills and he remains compliant with his medications.

Physical examination is normal except for right lower quadrant tenderness and associated fullness. There is no guarding or rigidity, and bowel sounds are present. A barium enema demonstrates a "string sign" in the ileal area. (See Figure 4–5.) **In which of the following conditions is this sign most often seen?**

Figure 4–5.

(A) in the stenotic or nonstenotic phase of the disease
(B) in the stenotic phase only
(C) with ileal involvement
(D) with gastric involvement
(E) with rectal involvement

51. A 22-year-old woman presents with chronic diarrhea. She has no abdominal discomfort, feels well, and reports no weight loss or systemic symptoms. Physical examination reveals a healthy young woman who is 5'7" tall and weighs 170 lb. The complete physical examination is normal. **Which of the following is the most likely cause of a secretory diarrhea in this young woman?**

    (A) surreptitious use of stimulant laxatives
    (B) carcinoid tumor
    (C) ulcerative colitis
    (D) lactose deficiency
    (E) celiac disease

52. A 57-year old man comes to the office with a complaint of food "sticking on the way down." His past medical history includes hypertension, type 2 diabetes, and dyslipidemia. His physical examination is completely normal. **Which of the following characteristics suggests a benign problem is causing the dysphagia?**

    (A) severe weight loss in comparison to the degree of dysphagia
    (B) hoarseness following the onset of dysphagia
    (C) episodic dysphagia for several years
    (D) difficulty only with solids
    (E) hiccups

53. A 70-year-old man is investigated for symptoms of dysphagia. He complains that the symptoms occur only when eating solids, but not with liquids. There is no pain associated with swallowing and he reports no weight loss. His physical examination is normal. Investigations reveal a Zenker diverticulum of the esophagus. **Which of the following historical characteristics suggests a Zenker diverticulum?**

    (A) severe weight loss
    (B) greater problems with liquids than solids
    (C) hoarseness
    (D) worse in semirecumbent position
    (E) aspiration unrelated to swallowing

54. A 27-year-old man with HIV comes to the clinic with symptoms of pain every time he swallows (odynophagia). He is not on any antiretroviral therapy and otherwise feels well. Examination of the mouth and pharynx are normal. **Which of the following is the most likely diagnosis?**

    (A) midesophageal cancer
    (B) distal esophageal cancer
    (C) peptic stricture
    (D) candida infection
    (E) bacterial esophagitis

55. A 33-year-old woman was evaluated for symptoms of severe intense generalized pruritus. Her physical examination reveals multiple sites of excoriation. Laboratory investigations confirm the clinical diagnosis of primary biliary cirrhosis (PBC). She is now inquiring about available treatments for this condition, including if there is a cure for the disease. **Which of the following treatments is most likely to "cure" her PBC?**

    (A) ursodiol
    (B) methotrexate
    (C) azathioprine
    (D) liver transplantation
    (E) glucocorticoids

56. A 47-year-old woman complains of food sticking every time she eats anything solid. She has lost 10 lb since the symptoms started, and points to her midthorax as the site where she feels the food is sticking. **If this is due to mechanical obstruction, this historical information suggests which of the following locations?**

    (A) at the location the patient points to
    (B) at or above the location the patient points to
    (C) below the location the patient points to
    (D) at or below the location the patient points to
    (E) the historical information is unhelpful in suggesting a location

57. A 52-year-old man is experiencing episodes of severe chest pain and associated dysphagia. He is seen twice in the emergency room, and both times the symptoms have responded to sublingual nitroglycerin. He then has a full cardiac evaluation including electrocardiogram (ECG), cardiac biomarkers, and an exercise stress test, that are all normal. His symptoms persist, and he undergoes a barium swallow which is diagnostic for this clinical condition. **Which of the following is the most likely diagnosis?**

    (A) herpetic infection of the esophagus
    (B) a motor disorder of the esophagus
    (C) midesophageal cancer
    (D) peptic stricture
    (E) external esophageal compression

58. A 16-year old girl is referred to your family practice for on-going follow-up. She is a recent immigrant from Southeast Asia, and is taking isoniazid (INH) for latent tuberculosis infection. She feels well and reports no constitutional symptoms. Routine blood tests are unremarkable, except for an elevated direct bilirubin. Other liver enzymes and function tests are completely normal. **Which of the following is the most likely diagnosis?**

    (A) hemolytic anemia
    (B) INH toxicity
    (C) Crigler–Najjar syndrome type I
    (D) rifampin toxicity
    (E) Rotor syndrome

59. A 45-year-old woman presents to the emergency department with a 1-week history of jaundice, anorexia, and right upper quadrant discomfort. On examination she is icteric, with a tender right upper quadrant and liver span of 14 cm. There is no shifting dullness or pedal edema and the heart and lungs are normal. On further inquiry, she reports consuming 1 bottle of wine a day for the past 6 months. **Which of the following laboratory tests is most characteristic of a patient with jaundice secondary to alcoholic hepatitis?**

    (A) ratio of AST:ALT is 3:1 and the AST is 500 U/L
    (B) ratio of AST:ALT is 2:1 and the AST is 250 U/L
    (C) ratio of AST:ALT is 1:1 and the AST is 500 U/L
    (D) ratio of AST:ALT is 1:1 and the AST is 250 U/L
    (E) ratio of AST:ALT is 1:3 and the AST is 750

60. **Which of the following medications causes predictable, dose-dependent hepatocellular injury?**

    (A) morphine
    (B) INH
    (C) gold
    (D) acetaminophen
    (E) acetylsalicylic acid (ASA)

61. A 22 year-old-woman is brought to the emergency room 2 hours after ingesting 30 tablets of acetaminophen (500 mg/tab). Her past medical history is significant for depression, but this is the first self-harm attempt. She is currently not on any other medications and denies any co-ingestions.

    On physical examination she is alert and oriented, the blood pressure is 110/74 mm Hg, heart rate 88/min, and respiratory rate 12/min. The heart and lung exam is normal, and the abdomen is soft, with a nontender liver on palpation. She is admitted to the hospital for further management of an acetaminophen overdose. **Which of the following is the mostly likely mechanism of acetaminophen hepatotoxicity?**

    (A) an allergic mechanism
    (B) an active metabolite
    (C) a reaction with hepatic glycogen stores
    (D) direct toxicity of the parent compound
    (E) circulating immune complexes

62. **Blood-filled lesions in the liver (peliosis hepatis) are most likely to be seen with which of the following medications?**

(A) methyltestosterone

(B) oral contraceptives

(C) trimethoprim-sulfamethoxazole

(D) chlorpromazine

(E) erythromycin

63. A 24-year-old man with a history of depression is brought to the emergency room because of a drug overdose. He is experiencing some nausea and vomiting, but no other symptoms. Physical examination and vital signs are normal. Six hours prior to presentation, he intentionally took 40 tablets of acetaminophen (500 mg/tablet). Baseline acetaminophen level, liver enzymes and function are drawn, and he is admitted to the hospital. **Which of the following is the most appropriate next step in management?**

(A) give ethanol to compete with the parent drug for metabolism, therefore preventing formation of toxic metabolites

(B) give Narcan to block its actions directly

(C) give intravenous prostacyclins to maintain cellular integrity

(D) give *N*-acetylcysteine to allow binding of the toxic metabolite

(E) give glucocorticoids to block the immune cascade

64. A 16-year-old girl is referred to the office because of chronic diarrhea and weight loss. She is experiencing large-volume watery diarrhea that is painless. The symptoms persist even when she is fasting, and there is no relationship to foods or liquids. She is not on any medications, and there is no travel history or other constitutional symptoms. Her physical examination is normal. **Which of the following is the most likely diagnosis?**

(A) partial small bowel obstruction

(B) partial large bowel obstruction

(C) osmotic diarrhea

(D) secretory diarrhea

(E) inflammatory bowel disease

65. A 52-year-old man has suffered with chronic diarrhea for several years, but has refused to see a doctor. He finally comes because he is having trouble driving at night, because of difficulty seeing. Physical examination reveals a slender, pale, unwell-looking man. He has a microcytic anemia, slight elevation in the INR, low ionized calcium, and albumin levels. **Which of the following is the most likely cause for his diarrhea?**

(A) malabsorption

(B) osmotic diarrhea

(C) secretory diarrhea

(D) inflammatory bowel disease

(E) colonic tumor

66. A 49-year-old woman is being investigated for chronic diarrhea and weight loss. Malabsorption is suspected. **Which of the following investigations is most likely to make a definitive diagnosis?**

(A) presence of fecal osmotic gap

(B) D-xylose test

(C) stool fat measurements

(D) Schilling test

(E) mucosal biopsy

DIRECTIONS (Questions 67 through 71): The following group of numbered items is preceded by a list of lettered options. For each question, select the one lettered option that is most closely associated with it. Each lettered option may be used once, multiple times, or not at all.

Questions 67 through 71: For each patient with gastritis, select the most likely mechanism of injury.

(A) bile acid reflux implicated in pathogenesis

(B) immune or autoimmune pathogenesis suspected

(C) ischemia of the gastric mucosa implicated in the pathogenesis

(D) associated with *Helicobacter pylori* infection

(E) unknown mechanism

(F) interruption of prostaglandin synthesis

67. A 67-year-old man is admitted to the intensive care unit (ICU) because of respiratory failure from pneumonia. He requires artificial ventilation and inotropic support. On the third day in the ICU, he develops melena and a drop in his hemoglobin. Urgent upper endoscopy is performed and it reveals three gastric ulcers in the fundus and body of the stomach. Appropriate treatment is started.

68. A 70-year-old man has a long history of heartburn and dyspepsia. He has tried many medications but the symptoms always return. His upper endoscopy is normal with no ulcers. Routine biopsies of the gastric mucosa report "gastritis."

69. A 57-year-old woman experiences frequent symptoms of heartburn. She reports no weight loss, diarrhea, or dysphagia symptoms. Past medical history is significant for vitamin B_{12} deficiency treated with monthly injections. She appears well, and the examination is normal, except for some patches on her arms where she has lost all the skin pigmentation. Her upper endoscopy is normal, except for gastric biopsies commenting on gastritis.

70. A 54-year-old man is investigated for weight loss, epigastric pain, nausea, and vomiting. He appears ill; on examination, there is epigastric tenderness and marked peripheral edema. Upper endoscopy reveals large mucosal folds in the body and fundus of the stomach. Biopsies are consistent with a diagnosis of Ménétrier disease.

71. A 65-year-old man has developed abdominal pain, early satiety, nausea, and vomiting. He reports no weight loss or change in bowel habits. He had a partial gastrectomy 30 years ago for a bleeding gastric ulcer. Upper endoscopy finds erythema of the gastric remnant, and biopsies report epithelial injury and minimal inflammation (gastritis).

Answers and Explanations

1. **(E)** Carcinoid tumors account for up to 75% of all GI endocrine tumors. They are frequently multiple. Primary carcinoid tumors of the appendix are common but rarely metastasize. Those in the large colon may metastasize but do not function. Carcinoids are the most common GI endocrine tumors. They arise from neuroendocrine cells most commonly in the GI tract, pancreas, or bronchi. GI carcinoids cause abdominal pain, bleeding, or even obstruction (usually via intussusception). Carcinoid syndrome is characterized by flushing, diarrhea, and valvular heart disease. *(Fauci, Chapter 344)*

2. **(C)** Adenocarcinoma of the small bowel accounts for about 50% of malignant tumors of the small bowel. They are most commonly found in the distal duodenum and proximal jejunum. Hemorrhage, or obstruction, is the most common presenting symptom. X-ray findings can mimic chronic duodenal ulcer disease or Crohn disease. *(Fauci, Chapter 87)*

3. **(D)** There is one unique form of lymphoma called IPSID or Mediterranean lymphoma. It diffusely involves the small intestine and usually presents with diarrhea and steatorrhea. Oral antibiotics, early in the disease, provide some benefit, suggesting a possible infectious component to the disorder. Antibiotics and chemotherapy are frequently combined. *(Fauci, Chapter 87)*

4. **(E)** Appendiceal tumors make up nearly half of all carcinoid tumors and are a frequent finding in routine appendectomy specimens. They are usually small, solitary, and benign. Even if they invade locally, they rarely metastasize. *(Fauci, Chapter 344)*

5. **(D)** Primary small bowel lymphoma is more common in the settings of celiac disease, regional enteritis, congenital immune disorders, prior organ transplantation, autoimmune disorders, and AIDS. *(Fauci, Chapter 87)*

6. **(E)** Carcinoid tumors are most frequently found in the distal ileum. Adenocarcinomas are characteristically more proximal. The ileum has more lymphatic tissue, than the rest of the small bowel, so lymphoma is more common here than in the jejunum or duodenum. However, there is not as strong a predilection for the distal ileum as there is for carcinoids. *(Fauci, Chapter 87)*

7. **(A)** Acquired lactase deficiency is very common in GI diseases with evidence of mucosal damage. Examples include celiac and tropical sprue, viral and bacterial infections, giardiasis, cystic fibrosis, and ulcerative colitis. It is not caused by a hypersensitivity reaction. *(Fauci, Chapter 288)*

8. **(A)** This syndrome is likely celiac disease, but a clinical and histologic improvement with a gluten-free diet would be required for confirmation. The decrease in pancreatic enzyme production is secondary to decreased intestinal secretion of hormones that stimulate the pancreas. Dermatitis herpetiformis might be related to celiac disease. Although gross malabsorption is the classical description of celiac disease, it can present with isolated deficiencies such as iron deficiency anemia. *(Fauci, Chapter 288)*

9. **(G)** Whipple disease is caused by infection with a Gram-positive bacillus called *Tropheryma whippelii*. The disease, previously invariably fatal, can be controlled with long-term antibiotic therapy (at least 1 year), and some patients seem to be cured. Arthritis and central nervous system (CNS) involvement are other manifestations of this rare disease. *(Fauci, Chapter 288)*

10. **(B)** Zollinger–Ellison syndrome is caused by a non beta islet cell tumor of the pancreas. It may be associated with the syndrome of multiple endocrine neoplasia, type I (MEN I). The syndrome should be suspected in patients with multiple ulcers, ulcers resistant to therapy, ulcers in unusual locations, strong family history of ulcers, unexplained diarrhea, or evidence of MEN I. *(Fauci, Chapter 287)*

11. **(D)** Diverticula are present in over 50% of octogenarians. Most patients remain asymptomatic. They are most common in the sigmoid colon and decrease in frequency in the proximal colon. The relative scarcity of diverticula in underdeveloped nations has led to the hypothesis that low fiber diets result in decreased fecal bulk, narrowing of the colon, and an increased intraluminal pressure to move the small fecal mass. This results in thickening of the muscular coat, and eventually herniations or diverticula of the mucosa at the points where nutrient arteries penetrate the muscularis. Surgery is not indicated unless the patient develops diverticulitis and complications, and laxatives or stool softeners are not part of the medical management of asymptomatic diverticular disease. *(Fauci, Chapter 291)*

12. **(C)** Amylase accumulates in the setting of renal failure, and thus becomes a less-valuable diagnostic test (false positive). Numerous other conditions involving the pancreas, the gut, and the salivary glands can raise amylase levels. Sulfonamides cause pancreatitis; therefore, an elevated amylase is not confusing, but rather a useful test for pancreatitis in patients taking the drug. Morphine can elevate amylase levels in the absence of pancreatitis. *(Fauci, Chapter 306)*

13. **(D)** This presentation is typical of esophageal cancer. Lesions in the upper two-thirds of the esophagus are squamous, but in the distal esophagus, most are adenocarcinomas. The adenocarcinomas develop more commonly from columnar epithelium in the distal esophagus (Barrett esophagus). Adenocarcinomas of the esophagus have the biologic behavior of gastric cancers. The incidence of squamous cell cancer of the esophagus is decreasing while adenocarcinoma is increasing. Currently, over 50% of esophageal cancer is adenocarcinoma. The 5-year survival for esophageal cancer is <5%. Combination therapy seems to be more effective than surgery alone. *(Fauci, Chapter 87)*

14. **(D)** Fat malabsorption demonstrated on stool collection for 72 hours is the gold standard, but does not indicate the exact cause. The Schilling test is useful in testing for vitamin B_{12} absorption, and not indicated in this patient unless the diagnosis of B_{12} deficiency is made. X-rays can be helpful in diagnosing underlying disorders, but are nonspecific. Small intestinal biopsy is useful in determining the cause of malabsorption (like celiac disease or IBD) once the diagnosis of malabsorption is confirmed. *(Fauci, Chapter 288)*

15. **(A)** The antibody can be demonstrated in 80%–90% of patients, usually late in convalescence, and indicates relative or absolute immunity. In contrast, HBsAg occurs very early and disappears in <6 months. Persistence of HBsAg indicates chronic infection. The pattern in this patient is also seen postvaccination, and perhaps as a consequence of remote infection. *(Fauci, Chapter 298)*

16. **(D)** Gilbert syndrome may be associated with impaired hepatic uptake of bilirubin. It is caused by hereditary decrease in the activity of glucuronosyltransferase in the uridine diphosphate glycosyltransferase 1 (UGT1) family. More severe enzyme deficits are the cause of the two variants of Crigler–Najjar syndrome and usually present in the neonatal period with very high elevations in unconjugated bilirubin,

making it not the correct answer in this patient. She does not have Dubin–Johnson or Rotor syndrome since both of these entities have elevations of conjugated bilirubin. *(Fauci, Chapter 297)*

17. **(A)** Intestinal polyposis is a possible indication of Peutz–Jeghers syndrome associated with dark brown spots on the lips and palate. There is characteristic distribution of pigment around lips, nose, eyes, and hands. Tumors of the ovary, breast, pancreas, and endometrium are associated with this syndrome. The other syndromes listed do not have the characteristic pigment changes described in this patient. *(Fauci, Chapter 54)*

18. **(B)** Despite some decline, distal tumors are still the most common. The fact that up to 60% of tumors are located in the rectosigmoid is the rationale for screening via flexible, fiberoptic sigmoidoscopes. Occult blood testing and colonoscopy are other possible screening techniques. *(Fauci, Chapter 87)*

19. **(E)** This pattern of symptoms is characteristic of afferent loop syndrome. It is caused by distention and incomplete drainage of the afferent loop and requires surgical correction. Bacterial overgrowth of the afferent loop is more common. Its clinical presentation includes post-prandial abdominal pain, bloating, diarrhea, fat, and vitamin B_{12} malabsorption. His symptoms are not characteristic of the dumping syndrome (early or late), and bile acid reflux can present with similar symptoms but is much less common than afferent loop syndrome. *(Fauci, Chapter 287)*

20. **(B)** Pancreatitis in AIDS patients can be caused by cytomegalovirus and cryptosporidium as well as *M avium* complex. Drugs are another cause of AIDS-related pancreatitis. The other organisms are not associated with pancreatitis in HIV-positive patients. *(Fauci, Chapter 307)*

21. **(B)** Hepatoma is the most likely diagnosis in this man and AFP elevations, over 500–1000 mg/L in the absence of a colonic tumor (or pregnancy), suggest hepatoma. In China, it is estimated that the lifetime risk of hepatoma in people with chronic hepatitis B is close to 40%. Paraneoplastic syndromes are not common but include erythrocytosis, hypercalcemia, and acquired porphyria. Elevations in AST, ALT, ALP, and bilirubin may be present in this man but are not diagnostic of the underlying hepatoma. *(Fauci, Chapter 88)*

22. **(D)** In uncomplicated ascites, the difference between plasma albumin and ascitic fluid albumin is >1.1 g/dL. Ascitic fluid (in uncomplicated) cirrhosis of the liver shows a specific gravity <1.016, protein is <25 g/L, and the gross appearance is straw-colored. In spontaneous bacterial peritonitis, the fluid may be cloudy, with elevated number of white cells >500 or >250 neutrophils. *(Fauci, Chapter 302)*

23. **(D)** Common duct stones can be painless, or may give rise to severe pain, chills, and fever. The jaundice is generally conjugated hyperbilirubinemia. Partial obstruction of the common duct produces variable amounts of jaundice and is influenced by the presence of concurrent hepatocellular disease or cholangitis. Although most such stones originate in the gallbladder, hemolytic disorders and parasitic infections can result in primary bile duct stones. *(Fauci, Chapter 305)*

24. **(E)** The most important mediator of the carcinoid syndrome is serotonin. Serotonin is rapidly metabolized to 5-HIAA, which is rapidly cleared by the kidneys. The measurement of 5-HIAA in the urine is thus the most useful diagnostic test. Its specificity is enhanced by an appropriate diet before testing. The syndrome is characteristic of carcinoid of midgut origin. The cardiac lesions are more common on the right side (hence murmur accentuation on deep inspiration). Foregut carcinoids (bronchus, stomach, duodenum) frequently are associated with wheezing. Serum noradrenaline and VMA levels are useful for confirming a clinical diagnosis of pheochromocytoma. Serotonin levels are not helpful in making the diagnosis of carcinoid. *(Fauci, Chapter 344)*

25. **(D)** These findings are characteristic of achalasia. Successful therapies include, balloon dilatation, nitroglycerine, nifedipine (a calcium channel blocker), botulinum toxin injected endoscopically, and esophageal myotomy (not excision). Anticholinergic medications and dietary changes do not provide much help. *(Fauci, Chapter 286)*

26. **(B)** These findings are characteristic of scleroderma, and esophageal symptoms should be treated with medications for acid suppression. If the disease is limited, the prognosis is not necessarily poor. The limited form is characterized by calcinosis, Raynaud's (often with distal ulceration), esophageal motility disorder, sclerodactyly, and telangiectasia (CREST syndrome). It has a female preponderance, and renal disease can be severe, but is not the most common cause of death. *(Fauci, Chapter 286)*

27. **(E)** Carcinoma has occurred in this patient with ulcerative colitis. The barium enema shows a long, constricting lesion in the transverse colon, with the whole colon devoid of haustral markings. There is no dilatation of the colon suggest this is toxic megacolon, and occasionally ischemic colitis can heal with stricture formation but the appearance of an "apple core" lesion in a patient with ulcerative colitis is cancer until proven otherwise. *(Fauci, Chapter 289)*

28. **(A)** In esophageal varices, the esophageal folds are thick and tortuous, giving rise to a wormy or worm-eaten appearance. The radiographic picture would vary with the severity of the varices, as well as the distention of the esophagus. When varices are severe, they should be appreciated in any projection. The left anterior oblique projection is most ideal for its demonstration. *(Fauci, Chapter 302)*

29. **(B)** Gallstones still remain the most common cause of pancreatitis. Other causes of acute pancreatitis are alcohol, metabolic factors (elevated triglycerides), and medications. In this patient, the history suggests biliary colic and that her pancreatitis is mostly the result of gallstones. *(Fauci, Chapter 305)*

30. **(A)** The image demonstrates an ulcer with raised margins and a central depression. It is likely due to the NSAIDs the patient is taking for his back pain. The ulcer could also be due to a malignancy and the difference between benign and malignancy may be difficult at times to establish on visual appearance. A biopsy is the gold standard of diagnosis. *(Fauci, Chapter 287)*

31. **(D)** *Helicobacter pylori* infection is the cause of most peptic ulcers, and the usual route of infection is via the water supply. Duodenal ulcer is clinically more common, although the prevalence on autopsy series is similar. Duodenal ulcer does not represent a malignant potential. Gastric ulcers are seen in an older population and can be malignant. Benign peptic gastric ulcers tend to be more distal. *(Fauci, Chapter 287)*

32. **(E)** Sugarless gums and candy often contain sorbitol, a sugar that is not absorbed in the gut. It thus produces an osmotic diarrhea if present in sufficient quantity. *(Fauci, Chapter 40)*

33. **(D)** Infection usually occurs early in life and is related to classic socioeconomic indicators such as poverty, domestic crowding, unsanitary living conditions, and unclean water. It is much more common in developing countries. *(Fauci, Chapter 287)*

34. **(E)** NSAIDs inhibit prostaglandins, which play an important role in maintaining gastroduodenal mucosal integrity and repair. *(Fauci, Chapter 287)*

35. **(D)** Antibiotic therapy for eradication of *H pylori* in combination with acid suppression with a proton pump inhibitor like omeprazole is the most effective treatment for duodenal ulcer disease. The most popular regimes include antibiotics and acid suppression medications. *(Fauci, Chapter 287)*

36. **(A)** Hepatitis A is the most likely viral hepatitis to be acquired by this traveler. Specific vaccines are available for hepatitis A and B. Hepatitis D is most frequently symptomatic in association with hepatitis B infection, so vaccination for hepatitis B will decrease the likelihood of

symptomatic hepatitis D infection. *(Fauci, Chapter 298)*

37. **(A or E)** Both hepatitis A and E are usually spread by the fecal–oral route. Hepatitis A is more common and the likely cause of this couple's infection. Hepatitis E is endemic in Central America but according to the CDC it is highly endemic in South-East Asia and North Africa, so that travel to those areas is more likely to result in infection with the E virus. Other forms of transmission are exceedingly uncommon. *(Fauci, Chapter 298)*

38. **(B or D)** Only hepatitis B and D are frequently spread by sexual transmission. It does not seem to occur with hepatitis E, and the evidence is equivocal for hepatitis A and C. *(Fauci, Chapter 298)*

39. **(C)** Chronic hepatitis C infection occurs in 80%–90% of patients. About 50%–70% will have evidence of chronic liver disease. In contrast, only 1%–10% of adults infected with hepatitis B will go on to chronic infection. *(Fauci, Chapter 298)*

40. **(B or C)** Interferon has been used in both hepatitis B and C infections. The response is better in hepatitis B infection. Combination therapy with interferon and ribavirin is more effective in hepatitis C. *(Fauci, Chapter 298)*

41. **(B)** In neonates, the transmission of hepatitis B results in a 90% probability of developing chronic infection. The ongoing infection (often resulting in hepatoma) is a major cause of morbidity and mortality in many parts of the world. *(Fauci, Chapter 298)*

42. **(A or B)** Immunoglobulin injection can provide prophylaxis against hepatitis A, and it is felt that hepatitis B immune globulin is protective for hepatitis B. *(Fauci, Chapter 298)*

43. **(D)** Hepatitis D is a defective ribonucleic acid (RNA) virus that requires the helper function of hepatitis B virus (or other hepadnavirus) for its replication and expression. *(Fauci, Chapter 298)*

44. **(C)** Hyperglycemia is very common in pancreatitis and is usually multifactorial in origin. Factors involved include decreased insulin release, increased glucagon release, and elevated adrenal glucocorticoids and catecholamines. Patients with acute pancreatitis can develop hypocalcemia (not hypercalcemia), and occasionally severe hypertriglyceridemia (not hypercholesterolemia) can be cause of pancreatitis. *(Fauci, Chapter 307)*

45. **(B)** The sclera are high in elastin content, which has an affinity for bilirubin. Therefore, jaundice is usually detected here first. Fluorescent lighting makes recognition more difficult. In some individuals, dark skin color makes jaundice more difficult to detect. *(Fauci, Chapter 43)*

46. **(A)** Hemolysis results in predominantly unconjugated bilirubin. Unconjugated hyperbilirubinemia is caused by overproduction, decreased uptake, or decreased conjugation. The other answers listed can also cause jaundice, but the elevation in bilirubin is predominantly conjugated (direct more than indirect). *(Fauci, Chapter 43)*

47. **(D)** Joint involvement in inflammatory bowel disease may involve sacroiliitis or specific large joint peripheral arthritis. The latter type of arthritis parallels the course of the bowel disease. The sacroiliitis (spondylitic) variety follows an independent course. Lymphoma of the small bowel, tropical sprue, and chronic pancreatitis are not known to have typical joint involvement. Amyloidosis does not cause joint involvement, but patients may complain of hand symptoms due to carpal tunnel syndrome. *(Fauci, Chapter 289)*

48. **(D)** This likely represents diarrhea secondary to *Clostridium difficile* infection as a complication of recent antibiotic therapy. It is mediated by toxins, not by direct bacterial invasion. Cephalosporins, because they are so widely used, are the most common cause of the disease. On a per case basis, however, clindamycin is the most likely antibiotic to cause the disease. Ischemic colitis is possible, especially if the patient has severe atherosclerotic disease,

but this diagnosis would only be considered if the *C difficile* toxin is negative. Finally, *C perfringens* is an anerobic microbe and does not usually cause diarrhea. *(Fauci, Chapter 123)*

49. **(E)** This patient may have primary biliary cirrhosis (PBC). A positive antimitochondrial antibody test is found in over 90% of symptomatic patients. The patient with PBC is typically a middle-aged woman with itching. Patients are often asymptomatic and diagnosed only on routine blood work, when an incidental elevated ALP is found on routine liver enzymes. The cause of PBC is unknown, but a disordered immune response is involved. The other investigations are not specific for any particular diagnosis in a patient presenting with her symptoms. They may be important to document liver function or structure but do not contribute to establishing a diagnosis. *(Fauci, Chapter 302)*

50. **(A)** The string sign represents long areas of circumferential inflammation and fibrosis. It is seen in the stenotic and nonstenotic phase of Crohn disease. In addition to the string sign, abnormal puddling of barium and fistulous tracts are other helpful x-ray signs of ileitis. Other radiologic findings in Crohn disease include skip lesions, rectal sparing, small ulcerations, and fistulas. *(Fauci, Chapter 289)*

51. **(A)** In this young woman, after considering other causes, surreptitious use of laxatives needs to be considered. Abuse of stimulant laxatives such as senna can cause a secretory diarrhea. Magnesium-based laxatives will cause an osmotic diarrhea. Although carcinoid tumor can cause diarrhea, it is an uncommon disorder and she should have other symptoms of carcinoid such as flushing or skin changes. Celiac disease and UC can cause diarrhea but would have associated weight loss or abdominal discomfort. Lactose deficiency does not cause a secretory diarrhea but an osmotic diarrhea. *(Fauci, Chapter 76)*

52. **(C)** Episodic dysphagia to solids of several years' duration suggests a benign disease, and is characteristic of a lower esophageal ring. Motor dysphagia presents with dysphagia to solids and liquids. Dysphagia due to obstruction starts with solids and can progress to liquids as well. Hoarseness following the onset of dysphagia can be caused by an esophageal cancer extending to involve the recurrent laryngeal nerve or because of laryngitis secondary to gastroesophageal reflux. Severe weight loss suggests malignancy, and hiccups are a rare occurrence in distal problems of the esophagus. *(Fauci, Chapter 38)*

53. **(E)** Aspiration, unrelated to swallowing, is seen in a Zenker diverticulum, achalasia, or gastroesophageal reflex. *(Fauci, Chapter 38)*

54. **(D)** Painful swallowing can be caused by candida or herpes infection of the esophagus, or pill-induced esophagitis. Patients with immunodeficiency states (eg, AIDS) may have herpetic, candidal, or CMV esophagitis, as well as tumors (lymphoma, Kaposi sarcoma). Candida infection is more common than the other etiologies listed, and therefore the most likely diagnosis. *(Fauci, Chapter 38)*

55. **(D)** In patients with end-stage liver failure, liver transplantation is "curative," since recurrence after transplantation is rare. There is no known effective therapy to prevent progression of liver disease in PBC. The other therapies listed have been reported as effective in small case series but not in controlled trials. Ursodeoxycholic acid seems effective in providing at least symptomatic improvement, and may even delay liver transplantation. Replacement of fat-soluble vitamins (eg, vitamin A to prevent night blindness) is an important part of therapy, as is replacement of calcium and vitamin D to prevent osteoporosis. *(Fauci, Chapter 302)*

56. **(D)** The history where the food stops or "sticks" is sometimes helpful. The site of obstruction is usually at or below where the patient says the sticking occurs. *(Fauci, Chapter 38)*

57. **(B)** Severe chest pain is characteristic of diffuse esophageal spasm and related esophageal motor disorders. The symptoms can mimic that of cardiac chest pain and can be difficult to distinguish one from the other, since both conditions

can respond to nitrates. Cardiac conditions should be ruled out before noncardiac conditions are considered. *(Fauci, Chapter 286)*

58. **(E)** Rotor syndrome is one of the two rare inherited disorders causing elevations in direct bilirubin. The other is Dubin–Johnson syndrome, and both have an excellent prognosis. Hemolytic anemia causes elevation in indirect bilirubin, and hematologic changes would be expected. INH causes elevation in liver enzymes, and although Rifampin can cause isolated hyperbilirubinemia, it is of the indirect kind. Crigler Najjar type I is a severe disorder of neonates with elevated indirect bilirubin. *(Fauci, Chapter 43)*

59. **(B)** In alcoholic hepatitis, the AST:ALT ratio is usually 2:1, and the level of AST is usually <300. When viral hepatitis or toxin-induced hepatitis causes jaundice, the AST:ALT ratio is usually 1:1, and the transaminases are usually >500. *(Fauci, Chapter 301)*

60. **(D)** Acetaminophen reliably produces hepatocellular damage when taken in large doses. Daily doses should not exceed 4 g a day, and accidental or intentional overdoses of 10–15 g will result in liver injury. Fatal fulminant disease is usually seen with ingestions over 25 g. *(Fauci, Chapter 299)*

61. **(B)** An active metabolite of acetaminophen is hepatotoxic. It is detoxified by binding to glutathione, and when hepatic glutathione stores are depleted, severe liver damage can occur. *(Fauci, Chapter 299)*

62. **(A)** Sinusoidal dilatation and peliosis can occur with anabolic steroid use but it is not a common occurrence. There have been deaths linked to peliosis. Anabolic steroids usually cause cholestasis and jaundice without inflammation. The other medications also cause various types of liver disease, but not peliosis. *(Fauci, Chapter 299)*

63. **(D)** *N*-acetylcysteine probably acts by providing a reservoir of sulfhydryl groups to bind the toxic metabolite of acetaminophen. Narcan is effective for narcotic overdose, and ethanol is the antidote for methanol intoxication. *(Fauci, Chapter 299)*

64. **(D)** Secretory diarrhea is caused by a derangement in fluid and electrolyte transport across the gut mucosa. The resultant diarrhea is watery, large volume, painless, and persists even when the patient fasts. If the symptoms were due to bowel obstruction she would be experiencing abdominal discomfort and likely reduced symptoms with fasting. Osmotic diarrhea improves with fasting, which is not the case with this patient. *(Fauci, Chapter 40)*

65. **(A)** His night blindness suggests vitamin A deficiency, which is more likely to occur with malabsorption. His anemia and general appearance are compatible with chronic inflammatory bowel disease as well, but the clinical and biochemical features of fat soluble vitamin deficiency (in this case vitamin A, D, and K) suggest malabsorption. *(Fauci, Chapter 288)*

66. **(E)** A small bowel mucosal biopsy will assist in determining the cause of malabsorption such as celiac disease. The osmotic gap is a characteristic of osmotic diarrhea in particular and useful in the diagnosis of malabsorption. Stool fat, D-xylose testing, and Schilling tests help establish the diagnosis of malabsorption, but not the etiology. The most common cause of such diffuse malabsorption, celiac disease, has a characteristic biopsy pattern with short or absent villi. Confirmation of the disease requires response to a gluten-free diet. *(Fauci, Chapter 288)*

67. **(C)** Acute erosive gastritis is most commonly seen in critically ill hospitalized patients. Ischemia of the gastric mucosa with breakdown of the normal protective barriers of the stomach is a key factor in the syndrome. Gastritis is classified based on the time course of the (acute or chronic), histologic features, and anatomical distribution. *(Fauci, Chapter 287)*

68. **(D)** Type B chronic gastritis is a more common cause of chronic gastritis. Chronic gastritis is classified based on anatomic site of involvement, Type B is an antral predominant form (*H pylori* related) and Type A refers to body

predominant form (autoimmune). It becomes more common with advancing age and is uniformly associated with *H pylori* infection. Eradication of *H pylori* produces histologic improvement, but is not routinely recommended unless peptic ulcer or mucosa-associated lymphoid tissue (MALT) lymphoma occurs. *(Fauci, Chapter 287)*

69. **(B)** Type A chronic gastritis may lead to pernicious anemia. Antibodies to parietal cells and to intrinsic factor are frequently seen in the sera, suggesting an immune or autoimmune pathogenesis. These patients can also have autoimmune thyroid disease and vitiligo. *(Fauci, Chapter 287)*

70. **(E)** Ménétrier disease is not a true gastritis, as inflammation is not present on histologic examination. It is characterized by large, tortuous gastric mucosal folds, and usually presents with abdominal pain. Protein-losing enteropathy often develops, resulting in hypoalbuminemia and edema. *(Fauci, Chapter 287)*

71. **(A)** Gastric surgery seems to accelerate the development of asymptomatic gastritis with progressive parietal cell loss. However, some patients develop bile reflux gastritis with symptoms of pain, nausea, and vomiting. *(Fauci, Chapter 287)*

Hematology
Questions

DIRECTIONS (Questions 1 through 6): For each of the questions in this section select the one lettered answer that is the best response in each case.

1. A 65-year-old man presents to the clinic for assessment of numerous symptoms which are worse in the winter months. He notices diffuse red patches which are not raised or painful and occasionally purple fingertips. Other symptoms include joint discomfort (arthralgia) and muscle weakness.

   On physical examination, the vital signs are normal, the heart sounds are normal, and the lungs clear. The joints are normal with no active inflammation, and the muscle strength is 4+/5. On his thighs and knees there are fine "lace"-like appearing skin changes that are consistent with livedo reticularis. Laboratory investigations reveal hemoglobin of 125g/L, a 2-fold elevation in ALT and AST, a positive hepatitis C virus antibody titer, and early renal impairment. **Which of the following is the most likely diagnosis?**

   (A) cold agglutinin disease
   (B) Henoch–Schönlein purpura
   (C) antiphospholipid antibody syndrome
   (D) cryoglobulinemia
   (E) cholesterol embolic disease

2. A 34-year-old man presents to the emergency department with symptoms of fatigue, weakness, nose bleeds, and palpitations with exertion. The symptoms started 1 week ago and are getting worse every day. He has no prior health issues and is not taking any medications.

On examination, he is pale, blood pressure 110/70 mm Hg, pulse 100/min, heart sounds are normal, lungs are clear, and he has multiple petechiae and bruises on his legs.

   His blood count is abnormal; hemoglobin 8.5 g/dL, white blood cells (WBCs) 4000/mL, platelets 50,000/mL, and there are blast cells in the peripheral blood. He is diagnosed with acute promyelocytic leukemia (AML-M3). (See Figure 5–1.) **Which of the following is a characteristic of this acute myelogenous leukemia?**

Figure 5–1. (Reproduced, with permission, from Lichtman MA, et al. *Williams Hematology*, 7th ed. New York: McGraw-Hill, 2006:Plate XVII-2.)

   (A) peak incidence in childhood
   (B) high leukocyte alkaline phosphatase
   (C) Philadelphia chromosome
   (D) Auer bodies in blast cells
   (E) response to vincristine and prednisone

3. A 62-year-old man reports early satiety, fatigue, and generally feeling unwell. The symptoms started gradually and are getting worse. He notes no chest discomfort, respiratory symptoms, or abdominal pain.

On physical examination, he appears pale, the vital signs are normal, and the pertinent findings are a large spleen, absence of lymph nodes, and normal heart and lungs.

His blood count is abnormal; the WBC is 50,000/mL with increased mature granulocytes, hemoglobin is 9.5 g/dL, and platelets are 450,000/mL. **Which of the following cytogenetic changes is most characteristic of his condition?**

(A) deletion of chromosome 14
(B) reciprocal translocation of 9 and 22 (Philadelphia chromosome)
(C) translocation of the renal artery stenosis (RAS) oncogene
(D) trisomy 21
(E) translocation of 8–14

4. An 18-year-old man is seen in the clinic for routine assessment. He reports no active symptoms, there is no past medical history and he is not taking any medications. He mentions that his brother has a "low blood count" that is hereditary but does not recall the name of the disorder.

His physical examination is entirely normal. A complete blood count reveals a hemoglobin of 10.5 g/dL and microcytic red cells on the blood film. A hemoglobin electrophoresis confirms the diagnosis of beta-thalassemia minor. **Which of the following findings is characteristic of this condition?**

(A) an increased amount of fetal hemoglobin (HbF) or hemoglobin A2 (HbA2)
(B) increased osmotic fragility of the red cells
(C) absent bone marrow iron
(D) increased macroglobulins in the serum
(E) small amounts of HbS

5. A 57-year-old man is seen in the clinic for symptoms of fatigue and shortness of breath on exertion. The physical examination is normal but a complete blood count reveals pancytopenia.

He is referred to a hematologist and a bone marrow aspirate and biopsy confirm the diagnosis of aplastic anemia. The best treatment option for him is an allogenic bone-marrow transplant and his sister is a human lymphocyte antigen (HLA)-matched donor. **Which of the following is the most likely complication of allogenic bone marrow transplantation?**

(A) graft-versus-host disease (GVHD)
(B) graft failure
(C) radiation sickness
(D) development of leukemia
(E) secondary skin cancer

6. A 19-year-old man is having recurrent bleeding occur in his knee when playing contact sports. He has no history of spontaneous bleeding, but his brother has similar problems. Consultation with a specialist reveals that he has "mild" hemophilia A. **Which of the following factor abnormalities is consistent with this diagnosis?**

(A) abnormal factor VIII function
(B) decreased levels of functional factor VIII
(C) decreased factor IX level
(D) decreased von Willebrand factor
(E) decreased factor IX level

DIRECTIONS (Questions 7 through 13): The following group of numbered items is preceded by a list of lettered options. For each question, select the one lettered option that is most closely associated with it. Each lettered option may be used once, multiple times, or not at all.

Questions 7 and 8: For each patient with a hematologic abnormality, select the most likely diagnosis.

(A) hyperthyroidism
(B) rectal cancer
(C) infectious mononucleosis
(D) acute myelogenous leukemia
(E) renal cell carcinoma
(F) acute lymphocytic leukemia

7. A 63-year-old man presents with headaches, itching, and feeling unwell. He appears plethoric, and the remaining examination is normal. On

laboratory investigations, he is found to have elevated hemoglobin of 18.5 g/dL, normal WBC, and normal platelet count. There is no palpable spleen or lymph nodes.

8. A 19-year-old college student develops a severe sore throat, cervical lymphadenopathy, and atypical lymphocytes on blood film. A heterophil antibody test is positive.

Questions 9 and 10: For each patient with anemia, select the corresponding clinical and laboratory findings.

(A) osteoblastic bone lesions
(B) increased spleen size
(C) her fertility is impaired
(D) increased osmotic fragility
(E) type III cryoglobulin
(F) increased plasma cells in bone marrow

9. A 19-year-old woman is found to be anemic with hemoglobin of 10.0 g/dL. She has target cells on the blood film, and is homozygous for HbC. She has no other clinical symptoms.

10. A 74-year-old woman is anemic with hemoglobin of 10.5 g/dL. She has symptoms of tingling in her feet and back discomfort. X-rays of her spine reveal osteopenia and multiple lytic lesions. She has an immunoglobulin G (IgG) spike on serum protein electrophoresis.

Questions 11 through 13: For each patient with a blood-count anomaly, select the corresponding clinical situation and/or laboratory finding.

(A) postsplenectomy
(B) increased numbers of reticulocytes
(C) thiamine deficiency
(D) acute hemorrhage
(E) low fecal urobilinogen
(F) immediate postoperative period
(G) acute lymphocytic leukemia
(H) iron deficiency

11. A 49-year-old woman feels unwell because of fatigue and shortness of breath on exertion. Her hemoglobin is 9.0 g/dL, the direct antiglobulin

test (Coombs) is positive, and she is suspected of having a hemolytic anemia.

12. A 69-year-old man presents with increasing symptoms of chest pain on exertion, but never at rest. He has a history of chronic stable coronary artery disease. Repeat evaluation now reveals a hypochromic microcytic anemia as the cause for his increased chest pain symptoms.

13. A 72-year-old woman is admitted to the hospital with an acute illness. Her platelet count is incidentally noted to be 800,000/mL.

DIRECTIONS (Questions 14 through 30): For each of the questions in this section select the one lettered answer that is the best response in each case.

14. A 7-year-old boy has severe microcytic anemia due to beta-thalassemia major (homozygous). He requires frequent blood transfusions (once every 6 weeks) to prevent the skeletal and developmental complications of thalassemia. **Which of the following medications is also indicated in the treatment of patients requiring frequent blood transfusions?**

(A) oral calcium supplements
(B) fresh frozen plasma (FFP)
(C) desferrioxamine
(D) penicillamine
(E) cryoprecipitate

15. A 45-year-old woman develops symptoms of shortness of breath on exertion, easy fatigue, and jaundice. On examination she is pale, and there is a palpable spleen, but no lymphadenopathy. Her hemoglobin is 9.0 g/dL, the reticulocyte count 9%, and the direct antibody test (Coombs) is positive. **Which of the following bone marrow findings is most likely to be seen in this patient?**

(A) megaloblastic changes
(B) giant metamyelocytes
(C) increased erythroid-to-myeloid ratio
(D) increased lymphocytes
(E) shift to left of the myeloid series

16. A 23-year-old woman of Italian extraction is found to have a hypochromic microcytic anemia of 10 g/dL. In addition, there is a fair degree of anisocytosis, poikilocytosis, and targeting on the blood film. The WBC is 9500/mL, the platelet count is 240,000/mL, and the reticulocyte count is 7%. The spleen is palpated 5 cm below the left costal margin. **Which of the following is the most appropriate treatment for her condition?**

    (A) splenectomy
    (B) removal of the abnormal Hb pigment
    (C) purely supportive
    (D) plasmapheresis
    (E) intramuscular iron

17. A 67-year-old man is complaining of fatigue. A routine complete blood count (CBC) reveals a platelet count of 850,000/mL, and the hemoglobin and WBC counts are normal. He reports no other symptoms, and his clinical examination is normal. **Which of the following characteristics is most likely to be helpful in differentiating essential (primary) from reactive (secondary) thrombocytosis?**

    (A) increased megakaryocyte number
    (B) increased total platelet mass
    (C) increased platelet turnover
    (D) normal platelet survival
    (E) thromboembolism and hemorrhage

18. A 19-year-old man is found to have a decreased eosinophil count. **Which of the following is the most likely cause?**

    (A) asthma
    (B) contact dermatitis
    (C) yeast infection
    (D) mycobacterial infection
    (E) prednisone administration

19. A 68-year-old man with aplastic anemia is due for another blood transfusion. He has had multiple blood transfusions in the past, but with the last transfusion, he developed fever and chills after the transfusion was started. Repeat cross-matching and testing at the time ruled out an acute hemolytic transfusion reaction. The next transfusion is ordered through a "filter" to prevent or minimize the febrile reaction. **Which of the following mechanisms is most likely to explain the effect of the filter?**

    (A) reducing bacterial transmission
    (B) reducing viral transmission
    (C) reducing parasite transmission
    (D) reducing leukocyte transfusion
    (E) reducing reticulocyte transfusion

20. A 19-year-old man is found to have low hemoglobin on routine screening. He feels well at the present time, but in the past he has had two presentations to the hospital for severe abdominal and back pain that resolved on its own with no specific diagnosis. His blood film is shown in Figure 5–2; the hemoglobin is 10 mg/dL, mean corpuscular volume (MCV) 80 fL, and reticulocyte count 0.04 (4%). **Which of the following is the most likely explanation for his previous episodes of abdominal pain?**

Figure 5–2. (Reproduced, with permission, from Kasper DL, et al. *Harrison's Principles of Internal Medicine*, 16th ed. New York: McGraw-Hill, 2005:596)

    (A) aplastic crisis
    (B) sequestration crisis
    (C) vaso-occlusive crisis
    (D) hemolytic crisis
    (E) adrenal crisis

21. A 23-year-old woman has symptoms of fatigue and not feeling well. She appears well and the physical examination is normal, but her hemoglobin is low at 9.8 g/dL with a mean corpuscular volume (MVC) of 76 fL. Her family history is positive for thalassemia. She also mentions a history of heavy menses in the past year. **Which of the following would be most helpful in distinguishing thalassemia from one of pure iron deficiency anemia?**

(A) peripheral blood smear
(B) osmotic fragility test
(C) Ham test
(D) Hb electrophoresis
(E) serum ferritin level

22. A 21-year-old woman is suspected of having mycoplasma pneumonia based on symptoms of a dry cough, fever, normal lung examination but abnormal chest x-ray with bilateral infiltrates. She is also anemic with hemoglobin of 10.5 g/dL, reticulocyte count 7%, and WBC 12,000/mL. Hemolytic anemia from cold agglutinins is suspected as the cause. **Which of the following tests will confirm an autoimmune cause of the anemia?**

(A) positive antinuclear antibody (ANA)
(B) positive rheumatoid factor
(C) polyclonal gammopathy
(D) presence of Heinz bodies
(E) positive Coombs test

23. A 59-year-old man presents to the emergency room with left face and arm weakness that lasts for 3 hours. He reports no other symptoms of palpitations, chest pain, or headache. Neurologic examination is now normal. A computerized tomography (CT) scan of the head, electrocardiogram (ECG), and laboratory workup are normal. He is started on clopidogrel, and referred for further evaluation as an outpatient. **Which of the following is the most likely mechanism of action on platelet function from this medication?**

(A) cyclooxygenase-1 inhibition
(B) modulation of cyclic adenosine monophosphate (cAMP) levels

(C) adenosine diphosphate (ADP) receptor blockade
(D) GPIIB-IIIA blocker
(E) cyclooxygenase-2 inhibition

24. A 23-year-old woman has symptoms of leg swelling and discomfort, but no chest pain or shortness of breath. She has no risk factors for a blood clot. On examination, the left leg is swollen when compared to the right. Leg Doppler ultrasound is positive for deep vein thrombosis in the left leg. Further investigations reveal decreased plasma antithrombin III (AT-III) levels. **Which of the following is the most likely clinical effect from the low AT-III levels?**

(A) aspirin sensitivity
(B) heparin resistance
(C) warfarin (Coumadin) resistance
(D) platelet dysfunction
(E) disseminated intravascular coagulation

25. A 4-month-old infant is anemic with a hemoglobin level of 9.5 g/dL and MCV 77 fL. The baby looks well, the height and weight growth parameters are normal, and she is breast-feeding well. **Which of the following is the most likely cause for her anemia?**

(A) inadequate dietary iron
(B) hemolysis
(C) late clamping of cord
(D) iron malabsorption
(E) folate deficiency

26. **Which of the following is the most likely effect of increased levels of red blood cell 2,3 diphosphoglycerate (2,3-DPG)?**

(A) hemolytic anemia due to sulfa drugs
(B) increased oxygen affinity
(C) decreased oxygen affinity
(D) loss of red cell energy
(E) multiple congenital abnormalities

27. A 63-year-old man is involved in a motor vehicle accident and is brought to the hospital. On examination, his blood pressure is 90/60 mm Hg, pulse 110/min, and his abdomen is distended and rigid. He has internal injuries and bleeding on an abdominal CT scan, and requires emergent blood transfusion on his way to the operating room. His blood group is AB. **Which of the following statements is not correct?**

   (A) he is a universal recipient
   (B) he has anti-A and anti-B in his serum
   (C) if a cross-match is not available; group O RBCs are universal
   (D) if insufficient AB blood is available, type A can be used
   (E) if insufficient AB blood is available, type B can be used

28. A 60-year-old man notices right-sided chest pain after sneezing. The pain is made worse with breathing, but he reports no fever, cough, or sputum production. Recently, he has been experiencing back discomfort and easy fatigue on exertion. On examination, the heart sounds are normal and lungs are clear. The left 6th rib is tender on palpation. X-rays of his chest are shown in Figure 5–3. **Which of the following is the most likely diagnosis?**

   (A) aneurysmal bone cyst
   (B) multiple myeloma
   (C) lymphosarcoma
   (D) prostatic metastases
   (E) hyperparathyroidism

29. A 36-year-old woman with sickle cell disease presents with increasing pain in her right hip. She has no fever, chills, back or other bone pain, and there is no history of any trauma.

   On examination, her temperature is 37.3°C, range of motion in the right hip is reduced, she walks with a limp, and the right leg is shorter than the left. Movements of the hip and walking on it are painful. X-rays of the hip are shown in Figure 5–4. **Which of the following is the most likely diagnosis?**

Figure 5–3.

Figure 5–4.

(A) avascular necrosis (AVN) of the femoral head

(B) osteomyelitis

(C) hip fracture

(D) septic arthritis

(E) multiple myeloma

30. A 30-year-old woman presents with increasing fatigue, but no other symptoms. Her past medical history is negative and she is not on any medications. About 3 weeks ago she had a "flu"-like illness that has now resolved.

On examination, the conjunctivae are pale, her sclera are icteric, the blood pressure 110/70 mm Hg, pulse 110/min, lungs clear, and heart sounds normal. Castell sign is negative and no spleen is palpable. Her hemoglobin is 9 g/dL, and the rest of the laboratory workup is shown in Table 5–1. **Which of the following is the most likely diagnosis?**

TABLE 5–1. CASE WORKUP

Blood film	Polychromatophilia, some spherocytes
Bilirubin	2 mg/100 mL total
	0.3 mg/100 mL direct
Haptoglobin	10 mg/100 mL
Lactate dehydrogenase	200 IU/L
Urine bilirubin	Negative

(A) iron deficiency

(B) congenital spherocytosis

(C) liver failure

(D) splenomegaly and hemolysis

(E) autoimmune hemolytic anemia

DIRECTIONS (Questions 32 through 41): The following group of numbered items is preceded by a list of lettered options. For each question, select the one lettered option that is most closely associated with it. Each lettered option may be used once, multiple times, or not at all.

Questions 31 and 32: For each mechanism of a prolonged bleeding time, select the most likely cause.

(A) aspirin

(B) naproxen

(C) tirofiban

(D) trimethoprim-sulfamethoxazole

(E) clopidogrel

(F) fish oils

(G) systemic lupus

(H) uremia

31. Inhibits platelet activation induced by ADP

32. Depletes platelet arachidonic acid

Questions 33 through 37: For each patient with a hemoglobin abnormality, select the most likely diagnosis.

(A) beta-thalassemia major

(B) HbH disease

(C) sickle cell disease

(D) HbC disease

(E) HbM disease

33. A 23-year-old man has recurrent episodes of mild back and chest pain, whenever he is ill. His physical examination is normal. The hemoglobin level is 9 g/dL, MCV 85 fL, and platelets 250,000/mL. His blood film shows characteristic red cell morphologic changes that have hemoglobin units polymerizing in long chains under hypoxic stress as the underlying mechanism.

34. A 32-year-old man has a mild anemia diagnosed on routine testing. He has no symptoms and feels fine. His clinical examination is normal, and a blood film reveals some target cells with some red cells having intraerythrocytic crystals.

35. A 4-month-old baby has developed feeding problems and diarrhea. Laboratory evaluation reveals severe anemia with hemoglobin of 7.5 g/dL. The blood film shows hypochromic microcytic cells and target cells. In this disorder, decreased beta-chain production leads to excess alpha-chain production and destruction of red cell precursors.

36. A 4-year-old boy has a chronic microcytic anemia, but no other symptoms. His physical examination is normal except for splenomegaly. His condition is due to decreased alpha-chain production, which leads to four beta-chain tetramer formation (HbH).

37. A 27-year-old woman complains of constant back pain. She recently had an episode of severe chest and back pain that required narcotic medications, blood transfusions, and lots of fluids to treat. On examination, she is afebrile, with midthoracic tenderness on palpation. X-rays of the spine reveal periosteal reaction of the eighth thoracic vertebra. She has a chronic blood disorder where bone infarction can occur that may be difficult to distinguish from osteomyelitis.

Questions 38 through 40: For each patient with a hematologic disorder, select the most likely complications or associated conditions.

(A) increased perioperative morbidity
(B) helmet cells and schistocytes are common
(C) occurs most commonly in the first trimester
(D) renal papillary necrosis
(E) cardiac arrhythmias
(F) increased HbH
(G) responds to folic acid
(H) paresthesias

38. A 63-year-old woman with lymphoma has been treated with vincristine for many months. She has now developed dose-limiting side effects from this drug.

39. A 19-year-old woman is positive for sickle cell disease.

40. A 24-year-old pregnant woman is found to be anemic.

DIRECTIONS (Questions 41 through 58): For each of the questions in this section select the one lettered answer that is the best response in each case.

41. A 32-year-old woman is confirmed as being 6 weeks pregnant. She feels well, and has no past medical history. This is her second pregnancy; the first pregnancy was uncomplicated and she delivered at term, but the baby was anemic due to beta-thalassemia. She is now worried that the current pregnancy may also be affected. **Which of the following methods is most likely to establish an accurate prenatal diagnosis?**

(A) fetal ultrasound at 12 weeks
(B) cord blood electrophoresis
(C) chorionic villus sampling
(D) buccal mucosal cytology of both parents
(E) electrophoresis of amniotic fluid

42. A 27-year-old female presents with easy fatigue and light-headedness. She also has a dry cough and fever for the past few days. On examination, she is pale, her lungs are clear, and the rest is normal. A chest x-ray (CXR) shows patchy bilateral infiltrates; the hemoglobin is 8.4 g/dL, reticulocyte count of 6%, and many spherocytes on the peripheral blood film. **Which of the following is the most likely significance of the spherocytosis on the blood film?**

(A) multiple long bone fracture
(B) hereditary elliptocytosis
(C) Coombs-positive hemolytic anemia
(D) glucose-6-phosphate dehydrogenase (G6PD) deficiency
(E) leukemia

43. A 25-year-old woman is pregnant for the first time. At prenatal assessment, she is found to have blood group A and Rh(D)-negative. Her husband is tested and he is Rh(D)-positive. **Which of the following is the most appropriate initial test to determine her risk for hemolytic disease of the newborn (erythroblastosis fetalis) due to Rh incompatibility?**

(A) anti-Rh(D) antibody in maternal serum
(B) direct Coombs test of maternal serum
(C) anti-Rh
(D) antibody in baby's serum
(E) ABO testing of the husband
(F) direct Coombs test of neonate serum after birth

44. A 63-year-old man presents with fatigue, shortness of breath on exertion, and easy bruising. He has no prior history of bleeding disorders, and is not taking any medications. On examination, his conjunctivae are pale, he has a palpable spleen, and there are multiple bruises and petechiae on his legs.

   A CBC reveals a hemoglobin of 8.3 g/dL, WBC of 2300/mL, and platelets of 30,000/mL. A blood film also shows multiple lymphocytes with prominent cytoplasmic projections. A bone marrow biopsy also shows similar cells in the marrow and marrow fibrosis. (See Figure 5–5.) **Which of the following is the most likely diagnosis?**

Figure 5–5. (Reproduced, with permission, from Lichtman MA, et al. *Williams Hematology*, 7th ed. New York: McGraw-Hill, 2006: Plate XXI-7)

   (A) lymphoma
   (B) myeloma
   (C) myelofibrosis and myeloid metaplasia
   (D) hairy cell leukemia
   (E) chronic myelogenous leukemia

45. A 22-year-old long-distance runner is found to be mildly anemic. His diet is adequate in caloric and vitamin intake, and there is no family history of hereditary anemias. His past medical history is negative and he is not taking any medications except for a daily multivitamin. He is asymptomatic; his stool is negative for occult blood, and the ferritin level is 200 ng/mL.

Which intervention is most likely to result in return of the hemoglobin to normal?

   (A) using more supportive footwear
   (B) iron replacement
   (C) folate replacement
   (D) decreasing his exercise program
   (E) investigating and treating gastrointestinal (GI) pathology

46. A 34-year-old woman notices blue toes and a lacy rash on her knees when outside in the winter months. She has chronic hepatitis C virus infection. She has also noticed weakness, joint discomfort, and red spots on her legs.

   On examination, she has livedo reticularis-type skin on her thighs, and areas of palpable purpura on her toes. She has abnormal proteins detected in her serum. **Which of the following is the most likely mechanism for the vessel injury seen in this condition?**

   (A) breakdown of erythrocytes
   (B) medium vessel vasculitis
   (C) aggregation of abnormal platelets
   (D) temperature-dependent antibodies
   (E) cold precipitable proteins

47. A 49-year-old man presents with jaundice, nausea, and vomiting. He has a history of chronic alcoholism, and is currently drinking over 1 bottle of red wine a day. On physical examination, he is jaundiced and pale with a large tender liver.

   Laboratory data include hemoglobin of 9 g/dL, WBC of 4200/mL, and platelet count of 80,000/mL. His liver enzymes and bilirubin are also elevated. Ultrasound of the abdomen reveals liver enlargement with no bile duct obstruction, a normal size spleen, and no ascites. **Which of the following cells are affected by the toxicity of chronic alcoholism on the bone marrow?**

   (A) developing erythrocytes and myelocytes
   (B) mature polymorphonuclear leukocytes
   (C) mature red cells
   (D) mature platelets
   (E) eosinophils

48. A 22-year-old medical student donates his blood as part of a clinical study. He is discovered to have persistent HbF (fetal hemoglobin) levels. He feels well, and his clinical examination is normal. **Which of the following features about this condition is most likely true?**

(A) cause of sickling red cells

(B) disease of infants only

(C) variant of thalassemia major

(D) anemia exacerbated by fava beans

(E) benign genetic abnormality

49. A 19-year-old man had his spleen removed 1 year ago after a motorcycle accident. He returns for routine follow-up and has fully recovered after his accident. A routine complete blood count is performed. (See Figure 5–6.) **Which of the following findings on the blood film are most consistent with a previous history of splenectomy?**

Figure 5–6.

(A) increase in macrophages

(B) leukopenia

(C) polycythemia

(D) increased reticulocytes

(E) red cells with nuclear fragments

50. A 49-year-old man is involved in a motor vehicle accident, resulting in large amounts of blood loss and hypotension. He is initially given normal saline at the accident site, and on arrival at the hospital, the trauma team orders an emergent blood transfusion with type O "universal donor" packed red cells. **Which of the following is a possible complication of unmatched type O blood?**

(A) type O donors have a higher incidence of hepatitis C virus

(B) type O donors have a shorter survival time when transfused than do other cell types

(C) at times type B blood may be mistyped as type O

(D) type O donors may have high titers of anti-A and anti-B in their plasma

(E) conversion of the recipient to type O blood

51. A 9-year-old boy presents with fever, feeling unwell, and easy bruising on his legs. On examination, he is pale, blood pressure 100/60 mm Hg, pulse 100/min, and temperature 37.8°C. His lungs are clear, abdomen is soft with a palpable spleen, and there are petechiae and bruises on his legs. His CBC reveals a hemoglobin of 8.5 g/dL, WBC of 17,000/mL, and platelets of 30,000/mL. A blood film reveals neutropenia and leukemic lymphoblasts. **Which of the following is the most appropriate initial diagnostic test to confirm the diagnosis?**

(A) monospot test

(B) bone-marrow aspirate and biopsy

(C) CT scan abdomen

(D) chest x-ray

(E) lumbar puncture and cerebrospinal fluid (CSF) fluid for cytology

52. A 50-year-old White woman presents with a 3-week history of tiredness and pallor. A family member has noted some yellowness of her eyes, but she denies darkening of the urine. Physical examination reveals only slight jaundice. Laboratory data include hemoglobin of 9 g/dL, reticulocyte count of 8%, a bilirubin in the serum of 2 mg/dL (indirect reacting), and some microspherocytes on peripheral smear. The direct antiglobulin test (Coombs) is positive. **Which of the following is the most likely cause for her anemia?**

(A) blood loss externally

(B) decreased red cell production

(C) ineffective erythropoiesis

(D) intravascular hemolysis

(E) extravascular hemolysis

53. A 57-year-old man, with a history of chronic alcohol ingestion, is admitted to the hospital with acute alcoholic intoxication and lobar pneumonia. Physical examination reveals pallor; a large tender liver; and consolidation of the right lower lobe. Laboratory data include hemoglobin of 7 g/dL, WBC of 4000/mL, and platelet count of 85,000/mL. **Which of the following is the most likely factor for the pancytopenia?**

(A) hemolysis

(B) hemobilia

(C) vitamin B$_{12}$ deficiency

(D) toxic marrow suppression

(E) hemoglobinopathy

54. An 82-year-old woman is brought to the hospital because of functional decline at home and an inability to care for herself. She has a prior history of hypertension and dyslipidemia, and her medications include hydrochlorothiazide and atorvastatin.

   She looks disheveled, pale, and has muscle wasting; her heart and lungs are clear and there are no focal neurologic findings. Her hemoglobin is 9 g/dL, MCV 105 fL, WBC 4500/mL, and platelets 100,000/mL. The blood film shows macrocytic RBCs and hyper-segmented neutrophils. **Which of the following vitamin deficiencies is most likely responsible for her pancytopenia?**

(A) B$_{12}$ (cyanocobalamin)

(B) folate

(C) pyridoxine

(D) thiamine

(E) riboflavin

55. A 39-year-old man with chronic alcoholism is brought to the hospital after a fall, while intoxicated. He has completely recovered except for a bruise on his shoulder. His only abnormality is a low hemoglobin of 9.6 g/dL, the platelets and WBC are normal. Additional tests including ferritin, vitamin B$_{12}$, and folate are all

normal. **Which of the following findings is most likely to be seen on his peripheral blood film?**

(A) macrocytosis

(B) basophilia

(C) red cell fragments

(D) increased platelet adhesiveness

(E) atypical lymphocytes

56. A 56-year-old woman presents with feeling light-headed when standing up and 3 days of passing dark black stools. She has a past history of chronic viral hepatitis B, and has developed cirrhosis.

   On examination, she is alert, blood pressure is 90/60 mm Hg supine and 76/60 mm Hg standing. Her abdomen is distended with signs of ascites, it is nontender, and there are multiple bruises on the legs. Her hemoglobin is 9.0 g/dL, platelets 90,000/mL, albumin 3 g/dL, bilirubin 1.3 mg/dL, and international normalized ratio (INR) 2.5 (prothrombin time [PT] 25 seconds). **Which of the following coagulation factors are most likely deficient in this patient?**

(A) V and VIII

(B) VIII, IX, XI, and XII

(C) XIII

(D) II, V, VII, IX, X, and XI

(E) II, VII, IX, and X

57. An 18-year-old man, of Italian extraction, is found to have a hypochromic microcytic anemia of 10 g/dL. In addition, there are a fair number of anisocytosis, poikilocytosis, and target cells seen on the blood film. The WBC is 9500/mL, the platelet count is 240,000/mL, and the reticulocyte count is 7%. The spleen is palpated 5 cm below the left costal margin. **Which of the following is the most likely diagnosis?**

(A) sickle cell trait

(B) thalassemia minor

(C) HbS-C disease

(D) sideroblastic anemia

(E) hereditary spherocytosis

58. A 28-year-old man, originally from West Africa, is found on routine examination to have splenomegaly. His hemoglobin is 9.5 g/dL, and blood film examination reveals target cells. **Which of the following is the most likely abnormal hemoglobin in this man?**

(A) HbM
(B) HbS
(C) Hb Zurich
(D) HbC
(E) Hb Barts

DIRECTIONS (Questions 59 through 72): The following group of numbered items is preceded by a list of lettered options. For each question, select the one lettered option that is most closely associated with it. Each lettered option may be used once, multiple times, or not at all.

Questions 59 through 63: For each patient with a hypochromic microcytic anemia, select the most likely diagnosis.

(A) iron deficiency anemia
(B) beta-thalassemia trait
(C) anemia of chronic disease
(D) sideroblastic anemia

59. A 42-year-old man is feeling chronically fatigued. His hemoglobin is 11.5 g/dL, and the blood film is hypochromic and microcytic. The serum iron is increased, total iron-binding capacity (TIBC) is normal, ferritin is increased, and HbA2 is decreased.

60. An 18-year-old woman is feeling chronically fatigued. Her hemoglobin is 11.5 g/dL, RBC count 5,900,000/mL, and the blood film is hypochromic and microcytic. The serum iron is normal, TIBC is normal, ferritin is normal, and HbA2 is elevated.

61. A 67-year-old man presents with fatigue due to a low hemoglobin value of 9.2 g/dL. The blood film shows hypochromic microcytic cells. His serum iron is decreased, TIBC is increased, ferritin is decreased, and HbA2 is normal.

62. A 43-year-old man, in hospital for 2 weeks with pancreatitis, is anemic with hemoglobin of 9.7 g/dL and MCV 79 fL. The blood film shows slightly microcytic hypochromic red cells, and the reticulocyte count is 0.5 %. The serum iron is decreased, TIBC is decreased, serum ferritin is increased, and HbA2 normal.

63. A 52-year-old man is complaining of fatigue. His physical examination is normal, but his hemoglobin is low at 8.9 mg/dL. The reticulocyte count is 0.5 %, serum iron and TIBC are normal, and ferritin is elevated. A bone marrow aspirate reveals erythroid precursors that have accumulated abnormal amounts of mitochondrial iron.

Questions 64 through 68: For each of the following conditions, select the most likely RBC morphology.

(A) spherocytes
(B) schistocytes
(C) sickle cells
(D) burr cells
(E) agglutinated cells
(F) Heinz bodies

64. Found in severe liver disease.

65. Represent precipitated Hb.

66. Caused by loss of red cell membrane.

67. Caused by polymerization of an abnormal Hb.

68. Caused by trauma to red cell membranes.

Questions 69 through 72: For each patient with a bleeding disorder, select the most likely diagnosis.

(A) von Willebrand disease
(B) hemophilia A
(C) hemophilia B
(D) thrombotic thrombocytopenic purpura (TTP)

69. A 23-year-old man presents with prolonged nose bleeds. He has always noted easy bruising, and ongoing bleeding after minor cuts.

There is no prior history of surgery or dental procedures. His hemoglobin is 14.5 g/dL, platelets 200,000/mL, and PT/PPT is normal. Further testing reveals that the bleeding time is elevated; the factor VIII level is reduced, as is the ristocetin cofactor assay.

70. An 18-year-old man develops excessive bleeding 2 hours after wisdom tooth extraction. He has a history of easy bruising after playing sports, and of minor cuts that rebleed. His examination is normal, except for the tooth extraction site, which is still oozing blood. His hemoglobin is 14.8 g/dL, platelets 230,000 mL, PT is normal, and partial thromboplastin time (PTT) is elevated. A bleeding time is normal, factor VIII level is reduced, factor IX is normal, and ristocetin cofactor assay is normal.

71. A 19-year-old man is brought to the hospital after injuring his knee playing football. The knee is swollen and painful to move. He has no prior history of bleeding disorders. Arthrocentesis of the knee reveals 20 cc of blood. Further investigations show that his platelets are 170,000/mL, PT is normal, PTT is elevated, bleeding time is normal, factor VIII is normal, factor IX is reduced, and the ristocetin cofactor assay is normal.

72. A 27-year-old woman presents with nose bleeds, rash on her feet, and fevers. She looks unwell, pale, jaundiced, and there are multiple petechiae on her feet. The lungs are clear, heart sounds normal, and abdomen is soft with no palpable spleen or liver. Her bilirubin is 2 mg/dL (mostly indirect), aspartate amino transferase (AST), alanine amino transferase (ALT), alkaline phosphatase (ALP) are normal. The hemoglobin is 8.7 g/dL, platelets 24,000/mL, PT/PTT normal, and bleeding time is elevated. The blood film reveals anemia, thrombocytopenia, and red cell fragments.

Answers and Explanations

1. **(D)** The symptoms are typical of cryoglobulinemia. Cryoglobulins are antibodies that precipitate under cold conditions and are associated with several diseases. There are three main types of cryoglobulin syndromes based on the immunoglobulin composition of the precipitating antibody. Most cryoglobulinemic vasculitis is Type II or mixed and seen secondary to hepatitis C virus infection. Cold agglutinin disease would present with hemolytic anemia. The other syndromes would not generally be temperature sensitive, and do not have an association with hepatitis C virus infection. *(Fauci, Chapter 319)*

2. **(D)** The image shows Auer bodies in the blast cell, they are slender, pink staining rods containing lysozyme, and are exclusively seen in AML. Although similar to normal azurophilic granules in content and staining properties, they are distinguished by their gigantic size. Special stains can enhance the detection of Auer bodies. They are only seen in a minority of cases. The Philadelphia chromosome is a feature of choric myelogenous leukemia (CML), and a high leukocyte alkaline phosphatase level is seen in patients with a high WBC due to a leukemoid reaction. *(Fauci, Chapter 104)*

3. **(B)** This is a case of chronic myelogenous leukemia (CML). The reciprocal translocation involves the long arms of 22 and 9, and results in translocation of the ABL proto-oncogene from chromosome 9 adjacent to a portion of the BCR gene on chromosome 22. The resultant abnormal chromosome 22 is known as the Philadelphia (Ph1) chromosome. *(Fauci, Chapter 104)*

4. **(A)** An increased amount of HbF or HbA2 is present in patients with beta-thalassemia. As the hemoglobin beta-chains are decreased in beta-thalassemia, the excess alpha-chains combine with gamma- and delta-chains to make HbF and HbA2, respectively. Increased osmotic fragility of red cells is a feature hereditary spherocytosis and not thalassemia. Most patients with thalassemia have normal quantities of bone marrow iron, and HbS is not a feature of thalassemia but of sickle cell disease. *(Fauci, Chapter 99)*

5. **(A)** Graft-versus-host disease (GVHD) is a frequent complication of hematopoietic cell transplantation. It is caused by a reaction of immunologically competent donor-derived T cells that react with recipient tissue antigens. It can be acute or chronic. Numerous treatment regimens involving methotrexate, glucocorticoids, cyclosporine, and other drugs are used in treatment. Radiation sickness is a side effect of the preconditioning required prior to transplantation. Graft failure, development of leukemia, and secondary skin cancers are less common complications than GVHD in bone-marrow transplantation. *(Fauci, Chapter 81)*

6. **(B)** In hemophilia A, there are decreased levels of functioning factor VIII. This can be due to reduced amounts of normal VIII, the presence of a functionally abnormal protein, or a combination of both. The activated partial thromboplastin time (APTT) is prolonged, and the prothrombin consumption test is abnormal. The prothrombin time, thrombin clotting time, and bleeding time are usually normal. *(Fauci, Chapter 110)*

7. **(E)** Renal cell carcinoma, cerebellar hemangiomas, hepatoma, and giant uterine myomas are the tumors associated with secondary polycythemia. Endocrine disorders, hypoxia, and high-affinity hemoglobins can also cause secondary polycythemia. (*Fauci, Chapter 59*)

8. **(C)** Heterophil antibodies react against sheep red cells and are not absorbed by the guinea pig kidney. They are positive in patients with infectious mononucleosis. In 90% of cases, liver enzymes are elevated. Examination of the blood film reveals a lymphocytosis with atypical lymphocytes. (*Fauci, Chapter 174*)

9. **(B)** Hemoglobin C is abnormal hemoglobin where lysine has been substituted for glutamic acid at the sixth position of the beta-chain. Homozygous C red cells are often target-shaped with "extra" membrane to make them less osmotically fragile. However, cells containing principally HbC are more rigid than normal and their fragmentation in the circulation may result in microspherocytes. Intracellular crystals and oxygenated HbC can be seen. The spleen is invariably enlarged. Women can become pregnant and tolerate the pregnancy well. (*Fauci, Chapter 99*)

10. **(F)** Bone lesions in myeloma are destructive, but the alkaline phosphatase is usually normal, indicating little blastic activity. Osteolysis, when combined with immobilization, can lead to hypercalcemia. It is usually mediated by an osteoclast-activating factor from neoplastic myeloma cells in the adjacent marrow. Bone pain can be severe. Bence Jones proteinuria might be present in myeloma patients, increased plasma cells in the marrow are typical. If cryoglobulinemia occurs, it is type I. (*Fauci, Chapter 106*)

11. **(B)** Hemolytic anemias are not associated with erythroid hypoplasia of the marrow. Erythroid hyperplasia is present except during infections or insults that lead to regenerative crises. As a result, there is usually an increased number of reticulocytes and elevated fecal and urinary urobilinogen. Decreased RBC survival is a hallmark of the disease. (*Fauci, Chapter 101*)

12. **(H)** Microcytic hypochromic anemias are caused by disorders of iron, globin, heme, or porphyrin metabolism and are not seen in thiamine deficiency. (*Fauci, Chapter 97*)

13. **(D)** Both acute blood loss and chronic iron deficiency can increase platelets. Hemolytic anemia is associated with both increased reticulocytes and thrombocytosis. Thromboembolic or hemorrhagic phenomena are more common in essential thrombocytosis rather than secondary causes. (*Fauci, Chapter 109*)

14. **(C)** Iron chelation with desferrioxamine will reduce the toxicity from iron overload if given regularly in high doses. The most lethal toxicity of iron overload is iron infiltration of the myocardium, with resultant dysfunction and death. Penicillamine has no role in the treatment of thalassemia patients requiring frequent transfusions. As well FFP, and cryoprecipitate are not indicated in the management of patients with thalassemia as there are no defects in thrombosis or coagulation. (*Fauci, Chapter 99*)

15. **(C)** Bone marrow examination is most likely to show increased erythroid-to-myeloid ratio. Erythroid hyperplasia is common to all hemolytic anemias, and megaloblastic features only develop if they become folate deficient. A left shift only occurs if the bone marrow is under stress, like during a severe infection, and giant metamyelocytes or increased lymphocytes are not features of an autoimmune hemolytic anemia. (*Fauci, Chapter 101*)

16. **(C)** The present treatment of choice for thalassemia minor is purely supportive. Care is taken to watch for anemia during intercurrent illness, due to a regenerative crisis. The therapies that are listed have no role in the management of patients with thalassemia minor. (*Fauci, Chapter 99*)

17. **(E)** Reactive thrombocytosis is usually transitory, without thromboembolism, hemorrhage, splenomegaly, or leukocytosis. Causes of secondary thrombocytosis include chronic inflammatory disorders (eg, rheumatoid arthritis), acute inflammatory disease, acute or chronic

blood loss, and malignancy. Recovery from thrombocytopenia ("rebound") can also result in very high platelets. A common cause is withdrawal from alcohol. (*Fauci, Chapter 109*)

18. **(E)** Steroids cause decreased numbers of eosinophils to circulate, so that eosinophilia may be seen in Addison disease, for example. Beta-blockers may cause eosinophilia by blocking beta-adrenergic eosinopenia. Atopic and nonatopic chronic asthma are frequently associated with mild eosinophilia. Numerous allergic diseases, allergic rhinitis, atopic dermatitis, and urticaria can also cause eosinophilia. Parasites are the most common worldwide cause of eosinophilia, but other infections rarely cause it. (*Fauci, Chapter 61*)

19. **(D)** Febrile reactions to donor leukocytes may be severe and cause hypotension, especially in repeatedly transfused patients. Antibodies to platelets can also develop. Usually, at least seven transfusions are required to induce sensitization. Occasionally, blood products can be contaminated with bacteria during the blood collection process and result in host infection but this is less likely than febrile reactions to donor leukocytes. Reducing viral and parasitic transmission associated with blood transfusions is an on-going activity and current blood procurement and screening processes make the risk of transfusion associated infections low. (*Fauci, Chapter 107*)

20. **(C)** The painful crisis seen in patients with sickle cell disease is due to vaso-occlusive disease where microvascular ischemic injury occurs to tissues. Acute illness, dehydration, and infections are common precipitants for this type of crisis. Because sickle cell anemia is a chronic hemolytic anemia, the reticulocyte is chronically elevated, except in aplastic crises, and erythrocyte life span is shortened. Infection is the most common precipitant of an aplastic crisis, particularly those caused by parvovirus B19. Sequestration crisis (hemoglobin level <6 mg/dL) is sudden massive pooling of red cells in the spleen resulting in hemodynamic instability. Hemolytic crisis is the sudden further reduction in red-cell life span marked by falling hemoglobin, jaundice, and increased reticulocyte count. (*Fauci, Chapter 99*)

21. **(E)** A serum ferritin determination would be most helpful; in iron deficiency anemia the ferritin level is very low (< 20 ng/ml). Iron stores in thalassemia are usually normal or increased and the ferritin level is normal or increased. The blood film, Ham test, and osmotic fragility test will not confirm the diagnosis of thalassemia or iron deficiency. While Hb electrophoresis can be useful in the diagnosis of some thalassemias it will not determine if the patient is iron deficient. (*Fauci, Chapter 98*)

22. **(E)** The Coombs test is an excellent screen for autoimmune hemolytic anemia. The diagnosis of autoimmune hemolytic anemia requires demonstration of immunoglobulin and/or complement on the patient's RBC. The other tests are not helpful in making the diagnosis of autoimmune hemolytic anemia. (*Fauci, Chapter 101*)

23. **(C)** Clopidogrel selectively inhibits platelet activation induced by ADP. It works as an ADP-receptor blocker. Other antiplatelet drugs such as ASA are COX-1 inhibitors, and dipyridamole modulates cAMP levels. (*Fauci, Chapter 112*)

24. **(B)** Heparin appears to act as catalyst in the inactivation of thrombin and factors XA, IXA, XIA, and it requires antithrombin III to accomplish this. However, not all patients with thrombosis and heparin resistance have antithrombin III deficiency. (*Fauci, Chapter 111*)

25. **(A)** Iron deficiency is the most common cause of anemia in infancy. Sixty percent of body iron concentration at birth is contained in circulating Hb. Milk is a poor source of iron, so the most common cause of iron deficiency in infancy is prolonged breast or bottle feeding. Cereals are high in iron content. Hemolysis and folate deficiency as the cause of this baby's anemia would result in a normocytic or macrocytic anemia, and it is unlikely malabsorption is the cause since the baby is gaining weight and doing well clinically. (*Fauci, Chapter 98*)

26. **(C)** The 2,3-bisphosphoglycerate (2,3-BPG) binds to the central cavity of the heme molecule and changes the configuration in favor of oxygen release. The other common factors that affect oxygen affinity are temperature and pH. The oxygen affinity of Hb is easily characterized by P50; the oxygen tension at which Hb is half-saturated. *(Fauci, Chapter 99)*

27. **(B)** Group AB has neither anti-A nor anti-B antibodies, as both A and B antigens are on the red cells. Persons with type AB blood are considered "universal recipients." It is a rare blood group (only 2%–3% of population); if large amounts of blood are required in an AB individual, any type of blood (A, AB, B, O) can be used as long as the plasma is removed from the donor blood (in other words packed RBCs are used). *(Fauci, Chapter 107)*

28. **(B)** There is lytic destruction of the sixth rib with a pathologic fracture and an extrapleural mass. The most common manifestation of multiple myeloma is multiple, "punched-out" lesions in the flat and tubular bones. Some may appear as discrete lytic lesions and remain as solitary lesions. Hyperparathyroidism can cause significant bone mineral loss and fragility fractures but there are no lytic lesions seen on the x-rays. Prostate cancer metastasis is osteosclerotic not osteolytic as seen in this patient. Lymphosarcoma is a possibility but it is a rare malignancy compared to myeloma. *(Fauci, Chapter 106)*

29. **(A)** The diagnosis is AVN of the femoral head. Bone complications occur frequently in patients with sickle cell anemia. Infarcted areas of bone and bone marrow can become sites of infection (osteomyelitis) with *Staphylococcus aureus* or salmonella, but the lack of fever and clinical signs in this patient suggest AVN. Infarction of the femoral head nutrient artery leads to AVN and chronic joint pain. The humeral head is also at risk of AVN. Septic arthritis is a less common complication. *(Fauci, Chapter 99)*

30. **(E)** Autoimmune hemolytic anemia is the most likely diagnosis, based on the elevated indirect bilirubin, spherocytes on the blood film, low hemoglobin and low haptoglobin level.

Spherocytosis is seen as well in burn victims, in microangiopathic hemolysis, and in congenital spherocytosis. In liver failure, the elevated bilirubin is usually direct, and in splenomegaly causing hemolysis the spleen should be enlarged on clinical exam. Finally, iron deficiency does not cause a hemolysis-type presentation. *(Fauci, Chapter 101)*

31. **(E)** Clopidogrel is an ADP-receptor blocker, and inhibits platelet activation induced by ADP. This results in a prolongation of bleeding time that is greater than that produced by acetylsalicylic acid (ASA). The effects last for 4–10 days after discontinuation. Clopidogrel is a prodrug that relies on an active metabolite for its effect, and is marginally more effective than ASA for certain conditions like stroke and acute coronary syndrome. The effect on bleeding time is additive to that of ASA. *(Fauci, Chapter 109)*

32. **(F)** Fish oils cause a slight prolongation of the bleeding time. The mechanism is twofold: they reduce platelet arachidonic acid, and as well they compete with arachidonic acid for cyclooxygenase. Other foods that may affect platelet function include garlic, onions, and black tree fungus (found in Chinese cuisine). *(Fauci, Chapter 59)*

33. **(C)** A number of factors influence the rate and degree of HbS aggregation, including concentration of HbS in the cell, cellular dehydration, and the length of time in deoxy conformation. *(Fauci, Chapter 99)*

34. **(D)** The patients with homozygous HbC disease have mild hemolysis, splenomegaly, target cells, and HbC crystals. Unlike sickle cell disease, the prognosis is favorable. *(Fauci, Chapter 99)*

35. **(A)** In beta-thalassemia, there is excess production of alpha-chains, which precipitate and destroy red cell precursors. *(Fauci, Chapter 99)*

36. **(B)** HbH (four beta-chains) most commonly results from the compound heterozygous state for alpha thalassemia (–/-α). The phenotypic expression of the disease is quite variable. *(Fauci, Chapter 99)*

37. **(C)** In sickle disease, if the bone infarction occurs in proximity to a joint, an effusion can develop. The underlying pathology is a vaso-occlusive phenomenon. Bone infarction can appear like osteomyelitis (radiographically and clinically), which is problematic since patients with sickle cell disease are also at increased risk of osteomyelitis. *(Fauci, Chapter 99)*

38. **(H)** Neurotoxicity is the dose-limiting side effect of vincristine. Neurologic toxicity is usually the result of a cumulative dose and usually begins when the total dose exceeds 6 mg/m². Paresthesia of fingers, feet, and loss of deep tendon reflexes are the usual initial manifestation. Continual administration may lead to severe motor weakness, particularly in the elderly. Constipation can also occur as a result of autonomic neuropathy. Syndrome of inappropriate antidiuretic hormone (SIADH) with hyponatremia can occur. *(Fauci, Chapter 379)*

39. **(D)** The renal concentrating defect and positive sickle prep are constant, but occlusive phenomena in the kidney can result in hematuria from papillary necrosis. This occurs when the red cells are prone to sickle cell formation under hypoxic stress. *(Fauci, Chapter 99)*

40. **(G)** The megaloblastic anemia of pregnancy is the most common of all folate-deficient states. Dilutional anemia and iron deficiency also occur in pregnancy. In pregnancy, a low Hb concentration may simply be due to a disproportionate increase in plasma volume, rather than a true anemia. The exact hormonal mechanism is unknown. Folate levels fall during pregnancy; therefore, frank deficiency is most common in the third trimester. *(Fauci, Chapter 100)*

41. **(C)** Chorionic villus sampling in the first trimester with deoxyribonucleic acid (DNA)-based diagnosis has a high degree of accuracy. Cord blood electrophoresis is suitable for screening high-risk infants at birth. *(Fauci, Chapter 99)*

42. **(C)** Spherocytes are seen on the blood film in patients with moderate to severe hemolytic anemia. This patient has autoimmune hemolytic anemia due to cold agglutinins due to the pneumonia. Spherocytosis is not associated with G6PD deficiency, trauma, or leukemia. The typical changes in G6PD deficiency include the presence of Heinz bodies. The cell morphology is not usually changed unless hemolysis is very severe. In hereditary spherocytosis, the Coombs test is negative. *(Fauci, Chapter 101)*

43. **(A)** Testing the mother for the presence of Rh (D) antibodies (alloimmunization) is done by indirect Coombs test of the maternal serum with known Rh(D) positive cells. Prevention of Rh immunization by the administration of Rh antibody (via Rh immune globulin) has been an effective preventive measure for this disorder. This condition is usually associated with a positive Coombs test using the baby's RBCs and a positive indirect Coombs test using the mother's serum. ABO hemolytic disease of the newborn is clinically mild because the antigens are not fully expressed in utero. *(Fauci, Chapter 7)*

44. **(D)** This patient has hairy cell leukemia, which is a rare form of adult leukemia (2%–3%). The disease is characterized by "hairy" cells in blood and bone marrow, splenomegaly, and pancytopenia. The lymphocytes have characteristic cytoplasmic projections, which give the disease its name. Treatment with the purine analogue, such as cladribine, produces complete remission in hairy cell leukemia. Recombinant alpha-interferon is not as effective. *(Fauci, Chapter 105)*

45. **(D)** Most elite athletes have increases in both plasma volume and red cell mass, but the increase in plasma volume is greater, resulting in a dilutional-type anemia. This is physiologically beneficial (increased O_2 transport with increased blood fluidity), so there is no reason to cease exercising to correct the Hb. Supportive footwear will decrease the likelihood of "march" hemolysis, but this rarely causes anemia. Similarly, although 20% of long-distance runners have GI blood loss, this is rarely of a magnitude to explain anemia. *(Fauci, Chapter 58)*

46. **(E)** The syndrome is caused by cold-precipitable proteins (cryoglobulins) that are found in plasma or serum. These cryoproteins can be of three classes. Type 1 are single component (immunoglobulin G, M, or A [IgG, IgM, IgA]), Type 2 are called "mixed cryoglobulins" (usually IgG molecules complexed with IgM molecules having anti-IgG reactivity), and Type 3 are polyclonal immunoglobulins with anti-immunoglobulin activity. Cryoglobulinemia is small vessel vasculitis (not medium), and platelet aggregation is not an important mechanism for the vessel injury. (*Fauci, Chapter 319*)

47. **(A)** Alcohol is directly toxic to dividing and maturing cells, but may also affect neutrophil function. The hematologic effects of alcohol may be direct or indirect, via diet, infection, liver disease, and GI disease. The resulting hematologic abnormalities may be profound. (*Fauci, Chapter 387*)

48. **(E)** HbF is evenly distributed among red cells, unlike the increased F in other conditions. It is a heterogeneous condition, and can be classified into deletion and nondeletion forms. Clinically, it can have features similar to mild thalassemia. (*Fauci, Chapter 99*)

49. **(E)** The spleen normally functions to pit nuclei and their fragments from red cells. These nuclear fragments are called Howell–Jolly bodies. The spleen has immune functions and filter functions. It also enhances iron reutilization, and acts as a reservoir and blood-volume regulator. In disease states, it can be a site of extramedullary hematopoiesis. (*Fauci, Chapter 60*)

50. **(D)** Anti-A and anti-B in the donor plasma are usually absorbed in the recipient's tissues but have the capacity to harm recipient cells. Type O blood donors do not have a higher risk of hepatitis C, nor do type O red cells have a shorter survival time when transfused into non-type O recipients. (*Fauci, Chapter 107*)

51. **(B)** In acute lymphoblastic leukemia (ALL), a bone marrow analysis is the most important test in confirming the diagnosis. Once the diagnosis of ALL is established, CSF fluid (leukemic cells in the CSF can be identified in up to a third of *all* patients at diagnosis) and CXR are important tests in the workup of the patient. It is the most common malignancy in children under age 15 in the United States, accounting for 25% of all cancers in White children. It is less common in Black children. (*Fauci, Chapter 104*)

52. **(E)** This patient has autoimmune hemolysis and the red cell destruction is extravascular, usually occurring in the liver, spleen, or other reticuloendothelial sites. It liberates unconjugated bilirubin causing jaundice. Intrinsic causes of hemolytic anemia are usually inherited, and are a result of abnormalities of membranes, red cell enzymes, globins, or heme. Extrinsic hemolysis is a result of mechanical forces, chemicals or microorganisms, antibodies, or sequestration in the monocyte-macrophage system. (*Fauci, Chapter 101*)

53. **(D)** The pancytopenia in this individual is most likely due to the marrow suppressive effects of alcohol. Anemia without white cell or platelet involvement can be multifactorial in alcoholics and includes marrow suppression, GI bleeding, hemorrhagic diathesis, and nutritional deficiency. Hemolysis does not result in pancytopenia and only rarely will severe vitamin B12 deficiency cause pancytopenia. Hemoglobinopathy is not usually a feature of chronic alcoholism: it is usually an inherited condition. (*Fauci, Chapter 387*)

54. **(B)** The macrocytosis and hypersegmented neutrophils suggests a megaloblastic anemia due to either folate or vitamin B_{12} deficiency. Folate deficiency results from decreased intake and malabsorption. Body folate stores are meager (only 3 months on average, compared to a few years for vitamin B_{12}), and therefore easily depleted when intake is poor. Alcohol itself can depress folate levels acutely, and can also cause pancytopenia directly. (*Fauci, Chapter 100*)

55. **(A)** Macrocytosis is frequently seen in patients with chronic alcoholism for multiple reasons

including vitamin B$_{12}$ or folate deficiency, chronic liver disease, and also from the direct toxic effects of alcohol on red cells. Because both iron deficiency and folate deficiency are very common in alcoholics, a dimorphic blood film can also be seen (macrocytes, hypersegmented neutrophils, and hypochromic microcytes can be found) on the same slide. *(Fauci, Chapter 387)*

56. **(D)** Coagulation factors II, V, VII, IX, X, and XI would most likely be deficient. These are some of the factors that are synthesized in the liver. Factors II, VII, IX, and X are the vitamin K-dependent factors, which are also synthesized in the liver. *(Fauci, Chapter 110)*

57. **(B)** Thalassemia minor usually represents a heterozygous state and is often asymptomatic. Symptoms may develop during periods of stress such as pregnancy or severe infection. Hemoglobin values are usually in the 9–11 g/dL range. The red cells are small and poorly hemoglobinized. *(Fauci, Chapter 99)*

58. **(D)** HbC characteristically produces targeting in the peripheral blood and also hemoglobin crystals in the cells. HbC is found in 17%–28% of West Africans. Splenomegaly is a fairly constant feature, but most patients are quite asymptomatic. *(Fauci, Chapter 99)*

59. **(D)** Sideroblastic anemia is associated with an increased serum iron and ferritin. TIBC is generally normal. HbA2 is usually decreased. *(Fauci, Chapter 98)*

60. **(B)** The beta-thalassemia trait is characterized by normal iron studies and an elevated HbA2. *(Fauci, Chapter 99)*

61. **(A)** Iron deficiency is characterized by low serum iron and ferritin and an increase in TIBC. HbA2 is normal. *(Fauci, Chapter 98)*

62. **(C)** Anemia of chronic disease is characterized by decreased serum iron and TIBC, an elevated ferritin, and normal HbA2. *(Fauci, Chapter 98)*

63. **(D)** Erythroid precursors that have accumulated abnormal amounts of iron are called ringed sideroblasts. Sideroblastic anemia can be either inherited or acquired. Common acquired causes are ingestion of certain drugs, alcohol, or toxins such as lead or zinc. The beta-thalassemia trait is diagnosed by demonstrating an elevated HbA2, iron deficiency by iron studies and ferritin levels, and anemia of chronic disease by demonstrating a chronic disease. Sideroblastic anemia generally requires a bone marrow aspiration revealing ringed sideroblasts for diagnosis. *(Fauci, Chapter 98)*

64. **(D)** Burr cells and stomatocytes are found in severe liver disease and might result from abnormal membrane lipids. *(Fauci, Chapter 58)*

65. **(F)** Heinz bodies (precipitated Hb) are found in disorders with unstable Hb or after oxidant stress. *(Fauci, Chapter 99)*

66. **(A)** Spherocytes are caused by loss of membrane, as in hereditary spherocytosis or autoimmune hemolytic anemia. *(Fauci, Chapter 101)*

67. **(C)** Sickle cell disease results in polymerization of HbS and the characteristic sickle cells. *(Fauci, Chapter 99)*

68. **(B)** Schistocytes are caused by traumatic disruption of the red cell membrane (eg, microangiopathic syndromes). *(Fauci, Chapter 109)*

69. **(A)** von Willebrand disease is the most common inherited bleeding disorder. The abnormal plasma glycoprotein, von Willebrand factor (vWF), has two major functions: facilitating platelet adhesion and serving as a carrier for factor VIII. The disease is heterogeneous in its manifestations but can be very severe (type III disease). Evaluation reveals a prolonged bleeding time and decreased factor VIII activity. *(Fauci, Chapter 109)*

70. **(B)** Hemophilia A results from a deficiency or dysfunction of the factor VIII molecule. It is a sex-linked disease affecting 1 in 10,000 males.

The PTT is prolonged, but the bleeding time is characteristically normal. *(Fauci, Chapter 110)*

71. **(C)** Hemophilia B is clinically indistinguishable from hemophilia A and is also inherited via the X chromosome. The bleeding time is usually normal, but the PTT is usually elevated. Differentiation from hemophilia A requires factor assay. *(Fauci, Chapter 110)*

72. **(D)** TTP is a fulminant disorder that can be fatal. It has been associated with malignancy, pregnancy, metastatic cancer, and high-dose chemotherapy. Most often, the classical tests of hemostasis and platelet function are normal. The classical symptoms include fever, thrombocytopenia, microangiopathic hemolytic anemia, renal failure, and fluctuating neurologic defects. *(Fauci, Chapter 109)*

CHAPTER 6

Oncology
Questions

DIRECTIONS (Questions 1 through 30): For each of the questions in this section select the one lettered answer that is the best response in each case.

1. A 19-year-old man presents with multiple lymph nodes in his neck. He reports no current infectious symptoms, and his monospot test is negative. On examination, he has blanching skin lesions on his face and conjunctivae, multiple large lymph nodes in his neck, and poor coordination when tested by tandem walking.

   He has past history of poor coordination and walking difficulty as well as recurrent sinopulmonary infections. A biopsy of the lymph node is positive for lymphoma. He is diagnosed with a hereditary disorder that is autosomal recessive, and is associated with defective deoxyribonucleic acid (DNA) repair mechanisms. **Which of the following is the most likely diagnosis?**

   (A) neurofibromatosis
   (B) tuberous sclerosis
   (C) ataxia-telangiectasia
   (D) von Hippel–Lindau syndrome
   (E) Peutz–Jeghers syndrome

2. A 33-year-old male immigrant from Taiwan presents with increasing right upper quadrant (RUQ) pain. The pain is dull, and it does not radiate or change with eating. On examination, the abdomen is soft, there is a mass in the RUQ, and no ascites is clinically detected.

   He has a prior history of hepatitis B. His laboratory investigations reveal hepatitis B surface antigen (HBsAg) positive, hepatitis B surface antibody (HBsAb) negative, aspartate amino transferase (AST) 60 U/L, alanine amino transferase (ALT) 72 U/L, and an elevated alpha-fetoprotein level. (See Figure 6–1.) **Which of the following is the most likely diagnosis?**

Figure 6–1.

   (A) hepatic abscess
   (B) hepatocellular carcinoma (HCC)
   (C) metastatic cancer
   (D) hepatic hemangioma
   (E) liver cirrhosis

3. A 42-year-old man presents to clinic for assessment of concerns about radiation exposure. Ten years ago he worked at a nuclear power plant, and even though there were never any accidents or excess radiation exposure while he worked there, he wants to know his future cancer risk from daily background exposure. **Which of the following statements is correct?**

(A) malignancies occur within 10 years of exposure

(B) leukemia has the longest latency period of all malignancies

(C) large radiation exposure is required to develop a malignancy

(D) risk increases with advancing age at the time of exposure

(E) therapeutic radiation therapy given without chemotherapy does not increase the risk of a second malignancy

4. A 25-year-old woman has recently moved to a new city. She comes today for her first routine visit and annual physical assessment. She feels well, reports no new symptoms, and her past medical history is negative. Her only medication is the oral contraceptive pill; she is currently in university and drinks on a social basis. She reports smoking in her teens but quit 7 years ago. The physical examination is completely normal. She asks you about screening tests for cancer at her age. **Which of the following cancer screening tests are recommended for her age group?**

(A) mammography every 5 years

(B) Pap smear at least every 3 years

(C) stool for occult blood

(D) chest x-ray (CXR) every 3 years

(E) physical examination of the breast by a physician

5. A 25-year-old woman presents to the clinic for assessment of symptoms consisting of intermittent double vision and fatigue. Her symptoms are worse at the end of the day. She reports no other focal muscle weakness or sensory symptoms.

On examination, her eye movements, motor strength, and reflexes in the upper and lower limbs are normal. Repetitive handgrip exercises cause loss of strength in the grip. A CXR reveals an anterior mediastinal mass. **Which of the following is the most likely diagnosis of the anterior mediastinal mass?**

(A) teratoma

(B) thyroid

(C) thymoma

(D) lymphoma

(E) mediastinal cyst

6. A 64-year-old man presents with symptoms of difficulty swallowing and weight loss of 10 lb. He has no prior history of heartburn, stomach ulcers, or difficulty swallowing. He smokes 1 pack a day for the past 45 years and drinks approximately 5 oz of alcohol a day.

He is thin appearing, there are no oral lesions, and the remaining examination is normal. Esophagoscopy reveals a midesophageal narrowing with a ragged ulcerating lesion, and biopsies are taken. **Which of the following is the most likely diagnosis?**

(A) adenocarcinoma of esophagus

(B) esophageal web

(C) achalasia

(D) squamous cell carcinoma of esophagus

(E) esophageal leiomyoma

7. A 62-year-old man presents to the emergency department with a 1-day history of dark tarry stools and light-headedness. He also reports a 1-month history of intermittent abdominal discomfort and poor appetite. For the pain he takes ibuprofen on an as needed basis.

On physical examination, the blood pressure is 102/75mm Hg, heart rate is 110/min, and the abdomen is soft and nontender. He undergoes urgent upper endoscopy that finds an ulcerating lesion in his stomach and biopsies confirm gastric cancer. **Which of the following is a risk factor for carcinoma of the stomach?**

(A) *Helicobacter pylori* infection

(B) high socioeconomic status

(C) high-protein diet

(D) high alcohol consumption

(E) high-fat diet

8. A young man with leukemia is treated with methotrexate. **Which of the following is the mechanism of action of this drug?**

    (A) preventing absorption of folic acid
    (B) inhibiting dihydrofolate reductase
    (C) preventing formation of messenger ribonucleic acid (mRNA)
    (D) forming a cytotoxic metabolite
    (E) preventing proper functioning of membrane adenosine triphosphatase (ATPase)

9. A 52-year-old man presents with abdominal pain and weight loss. He describes a dull "gnawing" pain located in the epigastric region radiating to the back. The abdominal examination is normal with no hepatosplenomegaly or masses palpated. A computerized tomography (CT) scan of the abdomen reveals a 3-cm mass in the pancreas. **Which of the following statements regarding cancer of the pancreas is true?**

    (A) tumors of the pancreas are divided almost equally between those arising from the exocrine portion and those arising from the endocrine portion
    (B) most endocrine tumors of the pancreas are not symptomatic
    (C) the body of the pancreas is the most common site of malignancy
    (D) adenocarcinoma is the most common pancreatic cancer
    (E) extension is through local invasion; metastases are a late manifestation

10. A 73-year-old man was born in Taiwan and came to the United States 3 years ago. He is known to be HBsAg positive. **Which of the following findings suggests the development of HCC?**

    (A) hepatomegaly
    (B) hepatic bruits
    (C) ascites
    (D) jaundice
    (E) all of the above

11. A 47-year-old man presents to the emergency department complaining of dark black stools and vague crampy abdominal pain. On examination, he is pale, blood pressure 100/70 mm Hg, pulse 110/min, and the abdomen is soft and nontender. Rectal examination confirms melena, and the patient is transfused 2 units of packed red blood cells. Upper endoscopy does not identify the source of bleeding, so a small bowel barium study is ordered. It reveals a small bowel tumor. **Which of the following statements concerning small bowel tumors is correct?**

    (A) carcinoid is a common cause of small bowel tumors
    (B) malignant adenocarcinoma most frequently occurs in the duodenum
    (C) malignant tumors bleed more frequently than benign tumors
    (D) Peutz–Jeghers syndrome is characterized only by benign hamartoma
    (E) most primary gastrointestinal (GI) lymphomas are located in the colon

12. A 58-year-old man is newly diagnosed with colon cancer and undergoes surgical resection of the tumor. The pathology result reports no lymph node involvement, the lesion is 4 cm in size and involves the muscularis layer. His preoperative evaluation for distal metastases was negative. **Which of the following factors is most important in predicting prognosis and survival in patients with colon cancer?**

    (A) age under 40
    (B) male gender
    (C) rectal bleeding
    (D) small tumor size
    (E) depth of tumor penetration

13. A 64-year-old woman presents to the clinic because she is concerned about the development of an abnormal vaginal discharge and postmenopausal bleeding. She reports no pelvic pain, fever, or constitutional symptoms. Her medical history includes type 2 diabetes and hypertension that are well controlled on medical therapy.

    Pelvic examination reveals a bulky uterus and no adnexal masses. She undergoes a dilation and curettage (D&C), and the pathology is positive for adenocarcinoma. **Which of the following is correct about carcinoma of the uterine endometrium?**

    (A) not associated with diabetes mellitus and obesity
    (B) most common in postmenopausal woman
    (C) associated with multiparity
    (D) common in Jews and Muslims
    (E) associated with herpes simplex virus type 2 (HSV-2) infection

14. You are seeing a 62-year-old woman in the clinic with a family history of breast cancer. She is worried about her future risk of breast cancer, since her mother died of breast cancer at the age of 63. **Which of the following features is also a recognized risk factor for breast cancer?**

    (A) early onset of menopause
    (B) early onset of menarche
    (C) late-life radiation exposure
    (D) multiparity
    (E) early full-term pregnancy

15. A 67-year-old man complains of shortness of breath on exertion and right-sided chest pain. The pain is constant in nature; he has no fever or chills and no sputum production. On examination, air entry to the left lower lobe is reduced and the area is dull on percussion. The CXR reveals left lower lobe pleural effusion, pleural thickening with calcification (plaques), and lower lobe fibrosis. Further history from the patient is significant in that he is a lifetime nonsmoker, and that he worked as a pipe fitter until retiring 2 years ago. **Which of the following is the most likely diagnosis?**

    (A) adenocarcinoma
    (B) squamous cell carcinoma
    (C) sarcoidosis
    (D) lymphoma
    (E) mesothelioma

16. A 23-year-old man notices left leg pain after returning from a ski trip. The pain persists for 2 months, and he presents for medical evaluation after noticing a lump on his calf. On examination, there is a 2-cm nonmobile mass in his anterior shin. A magnetic resonance imaging (MRI) scan suggests the lesion is arising from the tibia, and a biopsy reveals osteosarcoma. **Which of the following statements about osteosarcoma is correct?**

    (A) distal bone sarcomas have a better prognosis
    (B) lung metastases are a late sign
    (C) local lymph node involvement is very common
    (D) articular cartilage is a common plane for tumor spread
    (E) skip metastases within the same bone are common and unrelated to prognosis

17. A 19-year-old woman notices axillary lymphadenopathy and presents for evaluation. She has noticed the lymph nodes for over a month, but there is no associated fever, chills, weight loss, or night sweats.

    On examination, she has multiple mobile nontender lymph nodes in both axilla, and no cervical or inguinal lymph nodes. The spleen is not palpable, and the rest of the examination is normal. A monospot test is negative, and a complete blood count (CBC) and biochemistry are normal. A biopsy of one lymph node reveals Hodgkin disease (HD), nodular sclerosing variety. A bone marrow biopsy is arranged. **Which of the following tests is also part of the routine staging evaluation for patients with HD?**

    (A) positron emission tomography (PET) scan
    (B) gallium scan
    (C) CT of chest, abdomen, and pelvis

(D) staging laparotomy

(E) bone scan

18. A 68-year-old man presents to the clinic for re-assessment of left axillary adenopathy and to review biopsy results. The lymph nodes were first noticed 6 weeks ago, and the clinical assessment and preliminary diagnostic tests are negative. Because the lymph node enlargement is persistent, he is referred to a surgeon for an excisional biopsy. The biopsy reveals a low-grade lymphocytic lymphoma. **Which of the following statements is correct?**

(A) staging in this type of disorder is not relevant

(B) if disease is widespread, early aggressive chemotherapy will result in an improved prognosis for survival

(C) the disease is likely to be widespread at the time of diagnosis

(D) untreated, the prognosis is measured in months

(E) his age is not a relevant factor in treatment

19. A 63-year-old man presents with a new skin rash on his chest. His past medical history is significant for stable angina, hypertension, and dyslipidemia. His review of symptoms is negative except for unintentional weight loss of 10 lbs over the past 3 months. On physical examination, the lesions on his anterior chest wall are well-defined red-colored plaques. A skin biopsy of the lesion is performed for diagnosis and it reveals lymphoma. Further diagnostic evaluation does not reveal any evidence of a visceral malignancy. **Which of the following characteristics about this disease is correct?**

(A) it is invariably a precursor to leukemia

(B) it is of T-cell origin

(C) it has no specific geographic distribution

(D) it has a high likelihood of cure

(E) it is related to sun exposure

20. A 65-year-old man presents to the emergency department complaining of hematuria and flank pain. He reports no fever, chills, or dysuria, but he has lost 15 lbs over the past 2 months. His medical history is significant for COPD and a 45-pack-per-year history of smoking.

On examination the abdomen is soft, no mass is felt, and there is no flank tenderness on percussion. His hemoglobin (Hb) is 17.5 g/dL, and his liver enzymes are normal. A CT scan of the abdomen reveals a mass in the left kidney with involvement of the renal vein. **Which of the following is the most likely diagnosis?**

(A) renal cyst

(B) renal cell carcinoma (RCC)

(C) renal metastases

(D) renal abscess

(E) lymphoma

21. A 53-year-old woman presents to the clinic for evaluation of a new left breast lump that she discovered 1 week ago. The nodule is not painful; she feels well and has no other symptoms. On physical examination the lump is palpable, and there are no axillary lymph nodes. The mammogram confirms the presence of a 1-cm breast mass which on biopsy is positive for invasive breast cancer. **Which of the following is the most appropriate local therapy for her tumor?**

(A) simple mastectomy with axillary dissection

(B) radiation therapy to breast and axilla

(C) local excision plus radiation therapy

(D) local excision and axillary dissection followed by radiation therapy

(E) local excision and axillary sampling

22. A 68-year-old woman presents to her attending physician feeling unwell and having lost 10 lbs. Her medical history includes hypertension, dyslipidemia, and depression. She is a life-time non-smoker and drinks alcohol on a social basis.

    Physical examination is positive for abnormal left axillary lymphadenopathy, and an enlarged nontender liver. Excisional biopsy of the lymph node reveals well-differentiated adenocarcinoma. Further diagnostic tests including colonoscopy, upper endoscopy, mammography, and CT imaging of the abdomen, chest, and pelvis does not reveal an obvious primary site for the cancer. There is evidence of liver and bone metastasis on the imaging studies. **Which statement concerning her further management is correct?**

    (A) the response rate for metastatic adenocarcinoma (well differentiated) of unknown primary site is so poor that no investigation or treatment is indicated

    (B) special tumor stains or markers might guide management

    (C) extensive workup, including colonoscopy, abdominal CT scan, and mammography will define subsets that benefit from treatment

    (D) special studies of the excised lymph node are not useful in determining the site of origin

    (E) metastatic breast cancer is the most common cause of adenocarcinoma of unknown primary site in women

23. A 47-year-old woman with cancer phobia comes to the office for counseling. **Which of the following statements is true?**

    (A) cancer is the most common cause of death in the United States

    (B) cancer is the most common cause of death in middle-aged women

    (C) incidence rates for cancer are generally higher in women than men

    (D) colon and rectum cancers have the highest mortality rate when considering both men and women

    (E) about 25% of all cancers in the United States are due to environmental factors

24. A 63-year-old man, with chronic heartburn symptoms for many years, presents for reevaluation because of increased abdominal discomfort. He is taking a proton pump inhibitor for his symptoms but experiences little relief. He undergoes upper endoscopy that reveals no masses or tumors, but there is esophagitis. Biopsy of the lower esophagus reveals columnar cells. **Which of the following statements is correct?**

    (A) it is a major risk factor for squamous cell cancer of the esophagus

    (B) it can be found in up to 20% of patients undergoing esophagoscopy for esophagitis

    (C) the histologic changes include development of keratinized squamous cells

    (D) medical control of reflux will decrease the likelihood of malignant changes

    (E) only 10% of patients with Barrett esophagus may develop malignancy

25. A 59-year-old man develops jaundice and pruritus. He has no abdominal pain, and on physical examination he is icteric, the liver span is 10 cm, and no masses are felt. Ultrasound reveals dilated intrahepatic bile ducts. He undergoes endoscopic retrograde cholangiopancreatography (ERCP), which suggests a cholangiocarcinoma. **Which of the following is the most likely predisposing factor for cholangiocarcinoma?**

    (A) smoking
    (B) excess alcohol intake
    (C) chronic hepatitis B virus (HBV) infection
    (D) history of ulcerative colitis or sclerosing cholangitis
    (E) gallstones

26. A 53-year-old woman notices a lump in her left breast. She reports no symptoms of breast discharge or previous breast disease. She is postmenopausal, menarche was at age 13, and her family history is negative for breast cancer.

    Physical examination reveals a 2-cm palpable lump in the left breast, which is mobile and nontender, and there are no axillary lymph nodes. The right breast and axilla are normal.

Biopsy of the lump is positive for breast cancer, and she undergoes a lumpectomy and lymph node dissection. **Which of the following factors is important in deciding about adjuvant therapy for breast cancer?**

(A) menopausal status

(B) tumor size

(C) endocrine receptor status

(D) lymph node status

(E) all of the above

27. A 45-year-old man is worried about a dark pigmented skin lesion on his arm. The "mole" is 3 mm wide, symmetric with a regular border and even pigmentation. He reports no change in size or other symptoms. (See Figure 6–2.) **Which of the following is the most appropriate next step in management?**

(A) observation only

(B) excisional biopsy

(C) punch biopsy

(D) chemotherapy, then surgical excision

(E) surgical excision and regional node dissection

28. A 73-year-old man presents with fatigue and multiple lymph nodes in his neck. On physical examination there are multiple large non-tender lymph nodes in his neck and axilla. The spleen is not palpable, and the remaining examination is normal. A biopsy of the lymph node reveals lymphocytic lymphoma. **Which of the following factors predicts poor prognosis?**

(A) no extranodal involvement

(B) poor performance status

(C) age <60

(D) low serum lactate dehydrogenase (LDH) levels

(E) fever and weight loss

29. A 74-year-old man has a high erythrocyte sedimentation rate (ESR) noted on routine blood work done during a yearly physical examination. He is asymptomatic and feels well; and his past medical history is only significant for hypertension and type 2 diabetes. His physical examination is normal. A follow-up protein electrophoresis reveals a monoclonal immunoglobulin G (IgG) spike. **Which of the following statements suggests multiple myeloma, rather than monoclonal gammopathy of unknown significance (MGUS) as the cause for the abnormal protein electrophoresis?**

(A) Bence Jones protein 2 g/day

(B) normal hemoglobin

(C) M component level of 2 g/dL

(D) bone marrow plasma cells of 5%

(E) normal serum calcium level

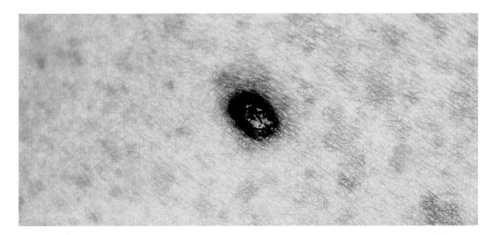

Figure 6–2. (Reproduced, with permission, from Wolff K and Johnson RA, *Fitzpatrick's Color Atlas & Synopsis of Clinical Dermatology*, 5th ed. New York: McGraw-Hill, 2005:175.)

30. A 23-year-old man is newly diagnosed with Hodgkin lymphoma. **Which of the following is the most likely presenting symptom of this type of lymphoma?**

    (A) coincidentally detected mediastinal mass
    (B) fixed tender inguinal lymph node involvement
    (C) mobile nontender cervical lymph nodes
    (D) fixed nontender axillary nodes
    (E) mobile tender axillary nodes

DIRECTIONS (Questions 31 through 63): The following group of numbered items is preceded by a list of lettered options. For each question, select the one lettered option that is most closely associated with it. Each lettered option may be used once, multiple times, or not at all.

Questions 31 through 37: For each type of cancer, select the most likely ethnic group.

    (A) Hispanic Americans
    (B) White Americans
    (C) Black Americans
    (D) Native Americans
    (E) Chinese Americans
    (F) Japanese Americans
    (G) Filipino Americans

31. Have the lowest cancer rates for both sexes.

32. Have very high rates of melanoma.

33. Have the highest rates for breast, corpus uteri, and ovarian cancers.

34. Have especially high rates for cervical cancer.

35. Have elevated rates for nasopharynx and liver cancers.

36. Have high rates for stomach cancer.

37. Have high cancer rates, at least partially, due to socioeconomic factors.

Questions 38 through 42: For each patient with cancer, select the most likely etiologic agent.

    (A) alcoholic beverages
    (B) alkylating agents
    (C) arsenic
    (D) asbestos
    (E) benzene
    (F) ultraviolet radiation
    (G) Epstein–Barr virus
    (H) hepatitis B virus (HBV)
    (I) human papillomavirus (HPV)
    (J) vinyl chloride

38. A 56-year-old man notices an ulcer on his tongue. The lesion persists for a month and becomes more painful and larger in size. There is a 5-mm pale lesion on the lateral border of his tongue, and the remaining examination is normal. A biopsy of the site is positive for squamous cell cancer.

39. A 68-year-old man complains of shortness of breath on exertion, but no fever, cough, or sputum. On physical examination, air entry is reduced to the right lower lobe and the area is dull on percussion. A CT scan of the chest reveals a pleural-based tumor in the right lower lobe, and areas of calcification on the pleura. A biopsy of the lesion is positive for mesothelioma.

40. A 64-year-old woman notices a nodule on her face that persists for more than a month. It appears as a raised lesion with small vessels on it. Excisional biopsy of the lesion confirms a diagnosis of basal cell carcinoma.

41. A 54-year-old woman has postmenopausal vaginal bleeding. There is no associated pain or systemic symptoms, and speculum examination reveals an irregular appearance to the cervix, which bleeds easily when samples are taken for a Pap smear. The diagnosis is cervical cancer.

42. A 58-year-old woman presents with RUQ abdominal discomfort. She has no history of

gallstones, and on examination, there is a firm mass in the RUQ. Ultrasound of the liver reveals a 6-cm solitary lesion in the liver, and her alpha-fetoprotein level is elevated.

Questions 43 through 47: For each of the following findings, select the most likely type of lung cancer.

(A) cancer metastatic to the lung

(B) squamous cell cancer of the lung

(C) adenocarcinoma of the lung

(D) small cell cancer of the lung

(E) large cell cancer of the lung

43. The most common type of lung cancer in the United States.

44. Has the best prognosis of all malignant lung cancers.

45. Most likely to cause nonmetastatic hypercalcemia.

46. Associated with syndrome of inappropriate antidiuretic hormone (SIADH).

47. Associated with myasthenic syndrome (Eaton–Lambert syndrome).

Questions 48 through 52: For each patient with an adverse reaction, select the most likely chemotherapeutic agent.

(A) methotrexate

(B) cytarabine

(C) 5-fluorouracil (5-FU)

(D) bleomycin

(E) doxorubicin

(F) pamidronate

(G) cisplatin

(H) busulfan

(I) cyclophosphamide

(J) vincristine

48. A 23-year-old man notices numbness in his hands and feet. On examination, there is distal loss of sensation to touch, and vibration in all four limbs. He recently finished chemotherapy for testicular cancer.

49. A 56-year-old woman is receiving chemotherapy for lymphoma for the past year. Her liver enzymes have been persistently elevated for the last 2 months. She has no prior history of chronic liver disease, and screening tests for viral hepatitis are negative. A liver biopsy indicates early hepatic fibrosis.

50. A 64-year-old man is receiving chemotherapy for squamous cell cancer of the lung. He has now developed erythema, induration, thickening, and eventual peeling of the skin on the fingers, palms, and soles of his feet.

51. A 54-year-old woman received adjuvant chemotherapy for breast cancer 1 year ago. She now presents with symptoms and signs of congestive heart failure. An echocardiogram confirms decreased left ventricular function.

52. A 34-year-old man is undergoing preconditioning high-dose chemotherapy for a bone marrow transplant. On the third day of treatment, he develops hematuria.

Questions 53 through 55: For each of the following statements, select the most likely type of thyroid cancer.

(A) anaplastic thyroid cancer

(B) follicular cancer of the thyroid

(C) lymphoma of the thyroid

(D) papillary cancer of the thyroid

(E) medullary thyroid cancer

53. Has the best prognosis of all thyroid malignancies.

54. Is proportionately more common in Blacks than Whites.

55. Is associated with a specific marker.

Questions 56 through 59: For each of the following statements, select the most likely type of Hodgkin disease (HD).

   (A) lymphocyte-predominant Hodgkin disease (HD)
   (B) nodular-sclerosing HD
   (C) mixed-cellularity HD
   (D) lymphocyte-depleted HD, reticular type
   (E) lymphocyte-depleted HD, diffuse fibrosis type
   (F) all variants of HD

56. The only form of HD more common in women.

57. Reed–Sternberg cells can be difficult to locate in this variant.

58. This variant has a particularly good outcome.

59. Can be accompanied by a nonnecrotizing epithelioid granulomatous reaction.

Questions 60 through 63: For each patient with metastatic cancer pain, select the most likely treatment choice.

   (A) nonsteroidal anti-inflammatory drugs (NSAIDs)
   (B) opioids
   (C) amphetamines
   (D) anticonvulsants
   (E) phenothiazines
   (F) butyrophenones
   (G) steroids

60. A 52-year-old woman has metastatic breast cancer with boney metastases. She is taking hydromorphone for the pain but is still experiencing back pain. She is reluctant to take more of the hydromorphone since she becomes very drowsy with higher doses. This group of medications is particularly useful for pain from bony metastases.

61. A 74-year-old man with metastatic prostate cancer develops shooting pains in his left leg and constant back pain. Further evaluation reveals a pathologic compression fracture of the lumbar spine and involvement of the nerve roots in his lower spine causing the pain. He is started on a medication to help reduce the symptoms, but a limitation of the drug is leukopenia and thrombocytopenia.

62. A 68-year-old woman was treated for melanoma 3 years ago. She now presents with constant headaches, nausea, vomiting, and left-sided weakness. A CT scan reveals two masses in the right parietal lobe consistent with metastatic melanoma. She is started on medication to help reduce her symptoms of headaches and nausea.

63. A 65-year-old man has metastatic lung cancer and severe bone and chest pain. He is started on morphine and ibuprofen to control the pain but is still not comfortable. Further gradual increases in the morphine dose achieve good pain control but he becomes drowsy on the appropriate dose and is unable to do much. He is started on a medication that can be useful in controlling opioid-induced sedation.

Answers and Explanations

1. **(C)** Ataxia-telangiectasia is inherited in an autosomal recessive manner. It is associated with non-Hodgkin lymphoma, acute lymphocytic leukemia, and stomach cancer. Associated immunoglobulin A (IgA) (± immunoglobulin E [IgE]) deficiency predisposes to infection as well. All the other conditions listed are inherited in an autosomal dominant manner, and a positive family history is much more likely. *(Fauci, Chapter 368)*

2. **(B)** Only the chronic carrier state increases HCC risk, not previous infection. The majority, but not all, of HCC associated with HBV occurs in the setting of cirrhosis (60%–90%). Because the latency period of HBV infection is 35 years, before HCC supervenes, early-life infection is strongly correlated with HCC. The chronic carrier state of HBsAg in endemic areas, such as Taiwan, is associated with a relative risk of over 100 for the development of HCC. Over half the chronic carriers of HBsAg in such a population will die of cirrhosis or HCC. In Taiwan, where childhood vaccination was introduced in 1984, the death rate from childhood HCC has already declined. The absence of fever or chills make hepatic abscess less likely and a hepatic hemangioma is usually not associated with an elevated alpha-fetoprotein level. The image does show multiple lesions consistent with metastasis but in this case the mets are due to HCC. *(Fauci, Chapter 88)*

3. **(C)** The amount of exposure determines the likelihood of developing malignancy. Radiation-induced malignancies tend to occur at the age where that particular malignancy would normally occur. Therefore, the latency period can be 40 years or more. The latency period tends to be shortest (5–7 years) for leukemia. The risk for most malignancies is greatest with early-life radiation, and evidence suggests that therapeutic radiation confers excess risk as well. *(Fauci, Chapter 88)*

4. **(B)** There is universal agreement on the need for regular Pap smears in young women. There is no need to screen for colon cancer (fecal occult blood) or lung tumors (CXR), particularly at this age. Mammography, if indicated for screening, would be only for older women. Many authorities recommend breast self-examination as well as physical examination by a physician. *(Fauci, Chapter 78)*

5. **(C)** All of the given responses are potential anterior mediastinal masses, but when an anterior mediastinal mass presents with myasthenia gravis, the diagnosis of thymoma is essentially established. Myasthenia gravis occurs as a paraneoplastic process of the thymoma. The ocular and muscle fatigue symptoms are characteristic of myasthenia. About 5%–10% of patients with thymoma will also have hypogammaglobulinemia. About 5% of patients with thymoma will have autoimmune pure red cell aplasia. *(Fauci, Chapter 97)*

6. **(D)** The history of weight loss and dysphagia suggests carcinoma of the esophagus, and squamous cell carcinoma is a disease that occurs in older men who drink and smoke heavily. Smoking and/or excessive drinking are considered etiologic factors in the development of squamous cell carcinoma. Adenocarcinomas arise within dysplastic columnar epithelium in

the distal esophagus, usually in the presence of chronic gastric reflux. *(Fauci, Chapter 87)*

7. **(A)** *H pylori* is another important risk factor, since it causes gastritis that eventually leads to chronic atrophic gastritis, metaplasia, dysplasia, and then carcinoma. Low dietary vitamin C, and high salt and nitrate consumption predispose to gastric cancer, as does ingestion of smoked foods. Smoking is a risk factor, but alcohol is not. *(Fauci, Chapter 87)*

8. **(B)** The mode of action of methotrexate is by tightly binding dihydrofolate reductase (DHFR), which maintains the intracellular folate pool in its fully reduced form as tetrahydrofolates. These compounds are required in the de novo synthesis of pyrimidines and purines. *(Fauci, Chapter 81)*

9. **(D)** Adenocarcinoma is the most common cancer of the pancreas. The proximal pancreas is the most common site, with only 20% occurring in the body and 5%–10% in the tail. About 95% of the tumors arise from the exocrine portion of the gland, and these are usually malignant. Most of the endocrine tumors are slow growing and usually present with symptoms related to the excess hormone such as insulin. Early development of metastases is characteristic of pancreatic adenocarcinoma. *(Fauci, Chapter 89)*

10. **(E)** For most patients, the development of HCC is the first manifestation of their underlying liver disease. The most common presentation is with RUQ pain, mass, and weight loss, but hepatic decompensation with jaundice and ascites is also common. About 25% of patients have hepatic bruits. *(Fauci, Chapter 88)*

11. **(B)** Adenocarcinoma, the most common malignancy of the small bowel, is most common proximally, particularly in the duodenum. Small bowel lymphomas are most common in the ileum, but the stomach is the most common site of GI lymphoma. Carcinoids usually present with local symptoms. Carcinoid syndrome is present only with hepatic metastases. Benign tumors bleed more frequently than malignant ones. Malignant adenocarcinomas can occur in Peutz–Jeghers syndrome. *(Fauci, Chapter 87)*

12. **(E)** Depth of tumor penetration (Dukes stage) is the most important prognostic factor in the 5-year survival in patients with colon cancer. Rectal bleeding is a good prognostic sign, perhaps because surface erosion leads to clinically visible bleeding and early detection of the cancer. Young age, male gender, and location in the rectum are not helpful for determining prognosis. Unlike most tumors, no correlation with tumor size and prognosis has been established for colon cancer. *(Fauci, Chapter 87)*

13. **(B)** Carcinoma of the cervix is common in young women. For endometrial cancer, the peak is from age 55 to 60. Endometrial cancer is associated with nulliparity, diabetes mellitus, and obesity. Cervical cancer is associated with human papilloma virus (HPV) infection. There is tremendous variation in incidence of cervical cancer based on geography, ethnicity, and sexual history. *(Fauci, Chapter 93)*

14. **(B)** Breast cancer risk is reduced by 20% for each year that menarche is delayed. Early menopause, natural or surgical, also decreases risk. Early (age 18 or 19) full-term pregnancy and multiparity decrease the risk. Radiation exposure is a risk factor primarily in adolescence and is marginal after the age of 40. In summary, there are 3 important dates in the assessing the risk of breast cancer: age of menarche, age of first full-term pregnancy, and age of menopause. *(Fauci, Chapter 86)*

15. **(E)** The history of being a pipe fitter suggests asbestos exposure, and the CXR finding of pleural plaques, and lower lobe fibrosis confirms prior asbestos exposure. The classic associated cancer is mesothelioma. However, in 30%–50% of cases, no history of asbestos exposure is apparent. The average age on presentation is 60, and this is typically many years after the exposure. The most common presenting symptoms are dyspnea and non-pleuritic chest pain. Smoking injury in patients with asbestos exposure increases the

risk of other lung cancers such as adenocarcinoma or squamous cell carcinoma. *(Fauci, Chapter 250)*

16. **(A)** Overwhelmingly, the major prognostic factor in osteosarcoma is location of the tumor. Pelvic and axial lesions do worse than those in the extremities, and survival is better in tibial tumors than femoral tumors. Lung metastases are very common. *(Fauci, Chapter 94)*

17. **(C)** CT imaging of the chest, abdomen, and pelvis is part of the staging workup for patients with HD. Other components of staging include CBC, lytes, LDH, CXR, and bone marrow biopsy. PET and gallium scanning are not always done, and are usually helpful at the completion of treatment to document remission. The purpose of staging laparotomy is to determine whether radiation alone will be used for treatment. As chemotherapy usage increases, the necessity for staging laparotomy decreases. *(Fauci, Chapter 105)*

18. **(C)** About 85% of low-grade lymphocytic lymphomas are widespread at the time of diagnosis. However, staging is still important as radiation therapy can be curative for localized (stage I, II) disease. Because the prognosis for this malignancy is measured in years, it has been difficult to demonstrate a survival benefit for aggressive chemotherapy. The poor prognosis for lymphoma in older patients might be a result of less-aggressive therapy. *(Fauci, Chapter 105)*

19. **(B)** Cutaneous lymphomas are of T-cell origin and are more common in other parts of the world, such as Japan. Patients with adult T-cell lymphoma-leukemia (ATLL) have acute fulminant courses characterized by skin invasion and leukemic cells. This syndrome is clearly related to human T-cell lymphotropic virus-I (HTLV-I), and there is a possibility that HTLV-I, or another retrovirus, might be the agent for mycosis fungoides and Sézary syndrome. ATLL responds poorly to treatment, and therapy for the low-grade malignancies controls symptoms but does not result in cure. *(Fauci, Chapter 105)*

20. **(B)** Age, history of smoking, and polycythemia in a patient with hematuria strongly suggests a renal cell carcinoma. The elevated hemoglobin represents increased erythropoietin production and is not related to prognosis. Involvement along the renal vein and metastases to the lung is also characteristic of renal cell carcinoma. The clinical features of elevated Hgb and involvement of the renal vein make the lesion seen on imaging RCC rather than lymphoma, renal abscess, or renal cysts. Elevated liver enzymes and weight loss can represent nonmetastatic effects of malignancy and can reverse with resection. Almost half of patients will have a palpable abdominal mass on presentation. The CT of the thorax is a useful test because three-quarters of those with metastatic disease will have lung metastases. *(Fauci, Chapter 90)*

21. **(D)** Breast-conserving surgery is now recommended for small tumors. Radiation therapy will decrease local recurrence rates. For tumors <1 cm, adjuvant therapy is indicated only if axillary nodes are positive. Therefore, in this case, an axillary dissection will provide important therapeutic information. However, this is an area of rapidly changing knowledge and practice. *(Fauci, Chapter 86)*

22. **(B)** Patients with adenocarcinoma of unknown origin are typically elderly and have metastatic tumors at many sites. Generally, the prognosis is poor, but some subsets, in which effective treatment is available, can be identified by clinical criteria with only moderate investigations. These include peritoneal carcinomatosis in women (responds to treatment for ovarian cancer), predominant skeletal metastases in men (can reflect prostatic cancer), and women with axillary lymphadenopathy (can reflect breast cancer). In the latter scenario, studies for estrogen and progesterone receptors are very useful in guiding therapy. *(Fauci, Chapter 95)*

23. **(B)** When men and women of all ages are considered, cardiovascular diseases are the most common cause of death. However, among women aged 35–74 years, cancer is the leading cause of death. Lung cancer is the number one

cause of death from cancer, when both men and women are considered. Men generally have higher incidence rates for cancer: breast, gallbladder, and thyroid cancers are the exceptions. It is felt that 75%–80% of all cancers in the United States are due to environmental factors. The environmental contribution is estimated by comparing age-adjusted US rates of specific cancers to the rates for the country with the lowest risk. *(Fauci, Chapter 78)*

24. **(B)** Barrett esophagus, characterized by a columnar cell-lined esophageal mucosa, is a major risk factor for adenocarcinoma of the esophagus. Although acid reflux may be a predisposing factor, there is no evidence that either medical or surgical antireflux measures alter the outcome. It is found in about 20% of patients undergoing endoscopy for esophagitis, and up to 50% may develop a malignancy. *(Fauci, Chapter 87)*

25. **(D)** In North America, primary sclerosing cholangitis and chronic ulcerative colitis are the most common predisposing factors. Worldwide, the presence of liver flukes (eg, *Clonorchis sinensis*) is the most likely pre-disposing factor for cholangiocarcinoma. Part of this increased risk is caused by the development of hepatolithiasis. The highest rate of cholangiocarcinoma is found in Southeast Asia. It is thought that liver flukes and a diet high in nitrosamine are the prime reasons for this. Cholelithiasis, alcohol, smoking, and chronic hepatitis B are not known to be risk factors. *(Fauci, Chapter 88)*

26. **(E)** The size of the tumor is a prognostic factor, as is knowing menopausal status, endocrine receptor status, and lymph node involvement. These four factors are used to decide who will benefit from adjuvant chemotherapy, radiotherapy, or tamoxifen treatment. *(Fauci, Chapter 86)*

27. **(A)** Observation alone is adequate for this lesion. The "ABCD" rules are helpful in distinguishing benign skin lesions from malignant melanoma. (A) asymmetry: benign lesions are symmetric; (B) border irregular: most nevi have clear-cut borders; (C) color variation: benign lesions have uniform color; (D) diameter: >6 mm is more likely to be malignant. In addition, recent rapid change in size is also helpful in distinguishing benign from malignant lesions. Thickness of the tumor is the most important prognostic factor in the majority of cases, and ulceration indicates a more aggressive cancer with a poorer prognosis. Although cumulative sun exposure is a major factor in melanoma (eg, more frequent near the equator), it cannot explain such things as the more common occurrence of some types in relatively young people. It is possible that brief, intense exposure to sunlight may contribute to, or initiate, carcinogenic events. *(Fauci, Chapter 83)*

28. **(B)** Prognosis of patients with non-Hodgkin lymphoma is best assessed with the International Prognostic Index. It is an index with 5 clinical risk factors that helps to predict the 5-year survival. Poor prognostic factors are: age >60 years; high serum LDH level; poor performance status (either Eastern Cooperative Oncology Group [ECOG] >2, or Karnofsky <70); Ann Arbor stage III or IV, or >1 extranodal involvement. *(Fauci, Chapter 105)*

29. **(A)** IgG spikes >3.5 g/dL or IgA >2 g/dL strongly suggest myeloma rather than monoclonal gammopathies of undetermined significance (MGUS). MGUS is suggested when the spike is <3.5 g/dL, the marrow has fewer than 10% plasma cells, and the Bence Jones proteinuria is <1.0 g/day. Depressed hemoglobin levels, elevated calcium levels, progressive bone lesions, and impaired renal function suggest more advanced stages of multiple myeloma. *(Fauci, Chapter 105)*

30. **(C)** The most characteristic presentation of Hodgkin disease is that of enlarged, superficial cervical or supraclavicular lymph nodes in a young person. The nodes are usually freely moveable, nontender, and not painful. Occult presentation with intrathoracic or intra-abdominal disease is unusual. *(Fauci, Chapter 105)*

31. **(D)** Native Americans of both sexes have low cancer rates, but cancer rates (for women) for stomach, biliary tract, cervix, and kidney are surprisingly high. *(Fauci, Chapter 79)*

32. **(B)** Whites have high rates for melanoma, lymphoma, leukemia, and lip cancer. *(Fauci, Chapter 83)*

33. **(B)** Whites have high rates for breast, corpus uteri, testis, bladder, brain, colon, and rectum cancer. *(Fauci, Chapter 79)*

34. **(A)** Although Hispanic Americans have relatively low cancer rates (66% of that for White Americans and 54% of that for Black Americans), they do have high rates for cancer of the cervix. *(Fauci, Chapter 93)*

35. **(E)** Chinese Americans have a rate of nasopharyngeal cancer 23 times greater than White Americans, and liver cancer rates 7 times greater than White Americans. *(Fauci, Chapter 84)*

36. **(F)** Japanese Americans have a threefold increase in stomach cancer rate compared to White Americans, but this is lower than rates in Japan. *(Fauci, Chapter 87)*

37. **(C)** The excess risk of cancers of the stomach, esophagus, lung, and cervix among Black Americans is diminished when socioeconomic variations are factored in. *(Fauci, Chapter 87)*

38. **(A)** Alcoholic beverages combine with tobacco smoking to increase cancer of the mouth and, by causing cirrhosis, can lead to liver cancer. *(Fauci, Chapter 84)*

39. **(D)** Asbestos exposure causes more deaths from lung cancer (twofold increase) than from mesothelioma (hundredfold increase) because the latter tumor is so rare. *(Fauci, Chapter 85)*

40. **(F)** Sun exposure severe enough to cause sunburn is associated with increased risk of melanoma, whereas other skin cancers are more related to cumulative exposure. *(Fauci, Chapter 83)*

41. **(I)** Although causation is not definite, a high proportion of cervical cancers reveal HPV-16 and HPV-18 on biopsy. HPV has also been isolated from vulvar, penile, and anal cancers. *(Fauci, Chapter 93)*

42. **(H)** Cirrhosis, related to chronic HBV infection, is a leading cause of HCC. *(Fauci, Chapter 88)*

43. **(C)** Adenocarcinoma is now the most common form of lung cancer, accounting for 40% of the total cases. *(Fauci, Chapter 85)*

44. **(B)** Because of its tendency for early exfoliation and obstruction, squamous cell cancer is often detected at an earlier stage. Even correcting for this, there is some suggestion that its prognosis is still better, perhaps because of its slow growth rate. *(Fauci, Chapter 85)*

45. **(B)** Nonmetastatic hypercalcemia occurs in up to 15% of all squamous cell cancers due to the production of parathyroid hormone-related peptide (PTH-rP). This is a paraneoplastic phenomenon. *(Fauci, Chapter 85)*

46. **(D)** SIADH occurs in up to 10% of all small cell cancers of the lung. SIADH, Cushing syndrome, and neurologic paraneoplastic syndromes usually occur with small cell lung cancer, not nonsmall cell lung cancer. *(Fauci, Chapter 85)*

47. **(D)** Eaton-Lambert syndrome is unusual, but small cell lung cancer causes the majority of cases that are paraneoplastic. *(Fauci, Chapter 85)*

48. **(G)** Cisplatin is used for the treatment of many different cancers including testicular cancer. Its major toxicities are renal, ototoxicity, myelosuppression, and peripheral neuropathy. The neuropathy is dose and duration dependent. *(Fauci, Chapter 81)*

49. **(A)** Liver toxicity is most common when methotrexate is used on a daily basis, such as for psoriasis. Myelosuppression and GI mucositis are the most common side effects in cancer therapy. *(Fauci, Chapter 81)*

50. (D) Although lung injury is the most serious complication of bleomycin, this unusual skin reaction is more frequent, occurring in almost 50% of patients. *(Fauci, Chapter 81)*

51. (E) Doxorubicin can cause a cumulative, dose-dependent cardiomyopathy that can result in congestive heart failure. However, an acute, non-dose-related myocarditis-pericarditis can also occur. It can cause arrhythmias, heart failure, or pericardial effusions. *(Fauci, Chapter 81)*

52. (I) Cyclophosphamide causes hemorrhagic cystitis in up to 10% of patients because active metabolites are excreted. Adequate hydration and frequent urination can decrease the frequency of this complication. *(Fauci, Chapter 81)*

53. (D) Papillary cancer has the best prognosis of all thyroid cancers. Although it is 7 times more common than follicular cancer, fewer people die from it. Even with follicular cancer, most patients will die of other diseases. In common with other thyroid cancers, age seems to be an independent risk factor for poor prognosis. *(Fauci, Chapter 335)*

54. (B) Although well-differentiated thyroid cancer is twice as common in Whites than in Blacks, the proportion that is follicular is more than twice as high in Blacks. *(Fauci, Chapter 335)*

55. (E) Serum calcitonin elevation is specific for medullary thyroid cancer and is the most specific tumor marker now available. When combined with provocative agents (eg, calcium, pentagastrin), it is also very sensitive. In the familial syndrome, provocative tests have been superseded by genetic studies. *(Fauci, Chapter 335)*

56. (B) Nodular sclerosing Hodgkin disease is more common in women, and is particularly common in younger age groups but can occur at any age. *(Fauci, Chapter 105)*

57. (A) In lymphocyte-predominant Hodgkin disease, multiple sections often have to be examined to find Reed–Sternberg cells. Some authorities question whether such cells are necessary for diagnosis of this form. Variants, often called lymphocytic and histiocytic (L&H), or popcorn cells, are often frequently found. *(Fauci, Chapter 105)*

58. (A) Most patients with lymphocyte-predominant Hodgkin disease have clinically localized disease and are asymptomatic; the prognosis is usually favorable. However, it accounts for only 4%–5% of cases. *(Fauci, Chapter 105)*

59. (F) This is a frequent accompaniment of Hodgkin disease and can be found in involved lymph nodes, and may be extensive enough to obscure the presence of Hodgkin disease. Rather than evidence of occult involvement, the presence of granulomas implies stage for stage, a better prognosis than those without this reaction. *(Fauci, Chapter 105)*

60. (A) Prostaglandins play a role in bone resorption in metastatic disease, perhaps explaining the effectiveness of NSAIDs for this type of pain. Aspirin has been shown to have an anti-tumor effect in an animal bone tumor model. *(Fauci, Chapter 11)*

61. (D) Carbamazepine is an anticonvulsant used widely as an adjuvant analgesic for neuralgic pain caused by either tumor infiltration or surgical nerve injury. Because cancer patients commonly have compromised hematologic reserve, leukopenia and thrombocytopenia caused by carbamazepine may limit its use. *(Fauci, Chapter 11)*

62. (G) Steroids are useful for controlling pain in patients with leptomeningeal metastases or headache from increased intracranial pressure. *(Fauci, Chapter 11)*

63. (C) Usually, sedation can be controlled by altering opioid dosage, or switching to a drug with a shorter half-life, as well as stopping other sedating medications. If this fails, amphetamine, methylphenidate, and caffeine can be used to counteract the sedative effect. *(Fauci, Chapter 11)*

CHAPTER 7

Neurology
Questions

DIRECTIONS (Questions 1 through 30): For each of the questions in this section select the one lettered answer that is the best response in each case.

1. A 69-year-old woman presents to the clinic with memory difficulty. The patient's daughter is concerned that her mother is having difficulty doing her finances, such as paying bills. Memory impairment testing reveals the poor ability to generate lists of words or copy diagrams (intersecting pentagons). Her remaining physical examination is normal. **Which of the following anatomic findings is most likely with her condition?**

   (A) atrophy of the medial temporal lobes
   (B) diffuse atrophy of the cerebral cortex and temporal lobes
   (C) cranial nerve involvement
   (D) transient episodes of hemiplegia
   (E) atrophy of the caudate

2. A 38-year-old man presents with involuntary facial grimacing, shrugging of the shoulders, and jerking movements of the limb. His father was similarly affected. There is also a history of mood changes for the past 3 months. On examination, he appears restless with intermittent slow movements of his hands and face. He has difficulty performing rapid finger movements, and tone is decreased in the upper and lower limbs. **Which of the following is most likely to represent the progression of his illness?**

   (A) a normal life span
   (B) a 50% chance of only male children being similarly affected
   (C) mental deterioration
   (D) eventual development of rigidity
   (E) development of hemiparesis

3. An 18-year-old woman presents to the emergency room because of a transient episode of blurry vision, followed by ataxia, dysarthria, and tinnitus. The symptoms lasted for 30 minutes and were then followed by a throbbing occipital headache. She had a similar episode a few months ago, and went to see her family doctor, who performed stroke investigations that were normal and no clear diagnosis was made. She was instructed to come to the hospital if the symptoms were to reoccur. She otherwise feels well, has no significant past medical history and is not taking any medications. Her physical examination is normal. **Which of the following is the most likely diagnosis?**

   (A) vertebral-basilar insufficiency
   (B) basilar artery dissection
   (C) classic migraine
   (D) ophthalmoplegic migraine
   (E) basilar migraine

4. A 6-month-old child presents with recurrent seizures and poor development. The evaluation reveals a baby with hydrocephalus, impaired movement of the extremities, hypotonia, and retinal abnormalities. A computerized tomography (CT) scan demonstrates large ventricles and calcified lesions. **Which of the following is the most likely diagnosis?**

   (A) Tay–Sachs disease

   (B) congenital hydrocephalus

   (C) kernicterus

   (D) toxoplasmosis

   (E) congenital neurosyphilis

5. A 74-year-old woman develops acute neurologic symptoms and presents to the emergency room. Her past medical history is significant for type 2 diabetes, hypertension, and dyslipidemia. An urgent magnetic resonance imaging (MRI) scan demonstrates acute occlusion in the right posterior cerebral artery. **Which of the following clinical symptoms is she most likely to have?**

   (A) homonymous hemianopia

   (B) total blindness

   (C) expressive aphasia

   (D) ataxia and dysarthria

   (E) a right-sided hemiplegia

6. A 53-year-old man presents to the clinic for assessment of symptoms of clumsiness with both hands. He gives examples such as difficulty doing up the buttons on his shirt or using his keys to open the door.

   On physical examination, the pertinent findings are fasciculations of his thigh and forearm muscles; diffuse muscle weakness grade 4/5, loss of muscle bulk, and increased tone in the upper and lower limbs. There is also generalized hyperreflexia, and positive plantar signs (Babinski) bilaterally. **Which of the following is the most likely natural progression of this condition?**

   (A) a long history of remissions and exacerbations

   (B) sensory loss in the distribution of peripheral nerves

   (C) focal seizures

   (D) a progressively downhill course

   (E) cogwheel rigidity

7. A 22-year-old woman presents to the emergency room with acute vision loss and pain in the left eye, but no other symptoms. On physical examination she appears well, blood pressure is 122/74 mm Hg, visual acuity in the affected eye is not possible, and she can only perceive movement and bright light. The direct pupillary reflex is absent but the indirect (consensual) response is normal. On funduscopy, the optic disc appears edematous. **Which of the following symptoms is also most likely present in a patient with this condition?**

   (A) limb weakness

   (B) hemiplegia

   (C) cervical myelopathy

   (D) sphincter impairment

   (E) seizures

8. A 63-year-old man presents to the emergency department because of transient symptoms of vertigo, slurred speech, diplopia, and paresthesias. He is symptom-free now, and clinical examination is entirely normal. His past medical history is significant for osteoarthritis, hypertension, and dyslipidemia. **Which of the following is the most likely cause for symptoms?**

   (A) posterior circulation transient ischemic attack (TIA)

   (B) anterior communicating artery aneurysm

   (C) hypertensive encephalopathy

   (D) pseudobulbar palsy

   (E) occlusion of the middle cerebral artery

9. A 75-year-old woman presents to the clinic because she is experiencing symptoms of visual change and facial weakness. On examination, the pupils are equal and reactive to light, the fundi appear normal, and there is a right homonymous visual field defect. There is also left-sided facial weakness with forehead sparing. **Which of the following is the most likely cause of the right homonymous hemianopia?**

(A) right optic nerve

(B) chiasm

(C) right optic radiations

(D) right occipital lobe

(E) left optic radiations

10. A 10-year-old boy is seen in the clinic for his annual assessment. He is doing well and reports no concerns. On physical examination, there are multiple tan-colored patches on his skin, and freckle-like skin changes in his armpit area. The remaining clinical examination is normal. **Which of the following conditions is also found in patients with this disorder as they get older?**

(A) bilateral eighth nerve tumors

(B) irregular small pupils

(C) multiple cutaneous and subcutaneous tumors

(D) cataracts

(E) hip involvement

11. A 56-year-old man is brought to the emergency department by his wife because of memory loss and difficulty walking. She has noticed personality changes, truancy from work, and lack of personal care over the past 1 year. On examination, he appears unkempt, smells of urine, and is uncooperative. He cannot recall the date or season, and gets angry when asked questions. His answers are often fabricated when checked with his wife.

The blood pressure is 150/90 mm Hg, pulse 100/min, and he is diaphoretic and tremulous. His gait is wide based, and motor strength and reflexes are normal. His ocular movements are normal but there is nystagmus on lateral gaze. In the past, he has had multiple admissions for alcohol withdrawal. **Which of the following is the most appropriate next step in management?**

(A) prophylactic phenytoin administration

(B) prophylactic diazepam administration

(C) prophylactic carbamazepine administration

(D) calcium administration

(E) steroid administration

12. A 60-year-old man is brought to the emergency department because of new symptoms of double vision and discomfort in his left eye. He reports no other neurologic symptoms. On physical examination, there is ptosis of the left eyelid, the eye is rotated down and out, and the pupil is 3 mm and reactive to light. The right eye is normal, and there are no other focal neurological deficits. **Which of the following is the most likely diagnosis?**

(A) fourth nerve palsy

(B) diabetic autonomic neuropathy

(C) third nerve palsy

(D) sixth nerve palsy

(E) seventh nerve palsy

13. A 48-year-old man complains of recurrent episodes of sudden-onset dizziness. He notices an abrupt onset of a "spinning" sensation when sitting up or lying down in bed. The symptoms last for 30 seconds and then resolve completely. He has no hearing change or other neurologic symptoms, and his physical examination is completely normal. A Dix–Hallpike maneuver reproduces his symptoms. **Which of the following is the most likely mechanism for his vertigo symptoms?**

(A) basilar migraine

(B) brain stem ischemic events

(C) benign cerebellar tumors

(D) calcium debris (calcium carbonate crystals) in the semicircular canals

(E) Meniere disease

14. A 40-year-old man is injured in a car accident and fractures his left elbow. He now complains of numbness of his fourth and fifth fingers, and weakness in his hand grip. Neurologic findings confirm weakness of handgrip with weakness of finger abduction and adduction, and decreased sensation over the fifth finger and lateral aspect of fourth finger. **Which of the following is the most likely diagnosis?**

(A) ulnar nerve injury

(B) radial nerve injury

(C) median nerve injury

(D) carpal tunnel syndrome

(E) axillary nerve injury

15. A 31-year-old woman complains of excessive sleepiness during the daytime for years despite adequate nighttime sleep. She has episodes of intense drowsiness 3–4 times a day, even when at work or while eating meals. She has sought medical attention in the past, after falling asleep while driving. She is slender and otherwise healthy and on no medications. **Which of the following treatments is most likely indicated for her condition?**

(A) a device providing continuous positive airway pressure (CPAP) at night

(B) oral surgery

(C) tracheostomy

(D) amphetamine type medication (modafinil)

(E) benzodiazepines at bedtime

16. A 43-year-old man presents to the emergency department with symptoms of difficulty in walking. The symptoms are gradually getting worse and he reports falling on numerous occasions. His past medical history is significant for chronic alcoholism and withdrawal. On physical examination, he appears unkempt, and there are multiple abrasions and bruises on the skin. He is not oriented to the day of the week, date, or month, but knows the year and location. His motor strength, reflexes, and ocular movements are normal. The gait is wide based, and there is loss of sensation in his feet up to the shins. **Which of the following is the most likely diagnosis?**

(A) Wernicke encephalopathy

(B) Wernicke–Korsakoff syndrome

(C) Alzheimer dementia

(D) Charcot–Marie–Tooth disease

(E) vascular dementia

17. A 59-year-old woman presents to the clinic for assessment of numbness and tingling in her feet. The symptoms started gradually and are now getting worse because of progression up her legs. On physical examination, there is decreased vibration and pain sensation in the feet up to the mid-shin, and loss of the ankle jerk reflexes. The sensory findings are symmetric. **Which of the following medical conditions is most likely to explain her peripheral nerve findings?**

(A) heart disease

(B) dermatomyositis

(C) hypothyroidism

(D) diabetes mellitus

(E) adrenal insufficiency

18. An 84-year-old man presents with progressive headaches, light headedness, drowsiness, and unsteady gait over 4 weeks. On examination, his blood pressure is 160/90 mm Hg, pulse 70/min, lungs clear, and he has no focal weakness. His gait is unsteady but sensation in the feet is normal. A CT scan reveals a partial hyperintense clot over the left cerebral cortex. **Which of the following is the most likely cause for this clot?**

(A) is venous in origin

(B) is arterial in origin

(C) is from injury to the middle meningeal artery

(D) is from a subarachnoid hemorrhage

(E) is from injury to the middle cerebral artery

19. A 68-year-old man presents to the clinic for evaluation of progressive hearing loss, ringing in his ears, and facial pain on the left side. The symptoms started 1 month ago. He has also noticed some difficulty with his balance, but reports no falls. Pertinent physical findings are an unsteady gait and decreased hearing in the

left ear. His eye movements, facial sensation, and facial movements are normal. An MR scan of the brain reveals a tumor at the cerebellopontine angle. **Which of the following cranial nerves is this tumor most likely to affect?**

(A) fourth cranial nerve

(B) sixth cranial nerve

(C) eighth cranial nerve

(D) tenth cranial nerve

(E) eleventh cranial nerve

20. A 25-year-old man presents to the out patient clinic complaining of feeling sleepy all the time, even during the daytime. The symptoms have persisted for years and are now brought to medical attention after falling asleep at work on multiple occasions. He is concerned that he might lose his job. He has no past medical history and is not taking any sedative medications. On physical examination, he is slender and the heart and lung exams are normal. Neurologic assessment reveals normal orientation, memory, concentration, and no focal deficits. **Which of the following symptoms might he also complain about?**

(A) excessive snoring (wife's report)

(B) automatic behavior (wife's report)

(C) restless sleep (wife's report)

(D) paresthesias

(E) morning headache

21. A 17-year-old woman presents to the clinic with symptoms of a fine tremor of her hands, weight loss, palpitations, and new amenorrhea. On physical examination, her blood pressure is 92/66 mm Hg, heart rate 110/min, and the tremor is best seen when her hands are stretched out. She is not on any medications and reports no alcohol use. **Which of the following is the most likely diagnosis?**

(A) hypopituitarism

(B) marijuana use

(C) hyperthyroidism

(D) myxedema

(E) iron overdose

22. A 19-year-old man presents to the clinic for evaluation of poor balance and difficulty running while playing sports. In the past year, he has also developed hand clumsiness and poor coordination. Physical examination reveals pes cavus, kyphoscoliosis, and both cerebellar findings and sensory loss in the legs. There is a positive family history of Friedreich ataxia. **Where are the pathologic changes seen in this condition?**

(A) spinal cord tracts

(B) basal ganglia

(C) cerebral cortex

(D) peripheral autonomic nerves

(E) peripheral motor nerves

23. A 24-year-old man is brought to the clinic by his family for assessment of jaundice, tremor, and personality changes. His past medical history is negative and he denies any recreational drug use. Physical examination reveals slowness of finger movements, rigidity, and coarse tremor of the outstretched hands. As well there is abnormal slow movement of the tongue and pharynx resulting in a change in speech and occasional difficulty swallowing. He is icteric, the liver span is 10 cm, and no spleen is palpable. **Which of the following findings is most likely seen in this condition?**

(A) a reduction of copper excretion in the urine

(B) an increase of the serum ceruloplasmin content

(C) no renal involvement

(D) retention of normal neurologic movements

(E) a peculiar greenish-brown pigmentation of the cornea

24. A 52-year-old man presents to the out-patient clinic complaining of episodes of severe unilateral, stabbing facial pain that is intermittent for several hours, and then disappears for several days. The pain is described as "electric shock-like" and only lasts a few seconds. Physical examination of the face and mouth is entirely normal. **Which of the following treatments is most effective for this condition?**

(A) morphine

(B) indomethacin

(C) cimetidine

(D) carbamazepine

(E) lidocaine (Xylocaine) gel

25. A 63-year-old woman presents to the emergency department complaining of nausea, vomiting, and dizziness, which started suddenly earlier in the day. She describes the dizziness as a to-and-fro movement of the room like as if she is on a boat. She has never experienced symptoms like these before. **Which of the following findings suggests the vertigo is central in origin?**

(A) deafness

(B) symptoms are more protracted but less severe

(C) unidirectional nystagmus

(D) visual fixation inhibits vertigo and nystagmus

(E) spinning sensation is toward the fast phase of nystagmus

26. A 30-year-old woman presents to the clinic complaining of double vision, and easy fatigue while exercising. The fatigue improves with resting, but it is interfering with her work. Physical examination reveals ptosis and impaired eye movements with normal pupillary response. The double vision is brought out by asking her to look at the ceiling, and after a sustained interval, the eyes slowly drift down. **Which of the following is the most likely diagnosis?**

(A) optic atrophy

(B) ophthalmic zoster

(C) paralysis agitans

(D) Horner syndrome

(E) myasthenia gravis

27. A 47-year-old woman presents to the clinic for assessment of increasing headaches and visual changes. She has no prior history of headaches or migraines, and her only significant past medical history is pre-eclampsia during her first pregnancy. After delivery, her blood pressure returned to normal. On examination, her pupils are normal and reactive to light, the extraocular movements are normal, but there are visual field defects of the outer half in both eyes (bitemporal hemianopsia). The remaining neurologic examination is normal. **Which of the following is the most likely diagnosis?**

(A) pituitary adenoma

(B) falx meningioma

(C) craniopharyngioma

(D) aneurysm of the internal carotid artery

(E) glioblastoma

28. A 45-year-old man presents to the clinic for evaluation of weakness in his arms and legs. The symptoms started gradually, and are now more noticeable and interfering with his ability to work as an electrician. On physical examination, the cranial nerves are normal, but there is weakness of his left handgrip and right leg quadriceps with loss of muscle bulk. There are obvious fasciculations over the left forearm and right thigh. Tone is increased in the arms and legs and the reflexes are brisk. **Which of the following is the most likely diagnosis?**

(A) amyotrophic lateral sclerosis (ALS)

(B) myotonic muscular dystrophy

(C) amyotonia congenita

(D) tabes dorsalis

(E) migraine

29. A 79-year-old woman is brought to the clinic for assessment of frequent falls. There is no loss of consciousness associated with the falls, and she reports no postural change or symptoms prior to the falls. She also describes difficulty in "getting going" when she starts walking and notices that her balance is "not right." Her gait is slow and shuffling on inspection. **Which of**

the following is the most likely finding in a patient with Parkinson disease?

(A) fine hand tremor with movement
(B) muscle atrophy
(C) akinesia
(D) pupillary constriction
(E) spontaneous remission

30. A 47-year-old man presents to the emergency room with symptoms of dizziness and difficulty walking. He describes his dizziness as a spinning sensation of the room with associated nausea and vomiting. **Which of the following findings suggests the vertigo is peripheral in origin?**

(A) optic neuritis
(B) tinnitus
(C) bidirectional nystagmus
(D) vertical nystagmus
(E) visual fixation does not affect vertigo or nystagmus

DIRECTIONS (Questions 31 through 39): The following group of numbered items is preceded by a list of lettered options. For each question, select the one lettered option that is most closely associated with it. Each lettered option may be used once, multiple times, or not at all.

Questions 31 and 32: For each patient with neurologic symptoms, select the most likely structural pathology.

(A) aqueductal stenosis
(B) infectious process
(C) enlarged foramina of Luschka
(D) agenesis of the corpus callosum
(E) acoustic neuroma

31. A 77-year-old woman presents with headaches and difficulty walking. She has an unbalanced gait and falls easily, especially when trying to walk upstairs. The tone is normal and there are no cerebellar findings. A CT scan reveals enlarged ventricles.

32. A 23-year-old woman presents with arm weakness, decreasing vision in her right eye, and difficulty with her balance. An MRI of the brain reveals multiple demyelinating lesions.

Questions 33 through 36: For each patient with altered level of consciousness, select the most likely diagnosis.

(A) basal ganglia hemorrhage
(B) cerebellar hemorrhage
(C) pontine hemorrhage
(D) lobar intracerebral hemorrhage
(E) cocaine-related hemorrhage
(F) subarachnoid hemorrhage
(G) arteriovenous malformation (AVM)
(H) hypertensive encephalopathy
(I) primary intraventricular hemorrhage

33. A 67-year-old man develops coma over a few minutes. He is unresponsive on arrival to the hospital. He has ataxic respirations and pinpoint, reactive pupils. Oculocephalic reflexes are absent. There is no motor response with noxious stimulation.

34. A 74-year-old woman develops occipital headache, vomiting, and dizziness. She looks unwell, her blood pressure is 180/100 mm Hg, pulse is 70/min, and respirations are 30/min. She is unable to sit or walk because of unsteadiness. Over the next few hours, she develops a decline in her level of consciousness.

35. A 52-year-old man, with poorly controlled hypertension in the past, presents with increasing headache, confusion, and vomiting. His blood pressure is 230/125 mm Hg, pulse 60/min, respirations 24/min, and there is papilledema. He has no focal deficits.

36. A 24-year-old man has a history of recurrent throbbing headaches. He suddenly develops mild right-sided weakness. His blood pressure in the past has been normal but is now slightly elevated.

Questions 37 through 39: For each patient with a neurologic condition, select the most likely associated findings.

   (A) hyperkalemia

   (B) weakness and atrophy of the hands

   (C) hypokalemia

   (D) hypercalcemia

   (E) convulsions

37. A 20-year-old man develops fatigue and severe muscle weakness of his limbs usually after eating a large meal. He is diagnosed with familial periodic paralysis.

38. An 11-year-old girl with a diagnosis of tuberous sclerosis.

39. A 23-year-old woman with impaired pain and temperature sensation in her arms but normal light touch. A CT scan reveals dilatation of the central part of the spinal cord in the cervical region (syringomyelia).

DIRECTIONS (Questions 40 through 55): For each of the questions in this section select the one lettered answer that is the best response in each case.

40. A 27-year-old woman complains of double vision and fatigue at the end of the day. Further history reveals difficulty in chewing food, and some weakness in climbing stairs. She has stopped running because of easy leg fatigue and leg weakness. The symptoms improve with resting.

    On examination, there is weakness of the eyelids, masticatory muscles, and thigh flexors. Her handgrip decreases with repetitive action. There is no sensory abnormality, and reflexes are normal. **Which of the following is the most likely diagnosis?**

   (A) hypercalcemia

   (B) myasthenia gravis

   (C) multiple sclerosis

   (D) thyroid storm

   (E) meningeal lymphoma

41. A 20-year-old man suffered a clinically significant closed head injury after a diving accident. He is left with minor memory impairment but makes a full recovery. A few months later, he has a witnessed loss of consciousness with some arm and leg twitching. After the event, he is disoriented for 2 hours and then gradually returns to baseline. There was no incontinence or tongue biting, and his examination is normal. **Which of the following is the most likely diagnosis?**

   (A) syncope

   (B) generalized seizure

   (C) focal seizure

   (D) cardiac arrhythmia

   (E) drop attack

42. A 22-year-old woman presents with fever, headache, and confusion. She has not been herself for the past 2 days, including not going to work and forgetting events. On examination, she is moving all her limbs, but not oriented to place or time. The remaining examination is normal. A CT scan shows bilateral, small, low-density temporal lobe lesions. Cerebrospinal fluid (CSF) shows mononuclear cell pleocytosis (increased cell count), increased protein, and normal glucose. The electroencephalogram (EEG) shows bilateral periodic discharges from the temporal leads and slow-wave complexes at regular intervals of 2–3/sec. **Which of the following is the most appropriate treatment for her condition?**

   (A) penicillin

   (B) chloramphenicol

   (C) acyclovir

   (D) erythromycin

   (E) steroids

43. A 67-year-old woman with hypertension presents with sudden onset of headache, vomiting, and left-sided weakness. On examination, she has weakness of the left side of her face, hand, and leg (graded 3 out of 5). The blood pressure is 180/100 mm Hg, heart rate 72/min, and respirations 20/min. **Which of the following is the most appropriate initial diagnostic test?**

(A) CT scan with contrast

(B) MR scan with gadolinium

(C) CT scan without contrast

(D) MR cerebral angiogram

(E) conventional cerebral angiogram

44. A 77-year-old woman develops acute hoarseness, difficulty swallowing, dizziness, and falling to the right side. On examination, there is decreased sensation to pain on the right side of her face and left side of her body. The palate and pharynx move very little on the right side, and there is loss of coordination of the right arm and leg. Motor power in the arms and legs is normal. While attempting to walk, she falls to the right side, and complains of vertigo. An MRI scan confirms the diagnosis of the ischemic stroke. **Which of the following is the most likely location of the stroke?**

(A) right medial medulla

(B) right lateral medulla

(C) right internal capsule

(D) right parietal cortex

(E) right cerebellum

45. A 27-year-old woman, a recent immigrant from the Caribbean basin, has had progressive leg weakness. Physical examination reveals increased tone of both legs with weakness, clonus, extensor plantar responses, and brisk reflexes. There is also loss of vibration and position senses in the feet. The upper extremities are normal. A clinical diagnosis of tropical spastic paraparesis (TSP) is made. **Which of the following is the most likely cause of this condition?**

(A) human immunodeficiency virus (HIV) infection

(B) cytomegalovirus (CMV) infection

(C) human T-cell lymphotropic virus (HTLV)-1 infection

(D) thiamine deficiency

(E) central nervous system (CNS) tuberculosis infection

46. A 40-year-old woman complains of episodes of severe unilateral, stabbing facial pain that is intermittent for several hours, and then disappears for several days. Physical examination is entirely normal. **Which of the following is the most likely diagnosis?**

(A) trigeminal neuralgia

(B) herpes zoster

(C) acoustic neuroma

(D) Bell palsy

(E) diabetic neuropathy

47. A 63-year-old man suddenly becomes acutely ill with headache and fever of 38.9°C. There is pain in the eye, and the orbits are painful to pressure. There is edema and chemosis of the conjunctivae and eyelids, and the eye bulbs are proptosed. Diplopia and ptosis are present, and the pupils are slow in reacting. **Which of the following is the most likely diagnosis?**

(A) cavernous sinus thrombosis

(B) chorioretinitis

(C) subarachnoid hemorrhage

(D) brain abscess

(E) none of the above

48. A 20-year-old woman presents to the emergency department with a history of rapid loss of vision in one eye. Examination reveals pain on movement of the eyeball. The appearance of the fundi is normal, but the afferent pupillary response is diminished. The indirect papillary response is normal and visual field assessment by perimetry shows a large central scotoma. **Which of the following is the most likely diagnosis?**

(A) optic atrophy

(B) papilledema

(C) retrobulbar neuritis

(D) amblyopia ex anopsia

(E) hysteria

49. A 67-year-old man has 2 episodes of numbness on the left side of his body, which last 5 minutes. He now experiences transient loss of vision in his right eye lasting 2 minutes. On examination, his blood pressure is 155/90 mm Hg, pulse 80/min regular, and visual fields, extraocular movements, and pupils are all normal. The remaining motor and sensory examination is also normal. **Which of the following is the most likely diagnosis?**

   (A) posterior cerebral artery insufficiency
   (B) parietal lobe neoplasm
   (C) parasagittal meningioma
   (D) AVM
   (E) right internal carotid artery atherosclerosis

50. An 18-year-old man is brought to the emergency department after developing symptoms of fever, headache, confusion, and generalized seizures. On examination, he is moving all his limbs, but incoherent. The neck is supple, heart and lungs are normal. A lumbar puncture is performed and the CSF shows mononuclear cell pleocytosis, increased protein, and normal glucose. A CT scan of the brain is normal and a clinical diagnosis of HSV encephalitis is made. **Which of the following is the most appropriate next step in management?**

   (A) angiography
   (B) observing response to therapy
   (C) cerebral biopsy
   (D) acute viral titers
   (E) CSF culture

51. A 24-year-old woman presents with foot and leg weakness that is progressively getting worse over the past 1 week. Initially, she developed tingling in her feet and noticed that they would drag, but now she has difficulty standing and walking due to the leg weakness. Three weeks ago she had a "chest cold," which resolved on its own. On examination, muscle bulk is normal, motor strength is 2 out of 5 in the quadriceps, and 1 out of 5 in the feet. Reflexes at the ankle and knee are absent, and sensation testing is normal. The upper limb examination is normal. The CSF protein is very high, glucose is normal, and cell count is slightly elevated.

Which of the following is the most likely diagnosis?

   (A) diabetic neuropathy
   (B) alcoholic neuropathy
   (C) Guillain–Barré syndrome
   (D) cyanide poisoning
   (E) poliomyelitis

52. A 37-year-old woman complains of drooping eyelids, double vision, and fatigue at the end of the day. Further history reveals difficulty in chewing food, and some weakness in climbing stairs. The symptoms improve with resting. On examination, there is weakness of the eyelids, masticatory muscles, and thigh flexors. Her handgrip decreases with repetitive action. There is no sensory abnormality, and reflexes are normal. Her chest x-ray (CXR) is shown in Figures 7–1 a and b. **Which of the following is the most likely diagnosis?**

Figure 7–1a.

Figure 7–1b.

(A) bronchogenic carcinoma

(B) Hodgkin disease

(C) teratoma

(D) thyroid tumor with retrosternal extension

(E) thymoma

53. A 79-year-old woman is seen in the office for "dizziness." **Which of the following findings would suggest true vertigo?**

(A) the patient is taking multiple antihypertensives

(B) the symptoms are worse on standing

(C) she has had 2 falls

(D) the room is spinning around her

(E) a prior Holter monitor was negative during episodes of dizziness

54. A 65-year-old woman comes to the clinic for assessment of recurrent episodes of dizziness and nausea. She describes an abrupt onset of a spinning sensation when moving her head. The symptoms last for 20 seconds and then completely resolve. She reports no hearing change or other neurologic symptoms, and her physical examination is completely normal. A Dix–Hallpike maneuver reproduces her symptoms. **Which of the following findings on vestibular testing favors the diagnosis of benign paroxysmal positional vertigo (BPPV) over central positional vertigo?**

(A) no latency period

(B) no fatigability

(C) habituation occurs

(D) mild vertigo

(E) symptoms consistently the same from one set of tests to the next

55. A 23-year-old man complains of intermittent double vision and fatigue. The symptoms are worse at the end of the day, and he has stopped working as a courier because of easy leg fatigue and weakness. He finds that the symptoms improve with resting. On physical examination, there is weakness of the eyelids, masticatory muscles, and thigh flexors. Having him look up at the ceiling for a long time brings on his double vision. There is no sensory abnormality, and reflexes are normal. **Which of the following treatments is contraindicated in this patient?**

(A) anticholinergic drugs

(B) surgery

(C) plasmapheresis

(D) cyclophosphamide

(E) high-dose prednisone

DIRECTIONS (Questions 56 through 75): The following group of numbered items is preceded by a list of lettered options. For each question, select the one lettered option that is most closely associated with it. Each lettered option may be used once, multiple times, or not at all.

Questions 56 through 60: For each patient with clinical symptoms and signs, select the most likely seizure type.

(A) simple partial seizure

(B) complex partial seizures

(C) tonic-clonic (grand mal) seizures

(D) absence (petit mal) seizures

(E) myoclonic seizures

(F) status epilepticus

56. A 55-year-old man presents with increasing shortness of breath, decreased urine output, malaise, nausea, and vomiting. He has a history of hypertension, chronic renal failure, and coronary artery disease. His laboratory data reveal very high urea and creatinine, consistent with acute on chronic renal failure. He also notes having intermittent "twitching" in his arms and legs that started recently.

57. A 24-year-old woman complains of having intermittent bouts of smelling burning rubber followed by lip smacking and chewing movements as observed by others. During these spells, she does not respond to questions. There has never been any complete loss of consciousness during these episodes either. An MRI of the brain reveals temporal lobe sclerosis.

58. A teenager has a long history of "daydreaming" in school. EEG reveals evidence of a generalized seizure disorder, but there has never been a history of convulsive muscular activity.

59. A 23-year-old woman has a history of repetitive involuntary movements of her right hand associated with abnormal facial movements. At times, the movements spread to involve the entire arm.

60. This form of epilepsy almost always starts in childhood.

Questions 61 through 65: For each type of seizure, select the most appropriate therapy.

    (A) phenytoin
    (B) carbamazepine
    (C) phenobarbital
    (D) primidone
    (E) sodium valproate (valproic acid)
    (F) ethosuximide
    (G) lorazepam
    (H) trimethadione

61. It is the drug of choice for absence attacks.

62. It is the drug of choice for myoclonic seizures.

63. It is the drug of choice for generalized tonic-clonic (grand mal) seizures.

64. It is the drug of choice for partial seizures.

65. It is the drug of choice for status epilepticus.

Questions 66 through 70: For each patient with a pupillary abnormality, select the most likely diagnosis.

    (A) essential anisocoria
    (B) Horner syndrome
    (C) tonic pupils (Holmes–Adie syndrome)
    (D) Argyll Robertson pupils
    (E) midbrain pupils
    (F) atropinized pupils
    (G) oculomotor palsy

66. A 63-year-old man is noticed to have asymmetric pupils. He is completely well and has no symptoms. On examination, the left pupil is small, round, and has a brisk response to light and near stimuli (accommodation). There is also ptosis of the left eyelid, but no other ocular movement abnormality or symptoms of double vision.

67. A 23-year-old woman is noticed to have irregular pupils on routine examination. She has 1 large pupil, which has minimal response to light stimulation, but it does respond to accommodation. The eye movements are normal and she experiences no double vision.

68. A 57-year-old woman presents for evaluation of memory loss. She is noticed to have small, irregular pupils that respond poorly to light but pupillary response to accommodation is normal.

69. A 24-year-old man notices different size pupils. The left pupil is 1 mm larger than the right. Both pupils respond normally to light and accommodation. The discrepancy in the pupils is still there in low, medium, and bright light conditions. He reports no other visual symptoms.

70. A 64-year-old woman is having double vision and severe headaches. On examination, the left pupil is dilated compared to the right, and the light response is diminished.

Questions 71 through 75: For each patient with muscle weakness, select the most likely anatomic site for the disorder.

 (A) anterior horn cell
 (B) peripheral nerve
 (C) neuromuscular junction
 (D) muscle

71. A 48-year-old man complains of muscle weakness in his right hand (dominant hand). On examination, the hand muscles are smaller than on the left, and the reflexes are decreased out of proportion to weakness.

72. A 26-year-old woman complains of early fatigue and weakness in doing strenuous activity. Her symptoms are worse near the end of the day. She appears well, muscle bulk, tone, and reflexes are normal. Handgrip strength decreases with repetitive testing.

73. A 63-year-old woman has noticed weakness in her right hand such that she is having difficulty writing and doing up buttons. On examination, there is marked atrophy of the forearm and hand muscles with fasciculations. Tone is increased and reflexes are brisk. Sensory testing in the hand is normal. There are also fasciculations on her thighs, which she has never noticed before.

74. A 49-year-old man notices weakness and numbness in his left hand. He had recently slipped on a wet floor and injured his elbow. Examination of the hand reveals predominantly weakness to abduction and adduction and sensory loss over the fourth and fifth fingers.

75. A 67-year-old man with lung cancer notices symptoms of weakness in his arms and legs. He describes difficulty in rising out of chair or going upstairs, but no pain or discomfort. On examination, proximal muscle strength is 4 out of 5 in the upper and lower limbs, but the reflexes, tone, and sensation are normal. He has a colored rash on his eyelids, and raised papules on his knuckles.

Answers and Explanations

1. **(B)** Alzheimer disease (AD) can be quite diffuse, but there is particular involvement of the medial temporal lobes and cortical association areas. The atrophy of the hippocampus is particularly marked. Microscopic examination reveals neurofibrillary tangles and amyloid plaques. Hemiplegia is not a feature of AD and suggests more vascular disease and vascular dementia. The cranials nerves are not involved in AD. *(Fauci, Chapter 365)*

2. **(C)** This is a case of Huntington chorea. It is an autosomal dominant gene (found on the short arm of chromosome 4), and male and female children are equally affected. Movement disorder, mental deterioration, and personality change are the hallmarks of the disease, but can be very subtle initially. The disease starts typically between ages 35 and 40 (although the variation is wide) and runs its course in about 15 years. The akinetic rigid variety (Westphal variant) of Huntington's typically has a childhood onset. *(Fauci, Chapter 367)*

3. **(E)** Basilar migraine can be very dramatic, and can resemble ischemia in the territory of the basilar posterior cerebral arteries. The visual symptoms of basilar migraine typically affect the whole of both visual fields, and can even cause temporary cortical blindness. There can also be an alarming period of coma or quadriplegia. The rapid recovery in symptoms in this patient followed by the pounding headache, her young age and lack of vascular risk factors make basilar migraine more probable than either vertebral-basilar insufficiency or basilar artery dissection. *(Fauci, Chapter 15)*

4. **(D)** Toxoplasmosis is the most likely diagnosis. The infection has a predilection for the CNS and the eye, and produces encephalitis in utero. Symptoms can be evident in the first few days of life. Infants born with active disease may have fever, rash, seizures, and hepatosplenomegaly at birth. *(Fauci, Chapter 207)*

5. **(A)** Occlusion of the right posterior cerebral artery is most likely to cause homonymous hemianopia. This artery conveys blood to the inferior and medial portion of the posterior temporal and occipital lobes and to the optic thalamus. Total blindness is usually not due to an ischemic stroke, unless it causes bilateral occipital cortex injury. Ataxia and dysarthria are more vertebral-basilar artery signs, and expressive aphasia is a cortical stroke sign due to middle cerebral artery territory involvement usually on the left side. Finally, a stroke in the right hemisphere will cause weakness on the left side of the body. *(Fauci, Chapter 364)*

6. **(D)** This man has amyotrophic lateral sclerosis (ALS). The disease causes neuronal loss in the anterior horns of the spinal cord and motor nuclei of the lower brain stem. The disease is one of constant progression, rather than remissions and exacerbations, and death usually occurs within 5 years. There is no sensory loss and no seizure diathesis, because only the motor system is involved. There can be signs of hyperreflexia and spasticity, depending on the balance of upper and lower motor neuron damage, but not cogwheel rigidity. *(Fauci, Chapter 369)*

7. **(A)** This patient has multiple sclerosis (MS). Weakness or numbness in one or more limbs is

the initial manifestation of disease in about half the patients. Other common initial presentations include optic neuritis (25%) and acute myelitis. Hemiplegia, seizures, and cervical myelopathy (in older patients) occur occasionally as the initial manifestation. Sphincter impairment usually occurs later in the disease. *(Fauci, Chapter 375)*

8. **(A)** Posterior circulation TIA is suggested by the constellation of symptoms (vertigo, dysarthria, and diplopia and the transient episode of his symptoms. The basilar artery is formed by the two vertebral arteries and supplies the pons, the midbrain, and the cerebellum. With vertebrobasilar TIAs, tinnitus, vertigo, diplopia, ataxia, hemiparesis, and bilateral visual impairment are common findings. This patient does not have occlusion of the middle cerebral artery since it results in cortical symptoms of motor and sensory loss on the contralateral side. This is also not hypertensive encephalopathy since it causes confusion, headache, nausea, vomiting, and focal neurologic signs. *(Fauci, Chapter 364)*

9. **(E)** The hemianopia is due to a lesion of the left optic radiations. The posterior cerebral artery arises from the basilar artery but is sometimes a branch of the internal carotid. With posterior cerebral artery lesions affecting the occipital cortex, it is possible for the hemianopia to be an isolated finding. *(Fauci, Chapter 364)*

10. **(C)** The two common forms of neurofibromatosis (NF-1 and NF-2) are genetically distinct. NF-1 is the type with multiple café au lait spots and is associated with axillary or inguinal freckling, iris hamartomas (Lisch nodules), peripheral neurofibromas, and boney abnormalities (including kyphoscoliosis). NF-2 is associated with CNS tumors, particularly bilateral eighth nerve tumors. Skin lesions are spare or absent, and early lens opacities can occur. *(Fauci, Chapter 54)*

11. **(B)** Prophylactic administration of diazepam in a withdrawing alcoholic can prevent or reduce severe syndromes such as delirium tremens (DTs). Prophylactic phenytoin, however, is not helpful. A calm, quiet environment with close observation and frequent reassurance is very important. Vitamin administration (especially thiamine) is important, but frequently, severe magnesium depletion slows improvement. *(Fauci, Chapter 387)*

12. **(C)** Third nerve palsy can result in ptosis of the eyelid. There is also loss of the ability to open the eye, and the eyeball is deviated outward and slightly downward. With complete lesions, the pupil is dilated, does not react to light, and loses the power of accommodation. In diabetes, the pupil is often spared. The sixth cranial nerve can also be affected by diabetes, but this is much less common. *(Fauci, Chapter 379)*

13. **(D)** This person has benign paroxysmal positional vertigo (BPPV), which is characterized by sudden-onset brief episodes of vertigo lasting less than a minute. The symptoms are usually brought on by head movement. The cause is commonly attributed to calcium debris in the semicircular canals, known as canalithiasis. The debris is loose otoconia (calcium carbonate) within the utricular sac. Although BPPV can occur after head trauma, there is usually no obvious precipitating factor. It generally abates spontaneously and can be treated with vestibular rehabilitation. Basilar migraine can cause vertigo, but it is not brought on by movement, there is an associated headache and lasts longer than the 30 seconds noticed in this patient. Brainstem ischemic events or cerebellar tumors can cause vertigo but the symptoms are persistent and not intermittent. Finally, Meniere disease also causes vertigo but there is associated hearing changes, and the symptoms last longer than in BPPV. *(Fauci, Chapter 22)*

14. **(A)** Injury to the ulnar nerve results in impaired adduction and abduction of the fingers. The nerve is commonly injured in elbow dislocations and fractures. The fibers arise from the eighth cervical and the first thoracic segments. The ulnar is a mixed nerve with sensory supply to the medial aspect of the hand. *(Fauci, Chapter 376)*

15. **(D)** This woman does not have risk factors for sleep apnea (older age, snoring, obesity) and likely has narcolepsy. Adrenergic stimulant drugs such as modafinil, methylphenidate, or amphetamines help the sleepiness, and tricyclic compounds can help the cataplexy. Strategically planned naps can also be helpful. *(Fauci, Chapter 28)*

16. **(B)** The combination of symptoms is typical of chronic alcohol abuse. The mental symptoms are suggestive of Wernicke–Korsakoff syndrome. A distal limb sensory-motor neuropathy is also typical of alcoholism. Confusion, tremulousness, and disorientation are typical for acute alcohol intoxication. Wernicke encephalopathy is a symptom complex of ophthalmoplegia, ataxia, nystagmus, and acute confusional state. *(Fauci, Chapter 387)*

17. **(D)** These signs and symptoms develop in a fairly large percentage of patients with diabetes mellitus. Loss of proprioceptive sensation together with absent reflexes superficially resembles tabes dorsalis. If sensory loss is severe, Charcot joints can develop. Heart disease, adrenal insufficiency and dermatomyositis do not cause sensory loss symptoms of peripheral neuropathy. Hypothyroidism can cause an axonal pattern polyneuropathy but is not as common as seen in diabetes. *(Fauci, Chapter 379)*

18. **(A)** A subdural hematoma is almost always of venous origin and secondary to a minor or severe injury to the head, but may occur in blood dyscrasias or cachexia in the absence of trauma. Acute subdural hematomas commonly present with a fluctuating level of consciousness and significant cerebral damage. Chronic subdurals may also present with seizures or papilledema. Between 2 to 6 weeks after bleeding in the subdural space the clot becomes less dense as it starts to break down. *(Fauci, Chapter 259)*

19. **(C)** A vestibular schwannoma (formerly called acoustic neuroma) is most likely to lead to a palsy of the eighth cranial nerve. Deafness, headache, ataxia, tinnitus, and diplopia are seen, as well as facial paresthesias. Vestibular schwannoma represent 5%–10% of all intracranial tumors. They develop from Schwann cells and generally grow very slowly. They may be very large before symptoms develop. *(Fauci, Chapter 374)*

20. **(B)** The early age of onset and otherwise good health suggest a diagnosis of narcolepsy, which is usually accompanied by other symptomatology. Hypnagogic hallucinations are almost always visual. They occur most frequently at the onset of sleep, either during the day or at night. They are generally very vivid. Cataplexy is a brief loss of muscle power without loss of consciousness. The patient is fully aware of what is going on. The paralysis may be complete or partial. Automatic behavior with amnesia is a common manifestation of the narcolepsy cataplexy syndromes, occurring in 50% of cases. Automatic behavior can be confused with complex partial seizures. Paresthesias are not part of narcolepsy syndrome. Snoring, restless sleep, and morning headache suggest sleep apnea. *(Fauci, Chapter 28)*

21. **(C)** In hyperthyroidism, neurologic symptoms include tremors of the hands, exophthalmos, lid lag, stare, and muscle weakness. Muscle weakness of hyperthyroidism affects the pelvic girdle and, to a lesser extent, the shoulder girdle. Reflexes are normal or increased, and sensation is normal. It must be differentiated from myasthenia gravis, which may also accompany thyrotoxicosis. *(Fauci, Chapter 335)*

22. **(A)** This young man has Friedreich ataxia, associated with a gene defect on chromosome 9. The pathologic changes are found in the spinal cord tracts. Degeneration is seen in the posterior columns, the lateral corticospinal tract, and the spinocerebellar tracts. Ataxia, sensory loss, nystagmus, reflex changes, clubfeet, and kyphoscoliosis are the characteristic findings. The heart is frequently involved, and cardiac disease is a common cause of death. *(Fauci, Chapter 368)*

23. **(E)** In Wilson disease the corneal pigmentation (Kayser–Fleischer ring) is the most important diagnostic finding on physical examination. If

it is absent, any neurologic findings cannot be ascribed to Wilson disease. There is usually a reduction of the serum ceruloplasmin content. Signs and symptoms of injury to the basal ganglia are accompanied by cirrhosis of the liver. Renal involvement is characterized by persistent aminoaciduria. The most common neurologic finding is tremor. *(Fauci, Chapter 354)*

24. **(D)** This patient has trigeminal neuralgia. Carbamazepine (an anticonvulsant drug) is given in doses varying from 600 to 1200 mg/day. Phenytoin has also been used. The two drugs can also be used in combination. Operative procedures include alcohol injection of the nerve or ganglion, partial section of the nerve in the middle or posterior fossa, decompression of the root, and medullary tractotomy. Radiofrequency surgery can destroy pain fibers but spare motor fibers. The other treatment options are not considered effective for this condition. *(Fauci, Chapter 371)*

25. **(B)** In central vertigo, the vertigo can be mild and chronic. In peripheral disease, the symptoms are generally more severe, but finite (although often recurrent). A history of hearing changes is an important clue that the vertigo is peripheral in origin. The direction of nystagmus is not helpful in differentiating peripheral from central causes of vertigo. *(Fauci, Chapter 22)*

26. **(E)** In myasthenia gravis, weakness of the facial and levator palpebrae muscles produces a characteristic expressionless face, with drooping of the eyelids. Weakness of the ocular muscles may cause paralysis or weakness of individual muscles, paralysis of conjugate gaze, ophthalmoplegia, or a pattern similar to internuclear ophthalmoplegia. The presence of normal pupillary responses to light and accommodation with weakness of extraocular muscles, levators, and orbicularis oculi is almost completely diagnostic of myasthenia. *(Fauci, Chapter 381)*

27. **(A)** Adenomas of the pituitary gland constitute approximately 7% of intracranial tumors, with the chromophobic type being the most common. With macroadenomas, some degree of pituitary insufficiency is common, and half the patients have headaches. With microadenomas, the other pituitary functions may be completely normal. The clue here is the bitemporal hemianopsia which is characteristic of pituitary tumors but not glioblastoma, craniopharyngioma, meningioma, or an aneurysm of the carotid artery. *(Fauci, Chapter 333)*

28. **(A)** The most common initial symptom of ALS is weakness and wasting of the extremities. The fasciculations can be a very prominent part of the disease. This is rare in other neurologic disorders. *(Fauci, Chapter 369)*

29. **(C)** The characteristic triad in Parkinson disease (**t**remor, **r**igidity, **a**kinesia) has been expanded to include **p**ostural instability. This forms the mnemonic **TRAP**. Autonomic instability is also common. Findings on examination also include masklike facies, dysarthria, stooped posture, and abnormal gait. The tremor of Parkinson disease is present at rest but diminishes/resolves on active movement. Muscle atrophy, papillary changes, and spontaneous remission are not usual features of Parkinson disease. *(Fauci, Chapter 366)*

30. **(B)** Tinnitus and deafness may be found in peripheral vertigo, but not central. The nystagmus is usually unidirectional and is never vertical. Visual fixation inhibits vertigo and nystagmus during testing in peripheral vertigo. *(Fauci, Chapter 22)*

31. **(A)** Adults may develop hydrocephalus as a result of occlusion of CSF pathways by tumors in the third ventricle, brain stem, or posterior fossa. In adults, the symptoms of obstructive hydrocephalus include headache, lethargy, malaise, incoordination, and weakness. Seizures do not usually occur. Dementia, altered consciousness, ocular nerve palsies, papilledema, ataxia, or corticospinal tract signs may be present. *(Fauci, Chapter 365)*

32. **(B)** Myelin is a complex protein lipid carbohydrate structure, which forms part of the cell membrane of the oligodendroglia. Vascular lesions cause demyelination because of ischemia. Papovaviruses can cause progressive multifocal

leukoencephalopathy in patients with HIV infection, or less commonly, malignancy. Acute disseminated encephalomyelitis has been described after smallpox or rabies vaccination. Nutritional deficiencies can also cause demyelination (eg, pernicious anemia with vitamin B$_{12}$ deficiency). *(Fauci, Chapter 375)*

33. **(C)** Pontine hemorrhage is associated with impaired oculocephalic reflexes and small, reactive pupils. It generally evolves over a few minutes, usually with coma and quadriplegia. The prognosis is poor, and death often occurs within hours. *(Fauci, Chapter 268)*

34. **(B)** Cerebellar hemorrhage, when mild, may present with only headache, vomiting, and ataxia of gait. Patients may complain of dizziness or vertigo. The eyes may be deviated to the side opposite the hemorrhage. Nystagmus is not common, but an ipsilateral sixth nerve palsy can occur. This is the only type of intracerebral hemorrhage that commonly benefits from surgical intervention. *(Fauci, Chapter 364)*

35. **(H)** Hypertensive encephalopathy is an unusual complication of chronic hypertension and, nowadays, is almost never the initial presentation of hypertension. Intracerebral hemorrhage into the cerebellum, pons, and thalamus are usually due to spontaneous rupture of small, penetrating arteries and are also associated with hypertension. The lack of physical findings argues against one of these hemorrhagic processes. Cocaine-related hemorrhage is caused by acute hypertension. Subarachnoid hemorrhage is more likely caused by an aneurysm, and lobar intracerebral hemorrhage is frequently caused by nonhypertensive factors such as amyloid angiopathy, AVMs, and aneurysms. *(Fauci, Chapter 241)*

36. **(G)** AVMs are more frequently seen in men and, although present from birth, do not usually become symptomatic until later in life. The peak incidence of symptoms is between ages 10 and 30. The headaches can be similar to migraine, or it can be more diffuse. It can also present with seizure or rupture. Hemorrhage can be massive or minimal when rupture does occur. *(Fauci, Chapter 364)*

37. **(C)** The most common familial periodic paralysis syndrome is usually associated with low potassium, but there are less common forms characterized by high or normal potassium. It is characterized by recurrent attacks of weakness or paralysis of the somatic musculature, with loss of the deep tendon reflexes. Preventive therapy includes potassium supplementation and possibly a low-carbohydrate, low-salt, and high-potassium diet. Imipramine and acetazolamide are said to be useful in acute attacks. *(Fauci, Chapter 383)*

38. **(E)** Tuberous sclerosis is an autosomal dominant disease with a wide variety of clinical phenotypes. Lesions occur in the nervous system, skin, bones, retina, kidney, and elsewhere. The skin lesions include facial nevi (fibroma molluscum) and patches of skin fibrosis. Hard nodules are found throughout the brain. Seizures and mental retardation can occur. *(Fauci, Chapter 278)*

39. **(B)** Syringomyelia is characterized by a dissociated sensory loss. Atrophy of the muscles can result in a clawhand deformity. Fasciculations are commonly found. *(Fauci, Chapter 372)*

40. **(B)** The most common presenting symptoms relate to weakness of eye muscles, causing ptosis or diplopia. Difficulty in chewing, dysarthria, and dysphagia are also common. The differential diagnosis includes all diseases that cause weakness of oropharyngeal or limb muscles. These include the muscular dystrophies, ALS, and progressive bulbar palsies, among others. Most other conditions do not improve after injection of edrophonium or neostigmine, which can help differentiate myasthenia from other neuromuscular disorders. Hypercalcemia can cause weakness, but the symptoms are constant, and do not worsen with use or improve with rest. Multiple sclerosis causes focal neurologic deficits and not diffuse muscle weakness, and thyroid storm can cause a myopathy but again the weakness is constant and more prominent in proximal muscle groups. *(Fauci, Chapter 381)*

41. **(B)** This man had a posttraumatic generalized seizure. The prolonged confusion after the

event suggests seizure rather than syncope. In the majority of cases, seizures do not develop until several months after the injury, 6–18 months being the most common interval. The more severe the injury, the greater the likelihood of seizures. For severe injuries, some authorities recommend prophylactic anticonvulsants for 1–2 years. However, there is no firm evidence for this. *(Fauci, Chapter 363)*

42. **(C)** This patient has herpes simplex virus encephalitis. Acyclovir selectively inhibits viral deoxyribonucleic acid (DNA) polymerase. Acyclovir is currently the treatment of choice because of better efficacy and less toxicity than previous drugs. Because it is so nontoxic, therapy can be started even if the diagnosis is only presumptive. *(Fauci, Chapter 172)*

43. **(C)** CT scan without contrast is still superior to MRI in certain circumstances, particularly in the emergency setting, for diagnosing acute subarachnoid hemorrhage, intracerebral bleeding, fractures of the face, temporal bone, and base of the skull. A CT is useful in evaluating patients with osseous spinal stenosis and spondylosis, but an MRI is preferred if there are neurologic defects due to spinal cord compression. A CT scan with contrast is useful when the diagnostic possibility includes cerebral metastasis or brain abscess. *(Fauci, Chapter 362)*

44. **(B)** The lateral medullary syndrome (also known as Wallenberg syndrome) causes ipsilateral numbness but also contralateral involvement of pain and thermal sense by affecting the spinothalamic tract. It can be caused by occlusion of the vertebral arteries; posterior-inferior cerebellar arteries; and superior, middle, or inferior medullary arteries. Ipsilateral ataxia and falling to the side of the lesion are common. Ipsilateral paralysis of the tongue is characteristic of medial medullary syndrome, which also causes contralateral paralysis of arm and leg. Paralysis of the body is not characteristic of lateral medullary syndrome, but ipsilateral paralysis of palate and vocal cord does occur. Ipsilateral Horner syndrome, nystagmus, diplopia, vertigo, nausea, and vomiting are characteristic. *(Fauci, Chapter 364)*

45. **(C)** TSP is frequently associated with a retroviral (HTLV-1) infection that can be spread through blood transfusion, sexual contact, intravenous drug use, and vertical transmission from mother to child. It is slowly progressive, and bladder involvement is characteristic. Sensory symptoms are usually mild, and a true sensory level is almost never found. On occasion, cranial nerve findings, frontal release signs, and cerebellar signs (tremor, dysmetria) are present. *(Fauci, Chapter 182)*

46. **(A)** The cause of trigeminal neuralgia (tic douloureux) is unknown, although some cases may be caused by compression of the trigeminal nerve by arteries or veins of the posterior fossa. The pain occurs in paroxysms and is strictly limited to one or more branches of the fifth cranial nerve. Paroxysms may be brief or last up to 15 minutes. There is no objective sensory loss, but the patient may complain of hyperesthesia of the face. Watering of the eye on the involved side may occur during an attack. *(Fauci, Chapter 375)*

47. **(A)** Cavernous sinus thrombosis is usually secondary to traumatic, neoplastic, or suppurative processes in the orbit, the nasal sinuses, or the upper half of the face. The optic discs are swollen, and there may be numerous surrounding small or large hemorrhages if the orbital veins are occluded. Visual acuity is normal or moderately impaired. Involvement of the cranial nerves in the cavernous sinus (third, fourth, sixth, and V1 and V2 divisions of the fifth) causes diplopia, ptosis, and sensory loss on the face. *(Fauci, Chapter 371)*

48. **(C)** In the vast majority of cases, retrobulbar neuritis occurs as an episode in a demyelinating disease such as multiple sclerosis. It is the first manifestation of multiple sclerosis in 15% of cases and occurs at some point in 50% of all patients with the disease. The course of the retrobulbar neuritis is that of gradual spontaneous improvement. *(Fauci, Chapter 375)*

49. **(E)** Internal carotid artery insufficiency is the most likely diagnosis. Abnormalities are found in the extracranial arteries in more than one-half

of the patients with symptomatic cerebral infarction. Current treatment is carotid endarterectomy for severe stenosis and aspirin therapy for lesser degrees of stenosis. *(Fauci, Chapter 364)*

50. **(B)** The patient's findings strongly suggest herpes simplex encephalitis. This is generally caused by herpes simplex virus type 1 (HSVI). When the disease is suspected, appropriate antiviral therapy (acyclovir) should be started immediately. CT scan is not helpful in diagnosis because it becomes positive only late in the disease, but MRI scans may be helpful. Brain biopsy, once the diagnostic test of choice, is the most definitive test but is rarely performed. *(Fauci, Chapter 172)*

51. **(C)** Guillain–Barré syndrome often appears days to weeks after a viral upper respiratory or gastrointestinal (GI) infection. The initial symptoms are due to symmetric limb weakness. Paresthesias may be present. Unlike most other neuropathies, proximal muscles may be affected more than distal muscles early in the disease. Tendon reflexes are usually lost within a few days. Protein content of the CSF is usually high within a few days of onset. Diabetic and alcoholic neuropathy do not have an acute onset type presentation as this patient did. Cyanide poisoning can cause paralysis, but it is generalized not just localized to the lower limbs. *(Fauci, Chapter 380)*

52. **(E)** This patient has myasthenia gravis and the thymus tissue is often abnormal, with encapsulated tumors occurring in about 15% of cases. Almost all thymomas occur in patients over age 30. Even without thymoma, thymectomy can result in remission in patients with generalized myasthenia. Its benefit is delayed for months or more, so it is not an emergency treatment for myasthenia. *(Fauci, Chapter 381)*

53. **(D)** Vertigo is defined as an illusory or hallucinatory feeling of movement of the body or environment, usually spinning. Dizziness can be caused by multiple factors in the elderly, including orthostatic hypotension, hypoglycemia, and depression. *(Fauci, Chapter 22)*

54. **(C)** Patients with BPPV, in contrast to those with central positional vertigo, have a latent period from the time of onset of the offending position to development of symptoms. With maintenance of the position, patients with BPPV become less symptomatic (fatigability), and repeated positioning also lessens the symptoms (habituation). As well, in BPPV, although the symptoms are usually severe, they can be quite variable from one testing period to the next. *(Fauci, Chapter 22)*

55. **(A)** Anticholinergic drugs exacerbate the underlying defects in patients with myasthenia gravis. Cholinergic drugs are largely inhibitors of cholinesterase. Prednisone may improve as many as 80% of patients. Thymectomy helps patients with no thymoma, but thymoma patients do not do as well. Plasmapheresis benefits most patients but needs to be repeated at intervals. *(Fauci, Chapter 381)*

56. **(E)** Myoclonic seizures are sudden, brief, single, or repetitive muscle contractions involving one body part or the entire body. Loss of consciousness does not occur unless other types of seizures coexist. These seizures can be idiopathic or associated with Creutzfeldt–Jakob disease, uremia, hepatic failure, subacute leukoencephalopathies, and some hereditary disorders. Recent evidence has linked a variant form of Creutzfeldt–Jakob disease with bovine spongiform encephalopathy (BSE), a prion disease of cattle. This variant form usually presents with ataxia and behavior changes prior to myoclonus and dementia. *(Fauci, Chapter 367)*

57. **(B)** Complex partial seizures were once classified as temporal lobe epilepsy. Although the temporal lobe (especially the hippocampus or amygdala) is the most common site of origin, some seizures have been shown to originate from mesial parasagittal or orbital frontal regions. *(Fauci, Chapter 363)*

58. **(D)** Pure absence seizures consist of the sudden cessation of ongoing conscious activity without convulsive muscular activity or loss of postural control. They can be so brief as to be inapparent

but can last several minutes. There is usually no period of postictal confusion. *(Fauci, Chapter 363)*

59. **(A)** Simple partial seizures can occur with motor, sensory, autonomic, or psychic symptoms. When a partial motor seizure spreads to adjacent neurons, a "Jacksonian march" can occur (eg, right thumb to right hand and right arm to right side of face). Face and hand movements are frequently linked because their cortical controlling regions are adjacent. *(Fauci, Chapter 363)*

60. **(D)** Absence seizures almost always begin in young children (age 6–14). They may first present as learning difficulties in school. The EEG is diagnostic, revealing brief 3-Hz spike and wave discharges occurring synchronously throughout all the leads. *(Fauci, Chapter 363)*

61. **(E)** Valproic acid can be used for typical and atypical seizures, myoclonic seizures, and tonic-clonic seizures. It causes little sedation and does not impair cognition. However, the blood count and liver tests must be monitored for a time after initiation of therapy to ensure the safety of the patient. *(Fauci, Chapter 363)*

62. **(E)** Valproic acid is the drug of choice for atypical absence seizures and myoclonic seizures. *(Fauci, Chapter 363)*

63. **(A)** Phenytoin is the first choice for tonic-clonic seizures; it can cause gum hyperplasia and hirsutism, which are particularly unpleasant side effects. Lymphadenopathy, ataxia, incoordination, confusion, and cerebellar toxicity can also occur. Carbamazepine and valproic acid are also options for the initial treatment of tonic-clonic seizures. *(Fauci, Chapter 363)*

64. **(B)** Carbamazepine is the initial choice for partial seizures. Phenytoin is also an option. *(Fauci, Chapter 363)*

65. **(G)** Lorazepam or diazepam is the treatment of choice for status epilepticus. Diazepam intravenously (IV) at 2 mg/min up to 20 mg, or lorazepam IV (0.1 mg/kg) at no faster than 2 mg/min, is initially given followed by phenytoin loading (15–18 mg/kg) no faster than 50 mg/min. *(Fauci, Chapter 363)*

66. **(B)** Horner syndrome results in a small, round pupil on one side. Light and near reaction is brisk, and response to mydriatics and miotics is normal. The affected pupil will not dilate in the dark, so darkness accentuates the anisocoria. The syndrome is often idiopathic but can be caused by neoplasm, brain stem stroke, or carotid dissection. *(Fauci, Chapter 29)*

67. **(C)** The tonic pupil (Holmes–Adie syndrome) is caused by a parasympathetic lesion at or distal to the ciliary ganglion. The pupil is large and usually unilateral, with absent response to light. A bright room, by causing constriction of the normal pupil, accentuates the anisocoria. The tonic pupil can be associated with Shy–Drager syndrome, amyloidosis, or diabetes. However, it is most commonly seen in otherwise healthy young women. *(Fauci, Chapter 29)*

68. **(D)** Argyll Robertson pupils are small, irregular, and often bilateral. The response to light is impaired, but the response to near vision is preserved. Argyll Robertson pupils can be a manifestation of syphilis, a treponemal infection. It can also be associated with lesions of the dorsal midbrain (obstructive hydrocephalus, pineal region tumors) and after aberrant regeneration. *(Fauci, Chapter 29)*

69. **(A)** This patient has physiologic or essential anisocoria, which can be seen in up to 20% of the population at some time. Its hallmarks are a normal response to light and accommodation and the asymmetry is maintained in different lighting conditions. It can also be variable from day to day. *(Fauci, Chapter 29)*

70. **(G)** Compression of the oculomotor nerve (third cranial nerve) results in paresis of the oculomotor muscles supplied by the nerve and symptoms of double vision. The parasympathetic fibers running along the outside of the nerve are also affected resulting in dilation of the pupil. Increased intracranial pressure from any mass lesion (blood, abscess, or

tumor) leading to uncal herniation and compression of the nerve is the usual cause. *(Fauci, Chapter 29)*

71. **(B)** Peripheral nerve lesions result in reflex loss greater than the degree of weakness. Reflex loss is variable in anterior horn cell disease and decreased proportionately in muscle disease. In neuromuscular junction disorders, reflexes are characteristically normal. *(Fauci, Chapter 379)*

72. **(C)** Diurnal fluctuations and pathologic fatigue are common in disorders of neuromuscular transmission (eg, myasthenia gravis). *(Fauci, Chapter 381)*

73. **(A)** In diseases of the anterior horn cell (such as ALS), atrophy is marked and early. Muscle disease can result in marked atrophy, but much later in the course of the disease. Atrophy is generally moderate in peripheral nerve disease and absent in disorders of the neuromuscular junction. *(Fauci, Chapter 369)*

74. **(B)** Peripheral nerve disease is the most likely to cause distal weakness and is the only one of the four to also cause sensory symptoms. *(Fauci, Chapter 379)*

75. **(D)** Dermatomyositis is one of the inflammatory myopathies that has a characteristic rash on the eyelids (heliotrope) and knuckles (Gottron papules). It is associated with certain cancers as a paraneoplastic syndrome. The muscle enzyme creatine kinase (CK) is elevated is most cases, but the condition is painless. Symptoms are those of proximal muscle weakness, with normal reflexes and tone on examination. *(Fauci, Chapter 383)*

CHAPTER 8

Nephrology
Questions

DIRECTIONS (Questions 1 through 37): For each of the questions in this section select the one lettered answer that is the best response in each case.

1. A 25-year-old woman presents to the emergency department with symptoms of nausea and vomiting of 2 days duration. She is not on any medications and was previously well until now. The physical examination is normal except for a postural drop in her blood pressure from 110/80 mm Hg supine to 90/80 mm Hg standing. Her serum electrolytes are sodium 130 mEq/L, potassium 3 mEq/L, chloride 90 mEq/L, bicarbonate 30 mEq/L, urea 50 mg/dL, and creatinine 0.8 mg/dL. **Which of the following electrolytes is most likely to be filtered through the glomerulus but unaffected by tubular secretion?**

   (A) potassium
   (B) sodium
   (C) bicarbonate
   (D) urea
   (E) creatinine

2. Ten days after a kidney transplant, a 32-year-old man returns to the hospital with symptoms of fever, and decreased urine output. He reports no cough, sputum, or dysuria. An ultrasound of the transplant kidney shows allograft enlargement. **Which of the following is the most likely diagnosis?**

   (A) steroid hyperglycemia
   (B) erythrocytosis
   (C) hyperacute rejection
   (D) acute rejection
   (E) renal artery stenosis

3. A 19-year-old man presents to the emergency department with symptoms of malaise, nausea, and decreased urine output. He was previously well, and his physical examination is normal except for an elevated jugular venous pressure (JVP) and a pericardial rub. His electrolytes reveal acute kidney injury (AKI). **Which of the following findings on the urinalysis is most likely in keeping with acute glomerulonephritis (GN)?**

   (A) proteinuria
   (B) white blood cell casts
   (C) granular casts
   (D) erythrocyte casts
   (E) hyaline casts

4. A 24-year-old woman presents to the hospital with symptoms of nausea, vomiting, anorexia, and gross hematuria. She had a sore throat 2 weeks ago that resolved on its own. On physical examination, the blood pressure is 160/90 mm Hg, pulse 90/min, JVP is 7 cm, heart sounds are normal, there is 1+ pedal edema, and the lungs are clear. She has a renal biopsy **Which of the following electron microscopy findings on the renal biopsy is most likely in keeping with poststreptococcal GN?**

   (A) diffuse mesangial deposits
   (B) no deposits
   (C) electron-dense endothelial deposits
   (D) closed capillary lumen
   (E) subepithelial humps

5. A 74-year-old man is brought to the hospital because of urinary retention. His past medical history includes hypertension, and benign prostatic hypertrophy. A Foley catheter is inserted to relieve the obstruction, and 1500 cc of urine is emptied from his bladder. Over the next few hours, he has 200cc/h of urine output. **Which of the following urine electrolyte values is most likely in keeping with his diagnosis of post obstructive diuresis?**

(A) high sodium
(B) low potassium
(C) high specific gravity
(D) low pH
(E) osmolality >500 mOsm/kg

6. A 68-year-old woman uses large amounts of nonsteroidal anti-inflammatory analgesics for years to relieve symptoms of back pain due to arthritis. She now has an elevated urea and creatinine consistent with chronic kidney disease. **Which of the following changes in the kidney is most likely seen with her diagnosis?**

(A) glomerulosclerosis
(B) papillary necrosis and tubulointerstitial inflammation
(C) cortical necrosis
(D) tubular necrosis
(E) nephrolithiasis

7. A 64-year-old woman develops severe diarrhea 2 weeks after finishing antibiotics for pneumonia. She also notices decreased urine output despite drinking lots of fluids. On physical examination, there is a postural drop in her blood pressure, the JVP is low, and the abdomen is soft but diffusely tender. Despite giving 4 L of normal saline, her urine output remains low. The urinalysis is positive for heme-granular casts and the urine sodium is 42 mEq/L. **Which of the following medications should be held during the recovery phase of this woman's AKI?**

(A) acetaminophen
(B) metoprolol
(C) lorazepam
(D) enalapril
(E) simvastatin

8. A 64-year-old woman is seen in the clinic for routine assessment of her hypertension. On physical examination, the blood pressure is 130/78 mm Hg, heart rate 80/min, and the rest of the exam is normal. Routine electrolytes and renal function are checked and the only abnormal value is an elevated bicarbonate level of 34 mEq/L. **Which of the following is the most likely cause for her metabolic alkalosis?**

(A) diuretic use
(B) hyperkalemia
(C) mineralocorticoid deficiency
(D) diarrhea
(E) angiotensin-converting enzyme (ACE)-inhibitor use

9. A 32-year-old man with sickle cell anemia is seen in the clinic for routine follow-up. He feels well at the present time, but in the past he has had many sickle cell crises, which have resulted in kidney injury. **Which of the following renal abnormalities is most likely to be seen in him?**

(A) inability to acidify the urine
(B) granular casts
(C) inability to concentrate the urine
(D) pyuria
(E) salt-losing state

10. A 63-year-old man presents to the clinic with severe pain in his left big toe. The pain started suddenly the previous evening and there is no history of any trauma. He mentions this pain occurs frequently over the past 8 years, and the symptoms usually resolve with ibuprofen. On physical examination, the big toe is red, swollen, and very painful to move. Electrolytes reveal an elevated creatinine level. **Which of the following mechanisms is the most likely explanation for his renal impairment?**

(A) GN
(B) vascular injury
(C) uric acid kidney stones
(D) distal tubular atrophy
(E) renal parenchymal uric acid crystals

11. A 67-year-old man presents to the emergency department with symptoms of renal colic. Plain x-rays of the abdomen reveal no obvious renal stone. A CT scan of the abdomen is ordered to confirm the clinical diagnosis. **Which of the following coexisting medical conditions increases the risk of contrast-induced nephropathy?**

   (A) hyperparathyroidism
   (B) pyelonephritis
   (C) nephrolithiasis
   (D) renal cell carcinoma
   (E) multiple myeloma

12. A 64-year-old man presents to the hospital with symptoms of weight gain, shortness of breath, easy bruising, and leg swelling. On physical examination, the blood pressure is 140/80 mm Hg, pulse 100/min, JVP 4 cm, heart sounds normal, and lungs are clear. There is 3+ pedal and some periorbital edema. Investigations include a normal chest x-ray (CXR), an electrocardiogram (ECG) with low voltages, anemia, high urea and creatinine, and 4 g/day of protein excretion in the urine. A renal biopsy shows nodular deposits that have an apple-green birefringence under polarized light when stained with Congo red. **Which of the following is the most likely diagnosis?**

   (A) amyloidosis
   (B) multiple myeloma
   (C) diabetic nephropathy
   (D) minimal change disease
   (E) immunoglobulin A (IgA) nephropathy

13. A 74-year-old man presents to the clinic for assessment of symptoms of fatigue, shortness of breath on exertion, and back and rib pain that is made worse with movement. Investigations reveal he is anemic, the calcium, urea, and creatinine are elevated. X-rays reveal multiple lytic lesions in the long bones and ribs, and protein electrophoresis is positive for an immunoglobulin G (IgG) paraprotein. **Which of the following is the most likely mechanism for the renal injury?**

   (A) plasma cell infiltrates
   (B) tubular damage by light chains

   (C) glomerular injury
   (D) vascular injury by light chains
   (E) uric acid crystals

14. A 77-year-old man has a mass in his left lung that is suggestive of lung cancer. His baseline investigations reveal low serum sodium and normal serum calcium, urea and creatinine values. On physical examination, the JVP is 4 cm, heart sounds are normal, and the lungs are clear. The urine sodium is 64 mEq/L and the urine osmolality is 550 mOsm/kg. **Which of the following is the most likely diagnosis?**

   (A) nephrotic syndrome
   (B) syndrome of inappropriate antidiuretic hormone (SIADH) production
   (C) renal metastases from lung cancer
   (D) lung metastases from hypernephroma
   (E) renal tubular acidosis (RTA)

15. A 69-year-old man has lost a friend to prostate cancer, and would like to be evaluated for the disease. He has no urinary symptoms. **Which of the following tests is most likely indicated to screen him for prostate cancer?**

   (A) prostate ultrasound
   (B) digital rectal examination (DRE)
   (C) DRE and prostate specific antigen (PSA)
   (D) PSA
   (E) none of the above

16. A 63-year-old woman has Type 2 diabetes mellitus, which is well controlled. Her physical examination is positive for peripheral neuropathy in the feet and nonproliferative retinopathy. A urinalysis is positive for proteinuria. **Which of the following treatments is most likely to attenuate the course of renal disease?**

   (A) calcium channel blockers
   (B) ACE inhibitors
   (C) hepatic hydroxymethylglutaryl-coenzyme A (HMG-CoA) inhibitors
   (D) dietary carbohydrate restriction
   (E) weight reduction

17. A 32-year-old man has trace proteinuria on a dipstick urinalysis. A 24-hour urine collection reveals 380 mg/day of protein excretion in the urine. **Which of the following statements concerning this degree of proteinuria is correct?**

    (A) rarely requires any investigation
    (B) in systemic diseases, it has no prognostic values
    (C) can be caused by fever
    (D) is rarely reversible
    (E) always caused by tubular defects

18. A 56-year-old man is involved in a severe motor vehicle accident. He develops AKI after admission to hospital. One of the possibilities for his AKI is posttraumatic renal vein thrombosis. **Which of the following findings is most likely to suggest renal vein thrombosis?**

    (A) white cell casts on urinalysis
    (B) heme-granular casts
    (C) heavy proteinuria
    (D) urine supernatant pink and tests positive for heme
    (E) specific gravity >1.020

19. A 69-year-old woman presents to the emergency department with symptoms of left flank pain and hematuria. On physical examination, the blood pressure is 165/96 mm Hg, heart rate is 104/min, and the abdomen is soft and nontender. There is some left costo-vertebral angle tenderness on percussion. A computerized tomography (CT) scan of the abdomen reveals a 5-cm mass in the left kidney. (See Figure 8–1.) **Which of the following laboratory abnormalities might also be present?**

Figure 8–1.

(A) polycythemia
(B) thrombocytopenia
(C) hypocalcemia
(D) leukocytosis
(E) high renin hypertension

20. A 60-year-old woman with heart failure and normal renal function is started on furosemide (Lasix) 80 mg/day. She notices a good diuretic response every time she takes the medication. A few weeks later, she is feeling unwell because of fatigue and muscle weakness, but her heart failure symptoms are better. **Which of the following is the most likely explanation for her muscle weakness?**

    (A) hyponatremia
    (B) hypernatremia
    (C) hypokalemia
    (D) hyperkalemia
    (E) anemia

21. A 57-year-old man has an incidental finding of low serum sodium on routine laboratory testing. He clinically feels well, and the physical examination is completely normal. His serum osmolality is low (268 mOsm/kg), but his urine osmolality is high (510 mOsm/kg). **Which of the following is most likely to be found on further evaluation?**

    (A) massive edema
    (B) hyperkalemia
    (C) dehydration
    (D) elevated urea nitrogen
    (E) an intrathoracic lesion

22. A 78-year-old man is brought to the hospital because of persistent nausea and vomiting. On examination he appears dry, his abdomen is soft, and the JVP is not visible. Laboratory investigations reveal hypernatremia (158 mEq/L) and his calculated free water deficit is approximately 3 L. **What segment of the normal kidney is most of the water reabsorbed from?**

    (A) collecting ducts
    (B) proximal tubule
    (C) distal tubule
    (D) ascending loop of Henle
    (E) descending loop of Henle

23. A 64-year-old man is admitted to the hospital for the assessment of hematuria after being involved in a motor vehicle accident. His physical examination is normal. A CT scan of the abdomen is shown in Figure 8–2. **Which of the following is the most likely diagnosis?**

Figure 8–2.

    (A) renal cell carcinoma
    (B) kidney contusion and laceration
    (C) transitional cell carcinoma
    (D) renal hamartoma
    (E) renal hemangioma

24. A 64-year-old man presents to the clinic for assessment of symptoms of malaise, shortness of breath, edema, and poor urine output for 24 hours. His past medical history is not significant, and his only medication is daily aspirin. On physical examination, the JVP is 4 cm, heart sounds are normal, lungs are clear, and the abdomen is soft. A Foley catheter is inserted into his bladder for 200 cc of urine, which is sent for urinalysis. His urine output still remains low. **Which of the following is the most appropriate initial diagnostic test?**

    (A) renal ultrasound
    (B) blood cultures
    (C) urine cultures
    (D) inferior vena cavagram with selective renal venogram
    (E) blood urea nitrogen (BUN)/creatinine ratio

25. A 68-year-old woman presents to the clinic for evaluation of new symptoms of burning when voiding. She has no fever, chills, or back discomfort. Her urinalysis reveals numerous white cells and bacteria. **Which of the following medical comorbidities is most likely to coexist in this patient?**

    (A) anemia
    (B) exercise
    (C) diabetes mellitus
    (D) influenza
    (E) analgesic drug use

26. A 28-year-old woman presents to the emergency department with a recent episode of coughing up some blood, frequent nosebleeds, and now decreased urine output. On physical examination, a nasal mucosa ulcer is seen on inspection and the remainder of the examination is normal. Her urinalysis is positive for protein and red cells consistent with a GN. The CXR shows two cavitary lesions and her serology is positive for antineutrophil cytoplasmic antibodies (ANCA). **Which of the following is the most likely diagnosis?**

    (A) Wegener granulomatosis
    (B) bacterial endocarditis
    (C) Goodpasture syndrome
    (D) lupus erythematosus
    (E) poststreptococcal disease

27. A 42-year-old man notices leg and facial swelling but no other symptoms. His physical examination is pertinent for 3+ pedal edema including periorbital edema. A 24-hour urine collection reveals 5 g/day of proteinuria. **Which of the following is the most likely diagnosis?**

    (A) sickle cell disease
    (B) medullary sponge kidney
    (C) radiation nephritis
    (D) staphylococcal infection
    (E) amyloid disease

28. A 74-year-old woman develops acute sepsis from pneumonia and is admitted to the intensive care unit because of hypotension. She is started on antibiotics, and her blood pressure is supported with intravenous normal saline. Despite this she remains oliguric and develops AKI. Her urinalysis has heme-granular casts and the urine sodium is 56 mEq/L. **Which of the following is the most likely cause of her AKI?**

    (A) nephrotoxic antibiotics
    (B) acute infectious GN
    (C) acute tubular necrosis (ATN)
    (D) contrast nephropathy
    (E) cholesterol emboli

29. A 27-year-old woman who is 34 weeks pregnant is seen in the clinic for routine assessment. She reports that her feet are more swollen now then before, but otherwise feels well. Her pregnancy until now has been uncomplicated. On physical examination, the blood pressure is 145/92mm Hg, heart rate 88/min, the heart and lungs are normal, and there is 2+ pedal edema to her mid-shin. A urinalysis reveals proteinuria, but no casts or red cells. **Which of the following is not a risk factor for the development of this complication?**

    (A) first pregnancy
    (B) diabetes mellitus
    (C) twin pregnancy
    (D) extreme of reproductive age
    (E) human immunodeficiency virus (HIV) infection

30. A 30-year-old man presents to the emergency department for assessment of new symptoms of hematuria. The physical examination is normal except for an elevated blood pressure of 164/94 mm Hg. An ultrasound of the kidneys reveals multiple renal cysts in both kidneys. His father had a similar condition. **Which of the following is not associated with this syndrome?**

    (A) liver cysts
    (B) intracranial aneurysms
    (C) autosomal dominant inheritance
    (D) rheumatoid arthritis (RA)
    (E) progression to end-stage renal failure

31. A 15-year-old boy develops symptoms of renal colic. The stone eventually passes spontaneously, but it is not recovered. The urinalysis reveals hexagonal crystals, and a cyanide-nitroprusside test on the urine is positive. **Which of the following is the most likely diagnosis?**

    (A) cystinuria
    (B) thalassemia
    (C) hereditary glycinuria
    (D) primary hyperoxaluria
    (E) sarcoidosis

32. A 29-year-old man is seen in follow-up 1 year post-kidney transplant. He is doing well clinically and the transplant is functioning well, with no recent episodes of rejection or changes to his immunosuppressive medications. **Which of the following complications of transplantation is the most likely cause of death?**

    (A) atherosclerotic disease
    (B) opportunistic infection
    (C) metabolic bone disease
    (D) lung cancer
    (E) lymphoma

33. A 37-year-old man with HIV and chronic nephropathy presents to the emergency department with acute onset of shortness of breath, fever, chills and sputum production. On physical examination, the blood pressure is 105/74mm Hg, heart rate 110/min, and the temperature is 38.7°C. There are bronchial breath sounds and inspiratory crackles in the left lower lobe. A CXR confirms the diagnosis of left lower lobe pneumonia. **Which of the following antibiotics, if used, would require a major reduction in dosage?**

    (A) erythromycin
    (B) doxycycline
    (C) tobramycin
    (D) ceftriaxone
    (E) amphotericin B

34. A 63-year-old woman presents to the clinic for routine evaluation. She has diabetes for the past 12 years with complications of neuropathy and retinopathy. You decide to screen her for renal complications of diabetes. **Which of the following findings is not compatible with diabetic nephropathy?**

    (A) nephrotic range proteinuria
    (B) microalbuminuria
    (C) hypertension
    (D) red blood cell (RBC) casts in urine
    (E) renal tubular acidosis (RTA) type IV

35. A 24-year-old woman's urinalysis is positive for blood on dipstick measurement. This is repeated twice between menstrual periods and it remains positive. Microscopic evaluation reveals RBCs, some of which are deformed and some in the form of casts. **Which of the following is the most likely cause of the hematuria?**

    (A) urinary tract stones
    (B) GN
    (C) trauma
    (D) benign renal tumor

36. A 63-year-old man presents to the emergency room with symptoms of nausea, vomiting, and right upper quadrant abdominal pain. The physical examination suggests acute cholecystitis, and the diagnosis is confirmed by abdominal ultrasound. He is admitted to the hospital and undergoes an urgent cholecystectomy. The surgery is uneventful but two days post-op he becomes oligoric. **Which of the following findings would suggest that prerenal AKI is a major factor in the etiology?**

    (A) postural hypotension
    (B) fractional excretion of sodium is 3%
    (C) specific gravity is 1.012
    (D) the urine sodium is 30 mEq/L
    (E) heme-granular casts on urine microscopy

37. A 46-year-old woman with nausea and vomiting presents to the hospital because of lightheadedness when standing and decreased urine output. She looks unwell; the blood pressure supine is 96/65 mm Hg and 80/64 mm Hg when standing. Her abdominal, heart, and lung examinations are normal. **Which of the following laboratory values suggests prerenal azotemia in this patient?**

    (A) markedly elevated urea, unchanged creatinine
    (B) unchanged urea, elevated creatinine
    (C) little change in either creatinine or urea for several days after oliguria develops
    (D) urea/creatinine ratio of 10
    (E) urea/creatinine ratio of 25

DIRECTIONS (Questions 38 through 79): The following group of numbered items is preceded by a list of lettered options. For each question, select the one lettered option that is most closely associated with it. Each lettered option may be used once, multiple times, or not at all.

Questions 38 through 41: For each patient with polyuria and polydipsia, select the most likely diagnosis.

(A) central diabetes insipidus (DI)
(B) nephrogenic DI
(C) primary polydipsia
(D) osmotic diuresis
(E) hypercalcemia

38. A 21-year-old woman develops polydipsia and polyuria during pregnancy.

39. A 19-year-old man develops polyuria and polydipsia after a head injury.

40. A 19-year-old man and one of his two brothers have polyuria and polydipsia since birth. Neither his sisters nor his parents are affected.

41. A 27-year-old woman with well-controlled bipolar affective disorder, treated with lithium, develops polyuria and polydipsia.

Questions 42 through 46: For each patient with new symptoms, select the most likely acid base disorder.

(A) metabolic acidosis
(B) metabolic alkalosis
(C) respiratory acidosis
(D) respiratory alkalosis

42. A 19-year-old girl develops sudden-onset non-bloody diarrhea. She was previously well and is not taking any medications or traveled anywhere recently. Her abdomen is soft and nontender on examination, and the anion gap is normal.

43. A 75-year-old man develops acute confusion and drowsiness after a dental procedure. He has a history of severe chronic lung disease due to smoking. Earlier in the day, he had a tooth extraction and afterwards was given acetaminophen with codeine (Tylenol #3) for pain relief.

44. A 74-year-old woman has symptoms of shortness of breath on exertion and waking up at night. Her physical examination reveals a JVP at 8 cm, extra third heart sound, lung crackles, and pedal edema. She is started on furosemide 80 mg/day for heart failure, while further investigations are performed.

45. A 53-year-old woman is being treated for tuberculosis with INH and rifampin.

46. A 69-year-old woman is taking large amounts of aspirin for osteoarthritis, and now complains of ringing in her ears and nausea.

Questions 47 through 52: For each patient with increased urine output, select the correct diagnosis.

(A) nephrogenic DI
(B) central DI
(C) primary polydipsia
(D) solute diuresis
(E) recovery phase of ATN

47. A 42-year-old man presents to hospital with dark black-colored stools and passing out while getting up. On examination he is diaphoretic, blood pressure 80/50 mm Hg supine, pulse 120/min, and the DRE is positive for melena. He is resuscitated in the emergency room. He has low urine output and develops renal failure from ATN. A few days later, his urine output increases to 200 cc/h.

48. A 27-year-old woman presents because she is feeling unwell. Her examination is normal, but her serum sodium is 115 mEq/L. Her urine lytes: sodium 55 mEq/L, osmolality 100 mOsm/L. This condition causes the greatest amount of medullary washout.

49. A 64-year-old man develops severe diarrhea after returning from a foreign holiday. He is hypovolemic clinically and is given normal saline. His serum sodium is 125 mEq/L and

potassium is 2.5 mEq/L. He develops increased urine output with urine sodium of 10 mEq/L and osmolality of 200 mOsm/L. His polyuria can be caused by hypokalemia.

50. A 34-year-old man is brought for evaluation because of bizarre behavior. He comments that he is voiding all the time of clear water-like urine. He has a past history of schizophrenia for which he is taking a major tranquilizer.

51. A 38-year-old man is admitted to hospital for investigation of polyuria and a low serum sodium concentration. After a fluid deprivation test, there was no change in his urine osmolality. He was then given vasopressin (DDAVP) with no change in urine volume or urine osmolality after 2 hours.

52. A 67-year-old man is admitted to hospital after a stroke. He has swallowing difficulties, and a nasogastric feeding tube is inserted to provide high protein content nutrition. After starting the tube feeds, he develops large amounts of urine output. His serum sodium is normal, and the urine values are sodium 60 mEq/L and osmolality 420 mOsm/L.

Questions 53 through 58: For each patient with hyponatremia, select the most likely diagnosis.

   (A) congestive heart failure (CHF)
   (B) extrarenal sodium and fluid losses
   (C) SIADH
   (D) polydipsia
   (E) essential hyponatremia
   (F) renal failure
   (G) endocrine cause of hyponatremia
   (H) renal sodium and fluid losses
   (I) artifactual
   (J) osmotic
   (K) impaired diuresis

53. A 74-year-old man from a nursing home is not feeling well and is confused. He is not able to give any reliable history. His serum sodium is 120 mEq/L and osmolality is 265 mOsm/kg. On examination, his blood pressure is 100/50 mm Hg, pulse 100/min, and neck veins are not visible. His urine sodium is 40 mEq/L and urine osmolality is 330 mOsm/kg.

54. A 65-year-old woman is admitted to the hospital after a stroke resulting in left hemiparesis. She has no trouble swallowing and is on a full diet. One week later, on routine biochemistry, her sodium is 128 mEq/L and osmolality is 270 mOsm/kg. She has no symptoms and is euvolemic on clinical examination. Urine sodium is 40 mEq/L and urine osmolality is 450 mOsm/kg.

55. A 42-year-old man is on amitriptyline for depression. Recently he has been feeling more lethargic and unwell. His clinical examination is normal. Serum sodium is 125 mEq/L and osmolality is 260 mOsm/kg, and urine sodium is 40 mEq/L and osmolality is 450 mOsm/kg.

56. A 32-year-old man is feeling unwell and brought to the hospital. His serum sodium is 125 mEq/L. On examination, his blood pressure is 110/70 mm Hg, pulse 110/min supine, and sitting up causes him to feel lightheaded with a drop in his blood pressure. His urine sodium is 5 mEq/L and urine osmolality is 800 mOsm/kg.

57. A 57-year-old man is referred for assessment of his low serum sodium of 125 mEq/L. On examination, he has pitting edema and elevated neck veins. His urine sodium is 10 mEq/L and urine osmolality 350 mOsm/kg.

58. A 63-year-old man is feeling unwell with symptoms of increased thirst and voiding. He is not taking any medications and there is no past medical history. Physical examination is normal, but his serum sodium is 130 mEq/L and serum osmolality is 310 mOsm/kg.

Questions 59 through 63: For each patient with hypokalemia, select the most likely diagnosis.

   (A) lower gastrointestinal (GI) losses
   (B) prior use of diuretics
   (C) RTA
   (D) current use of diuretics
   (E) malignant hypertension
   (F) primary hyperaldosteronism
   (G) glucocorticoid excess

59. A 30-year-old woman is having symptoms of muscle weakness and fatigue. On examination, her blood pressure is 120/80 mm Hg, pulse 80/min, JVP 4 cm, heart sounds normal, and lungs clear. Her serum potassium level is 2.5 mEq/L, and bicarbonate 30 mEq/L. The urine potassium is 10 mEq/L.

60. A 55-year-old man is having symptoms of muscle weakness and fatigue. He has poorly controlled asthma and recently had an exacerbation. On examination, his blood pressure is 160/90 mm Hg, pulse 80/min, JVP 4 cm, heart sounds normal, and lungs clear. His serum potassium level is 2.5 mEq/L and bicarbonate 30 mEq/L. The urine potassium is 40 mEq/L. Plasma renin and aldosterone levels are low.

61. A 44-year-old woman is having symptoms of muscle weakness and fatigue. On examination, her blood pressure is 120/80 mm Hg, pulse 80/min, JVP 4 cm, heart sounds normal, and lungs clear. Her serum potassium level is 2.5 mEq/L, bicarbonate 18 mEq/L, and anion gap is normal. The urine potassium is 40 mEq/L.

62. A 30-year-old man is having symptoms of muscle weakness, fatigue, and headaches. On examination, his blood pressure is 180/100 mm Hg, pulse 80/min, JVP 4 cm, heart sounds normal, and lungs clear. His serum potassium level is 2.5 mEq/L and bicarbonate 30 mEq/L. The urine potassium is 40 mEq/L. Plasma renin is low and aldosterone is high.

63. A 60-year-old woman is having symptoms of muscle weakness and fatigue. On examination, her blood pressure is 110/80 mm Hg, pulse 100/min, JVP 1 cm, heart sounds normal, and lungs clear. Her serum potassium level is 2.5 mEq/L, bicarbonate 15 mEq/L, and anion gap is normal. The urine potassium is 10 mEq/L.

Questions 64 through 68: For each of the following medical conditions, select the associated acid base disturbances.

    (A) metabolic acidosis and respiratory acidosis

    (B) metabolic acidosis and respiratory alkalosis

    (C) metabolic alkalosis and respiratory acidosis

    (D) metabolic alkalosis and respiratory alkalosis

    (E) metabolic alkalosis and metabolic acidosis

64. Salicylate overdose.

65. Sepsis.

66. Chronic pulmonary disease on steroids.

67. Renal failure with vomiting.

68. Hepatic cirrhosis complicated by AKI.

Questions 69 through 73: For each patient with GN, select the most likely diagnosis on renal biopsy.

    (A) diffuse proliferative GN

    (B) crescentic GN

    (C) focal proliferative GN

    (D) membranoproliferative GN

    (E) minimal change GN

    (F) focal segmental GN

    (G) membranous GN

    (H) deposition diseases

    (I) nonimmune basement membrane abnormalities

69. A 14-year-old girl develops a rash, abdominal pain, and arthralgias. She is also experiencing some nausea, vomiting, and crampy abdominal pain. On examination, she has a palpable purpuric rash on her buttocks and lower legs, a tender abdomen, and no active joint inflammation. Her stools test positive for blood, and urinalysis reveals RBCs and RBC casts. Her renal function deteriorates rapidly over several days. A renal biopsy is performed.

70. A 28-year-old woman has noticed increasing lower limb swelling and shortness of breath. She has a 2-year history of facial rash, hair loss, arthralgias, and thrombocytopenia. On examination, her blood pressure is 150/90 mm Hg, pulse 80/min, there is a maculopapular rash on her face, JVP is 4 cm, heart sounds normal, lungs clear, and there is pedal and periorbital edema. Her creatinine is very high, a urinalysis reveals many RBCs and RBC casts. A renal biopsy is performed.

71. A 47-year-old woman with RA is being treated with nonsteroidal anti-inflammatory drugs (NSAIDs) and gold. She develops acute shortness of breath with hypoxemia and is admitted to the hospital. Admission urinalysis reveals 4+ proteinuria but no active sediment. A renal biopsy is performed.

72. A 19-year-old man, who is otherwise healthy, is found to have RBCs in his urine. There is no proteinuria. Evaluation of his family reveals that his mother also has hematuria. She has minimal renal impairment and, other than being hard of hearing, is in good health. A renal biopsy might show.

73. A 33-year-old man from Southeast Asia, without HIV infection, is diagnosed as having pulmonary tuberculosis. He is started on multiple medications, including INH and rifampin. Three months later, he has developed edema. Liver tests are normal, and serum creatinine is increased by 30% over baseline. Urinalysis reveals 4+ proteinuria. A renal biopsy is performed.

Questions 74 through 77: For each patient with a medical problem, select the most likely diagnosis or renal impairment.

   (A) polycystic kidney disease
   (B) medullary sponge kidney
   (C) medullary cystic disease
   (D) Bartter syndrome
   (E) congenital nephrogenic DI
   (F) cystinuria
   (G) Fanconi syndrome

74. A 14-year-old boy is short in height and has had several fractures with minimal trauma. Physical examination reveals prominent costochondral junctions and bowed legs. What could this syndrome be secondary to?

75. A 43-year-old man had a subarachnoid hemorrhage from an intracranial aneurysm 8 years ago. He has also had progressive renal impairment associated with hematuria. What is the most likely diagnosis?

76. An 18-year-old man is found to have metabolic alkalosis and hypokalemia. What could this be secondary to?

77. A 28-year-old man presents with a kidney stone. He is married to his first cousin, and 6 months earlier, his 8-year-old son had a kidney stone as well. What is the most likely diagnosis?

Questions 78 and 79: For each patient with AKI, select the characteristic urine electrolyte and microscopy findings.

   (A) urinary osmolality < 100
   (B) oxalate crystals in the urine
   (C) urinary sodium <20
   (D) fractional sodium excretion >1%
   (E) RBCs casts in the urine
   (F) heme-granular casts in urine

78. A 21-year-old woman presents with a 2-day history of abdominal pain, nausea, and vomiting. On examination, her blood pressure is 100/70 mm Hg, pulse 100/min, JVP is below sternal angle, and abdomen is diffusely tender. Her urine output is low and electrolytes reveal elevated urea and normal creatinine.

79. A 63-year-old woman presents with left arm swelling, redness, fever, and symptoms of lightheadedness. She has a prior history of hypertension and high cholesterol. On examination, her blood pressure is 80/50 mm Hg, pulse 120/min, there is a large area of cellulitis on her left arm, and she appears flushed. She is admitted to the intensive care unit for management of sepsis and hypotension. On the second hospital day, she still has a low urine output, despite a normal blood pressure and heart rate. Her urea and creatinine have doubled since admission.

Answers and Explanations

1. **(D)** Urea is filtered at the glomerulus, and thereafter, any movement in or out of tubules is a passive process depending on gradients, not secretion. Reabsorption of urea in the distal tubule and collecting duct, when urine flow is reduced, results in the disproportionate elevation of urea nitrogen over creatinine in prerenal azotemia. *(Fauci, Chapter 271)*

2. **(D)** Renal scans initially show a reduction in excretion with cortical retention. This is the most common type of rejection. Most acute rejections will respond to immunosuppressive agents if diagnosed early. In contrast, immediate nonfunction of a graft can be caused by damage to the kidney during procurement and storage. Such problems are becoming less frequent. Obstruction, vascular compression, and ureteral compression are other causes of primary nonfunction of a renal graft. *(Fauci, Chapter 276)*

3. **(D)** Both granular and erythrocyte casts are present, but the latter indicate bleeding from the glomerulus and are most characteristically seen. Red cells reach the urine probably via capillary wall "gaps" and form casts as they become embedded in concentrated tubular fluid with high protein content. Proteinuria is invariably present but is not as specific. White blood cell casts are indicative of interstitial nephritis or infection, and hyaline casts are nonspecific findings. *(Fauci, Chapter 277)*

4. **(E)** These humps are discrete, electron-dense nodules that persist for about 8 weeks and are highly characteristic of poststreptococcal GN. Light microscopy reveals diffuse proliferation, and immunofluorescence reveals granular immunoglobulin G (IgG) and C3. Most patients will recover spontaneously. *(Fauci, Chapter 277)*

5. **(A)** The urine contains large amounts of potassium, magnesium, and sodium. The large volume is often appropriate from the preexisting volume expansion that occurs during the obstruction and poor renal output. Careful attention to fluid and electrolytes is important after the obstruction is relieved, to prevent hypokalemia, hypomagnesemia, hyponatremia or hypernatremia, and volume depletion. The urine osmolality is low since ADH is decreased from the volume expansion prior to the insertion of the catheter and later if the diuresis continues once the patient is euvolemic it is indicative of tubular dysfunction from the prolonged post-renal obstruction. *(Fauci, Chapter 283)*

6. **(B)** She has analgesic nephropathy, and chronic analgesic ingestion may lead to papillary necrosis and tubulointerstitial inflammation. Complete understanding of the pathogenesis is lacking, and may vary with different analgesics. Depletion of reducing equivalents such as glutathione may also play a role. *(Fauci, Chapter 274)*

7. **(D)** Although all drugs should be reassessed at this time, and if appropriate, the dosage adjusted, drugs with known nephrotoxicity, such as ACE inhibitors and NSAIDs, should be stopped. *(Fauci, Chapter 273)*

8. **(A)** Diuretics are a common cause for metabolic alkalosis since many patients take these medications for hypertension or CHF. Diarrhea

causes a nonanion gap metabolic acidosis, and mineralocorticoid excess leads to metabolic alkalosis, primarily because of renal bicarbonate generation. ACE-inhibitors don't cause a metabolic alkalosis either. Other major mechanisms for metabolic alkalosis include extracellular fluid (ECF) volume contraction, potassium depletion, and increased distal salt delivery. Less common causes are Liddle syndrome, bicarbonate loading (posthypercapnic alkalosis), and delayed conversion of administered organic acids. *(Fauci, Chapter 48)*

9. **(C)** In sickle cell anemia, the kidney is characterized by an inability to concentrate the urine because of functional tubule defects that occur as a result of ischemic injury. Papillary necrosis may also occur in patients with homozygous sickle cell disease or sickle cell trait during a sickle crisis. Some patients can develop glomerular injury (focal and segmental glomerular sclerosis) after many years from the anemia-induced hyperfiltration that occurs. Pyuria is not a feature of sickle cell renal disease, during acute vaso-occlusive crisis patients might develop hematuria due to papillary necrosis. *(Fauci, Chapter 280)*

10. **(E)** The typical renal lesions in gout are urate crystals in the medulla or pyramids, with surrounding mononuclear and giant cell reaction. The degree of renal impairment, however, does not correlate with hyperuricemia, and the decline in renal function correlates with aging, hypertension, renal calculi, or unrelated nephropathy. A GN or vascular injury are not features of gouty nephropathy, and uric acid kidney stones can occur in individuals with hyperuricemia, but this usually presents with renal colic type symptoms. The nephropathy associated with chronic gout is insidious. *(Fauci, Chapter 279)*

11. **(E)** The danger of AKI after intravenous contrast for a CT scan has led to caution, especially in patients with multiple myeloma. The patient should not be dehydrated if CT contrast is necessary. The risk is also increased in patients with diabetes mellitus or chronic kidney disease. CT scan of the abdomen looking for renal stones is usually done without contrast. *(Fauci, Chapter 281)*

12. **(A)** Renal amyloidosis can be primary (AL) or secondary amyloidosis (AA). The hallmark finding, nephrotic syndrome, is present in 25% of patients at presentation and probably develops ultimately in over 50%. The apple-green birefringence deposits under polarized light are diagnostic of amyloidosis, and not seen in any other renal disease. *(Fauci, Chapter 324)*

13. **(B)** In multiple myeloma, tubular damage by light chains is almost always present. The injury is a direct toxic effect of the light chains or indirectly from the inflammatory response. Infiltration by plasma cells and glomerular injury is rare. Hypercalcemia may produce transient or irreversible renal damage as do amyloid and myeloma cell infiltrates. *(Fauci, Chapter 106)*

14. **(B)** The urine osmolality in patients with SIADH need not be hypertonic to plasma, but only inappropriately high compared with serum. The major characteristics of SIADH include hyponatremia, volume expansion without edema, natriuresis, hypouricemia, and normal or reduced serum creatinine level, with normal thyroid and adrenal function. *(Fauci, Chapter 46)*

15. **(C)** Although an elevated PSA (>4) has the best positive predictive value, combining it with DRE is probably the most effective screening process. *(Fauci, Chapter 91)*

16. **(B)** It is very likely that control of hypertension and excellent glucose control will slow the development and course of renal disease in Type 2 diabetes mellitus. ACE inhibitors seem to decrease proteinuria and slow progression of renal disease. As renal function deteriorates, limiting dietary protein intake can also be beneficial. Calcium channel blockers have no extra effect beyond their antihypertensive effect. *(Fauci, Chapter 277)*

17. **(C)** Persistent proteinuria should always be investigated and, if no cause can be found,

yearly follow-up instituted. Mild proteinuria has significant prognostic value in diabetes. Mild proteinuria can be caused by glomerular or tubular causes. Functional causes of proteinuria such as fever, orthostasis, exercise, and heart failure are usually reversible. *(Fauci, Chapter 45)*

18. **(C)** Renal vein thrombosis is associated with heavy proteinuria and hematuria. Flank pain and pulmonary embolism can also occur. *(Fauci, Chapter 280)*

19. **(A)** This patient likely has renal cell carcinoma (RCC). Polycythemia is caused by the production of erythropoietin-like factors. There is no relationship to hypertension. The tumor frequently presents as metastatic disease. Thrombocytopenia is not a feature of RCC, and hypercalcemia may occur if there is bone metastasis. High renin production does not occur in RCC either. *(Fauci, Chapter 91)*

20. **(C)** Hypokalemia can result in paralytic ileus, rhabdomyolysis, weakness, and cardiac repolarization abnormalities. It is a common complication along with hyponatremia of starting patients on diuretics. *(Fauci, Chapter 46)*

21. **(E)** This patient's lab values suggest SIADH. Intrathoracic lesions may be benign or malignant, and the latter may secrete a substance similar to vasopressin. Bronchogenic carcinoma is the most common intrathoracic lesion causing SIADH. Patients with SIADH are euvolemic to slightly hypervolemic with edema, and the urea is usually normal or reduced. Hyperkalemia is not a feature of SIADH. *(Fauci, Chapter 46)*

22. **(B)** The largest volume of water is reabsorbed in the nephron at the proximal convolution. Maximally concentrated urine depends on ADH, which allows distal convoluted tubes and collecting ducts to become permeable to water. *(Fauci, Chapter 271)*

23. **(A)** The diagnosis is renal cell carcinoma. There is marked hypervascularity of the left kidney. The arteries are irregular and tortuous, following

a random distribution. The kidney is enlarged and abnormally bulbous in the lower pole. CT scans have dramatically decreased the need for arteriography in evaluating renal lesions. *(Fauci, Chapter 90)*

24. **(A)** Renal ultrasound is an important test in the assessment of acute and chronic renal failure. The oliguria suggests that obstruction is a possible explanation for the renal failure. Imaging is very sensitive for obstruction, but if bladder obstruction secondary to a large prostate is suspected, bladder catheterization would be the first step. *(Fauci, Chapter 273)*

25. **(C)** Urinary tract infections (UTIs) are increased in diabetes mellitus as well as in pregnancy, sickle cell disease, polycystic disease, and structural abnormalities of the urinary tract. *(Fauci, Chapter 281)*

26. **(A)** Wegener is typically associated with antineutrophil cytoplasmic antibodies and respiratory epithelium involvement such as frequent nose bleeds or nasal ulcers. Numerous diseases are associated with renal and pulmonary manifestations, including lupus, Goodpasture syndrome, and microscopic polyangiitis. Right-sided bacterial endocarditis can cause renal and lung involvement but serology of ANCA is negative in endocarditis. This is less likely to be Goodpasture because of the nasal involvement. *(Fauci, Chapter 319)*

27. **(E)** In addition to amyloid disease, other conditions associated with nephrotic syndrome are secondary syphilis, malaria, and treatment with gold salts. Minimal change nephrotic syndrome, focal glomerular sclerosis, membranous nephropathy, and diabetic nephropathy are the primary renal diseases that present as nephrotic syndrome. Sickle cell disease, radiation nephritis, and staphylococcal infection can also cause renal disease but not nephritic range proteinuria (>3gm/day) *(Fauci, Chapter 277)*

28. **(C)** ATN is a common complication of prolonged hypotension and ischemic injury to the renal tubules. Heme-granular "muddy brown" casts are consistent with ATN. An

acute infectious GN will have an "active" urine sediment (red cells and/or red cell casts) which this patient did not, and contrast nephropathy is a possibility if she recently received IV contrast. Cholesterol emboli are common complication post angiographic procedures and usually there are eosinophils in the urine. *(Fauci, Chapter 273)*

29. **(E)** HIV is not associated with preeclampsia unless there is a preexisting renal disease. Diabetes mellitus, chronic hypertension, multifetal gestation, and prior preeclampsia are associated with preeclampsia. When toxemia occurs in the first trimester, however, hydatidiform mole must be considered. The clinical manifestations of severe preeclampsia include headache, epigastric pain, visual disturbances, and hypertension. *(Fauci, Chapter 7)*

30. **(D)** RA is not associated with polycystic kidney disease. It has an autosomal dominant inheritance and about 50% developed renal failure by age 60 years. Cysts are also seen in the liver (more common) and pancreas. Also 5%–10% of asymptomatic patients can have cerebral aneurysms. Renal transplantation is utilized in end-stage renal failure (ESRF). The transplanted kidney cannot be affected by the disease. *(Fauci, Chapter 278)*

31. **(A)** Cystinuria is a congenital disorder associated with decreased tubular resorption of cystine, arginine, ornithine, and lysine. Only cystine is insoluble and is the cause of renal calculi. The typical hexagonal crystals are most likely to be seen on an acidic early-morning urine specimen. A positive cyanide-nitroprusside screening test should be confirmed by chromatography. *(Fauci, Chapter 281)*

32. **(A)** The most common causes of death are cardiovascular and tend to occur earlier than in the general population. Increase in neoplasms in renal transplant recipients includes cervical carcinoma, lymphoma, and cutaneous malignancies. Osteoporosis and persistent hyperparathyroidism are other boney complications. Risk of infection is related to degree of immunosuppression. *(Fauci, Chapter 276)*

33. **(C)** Tobramycin which is an aminoglycoside requires dose reduction and caution when used in patients with CKD. Amikacin and vancomycin are the other antibiotics that require dose reduction in renal failure. Newer antibiotics are often used instead of aminoglycosides to reduce the risk of renal damage. *(Fauci, Chapter 127)*

34. **(D)** Red cell casts are not seen in diabetic nephropathy and suggest another acute GN process. Nephrotic range proteinuria, type IV RTA (hyporeninemic hypoaldosteronism), hypertension, and microalbuminuria are all complications of diabetic kidney disease. *(Fauci, Chapter 277)*

35. **(B)** The finding of red cell casts or dysmorphic red cells (best appreciated by phase microscopy) suggests the source of bleeding is glomerular in origin. Isolated hematuria is usually of urologic cause (eg, tumor, trauma, stone) but can also be of glomerular in origin. *(Fauci, Chapter 277)*

36. **(A)** Although evidence of volume contraction cannot confirm prerenal ARF, as this can progress into intrinsic renal failure, it suggests that prerenal factors are contributing. In prerenal ARF, specific gravity is usually >1.020 and sodium concentration is <10 mmol/L. The fractional excretion of sodium relates sodium clearance to creatinine clearance and is more sensitive than direct measurements of sodium excretion. In prerenal azotemia, sodium is avidly resorbed from glomerular filtrate, but not in intrinsic renal azotemia because of tubular epithelial cell injury. Creatinine is resorbed less efficiently in both conditions. Therefore, the fractional excretion of sodium is <1% in prerenal azotemia (often much less) whereas it is >1% in intrinsic renal azotemia. Fractional excretion of sodium (%) = UNa/PCr × PNa/UCr × 100. *(Fauci, Chapter 45)*

37. **(E)** The ratio of BUN/creatinine is usually <10–15 in intrinsic renal disease and >20 in prerenal azotemia. *(Fauci, Chapter 45)*

38. **(A)** Gestational diabetes can result in hyperglycemia and polyuria with subsequent polydipsia (osmotic diuresis). A primary deficiency in vasopressin can result from increased

metabolism by a placental enzyme and result in polyuria and polydipsia (called gestational DI). It resolves within a few weeks after delivery. *(Fauci, Chapter 334)*

39. **(A)** Head injury can result in central DI from injury to the pituitary or hypothalamus. This can develop abruptly or gradually. *(Fauci, Chapter 334)*

40. **(B)** Nephrogenic DI can be inherited on the X chromosome. Its X-linked recessive nature means that males are predominantly affected. Only women who are homozygous are affected. *(Fauci, Chapter 334)*

41. **(B)** Lithium is one of the drugs that cause nephrogenic DI. Hypercalcemia and hypokalemia can also cause the syndrome. *(Fauci, Chapter 334)*

42. **(A)** She has a nonanion gap metabolic acidosis because of bicarbonate loss from the diarrhea. The anion gap is calculated as the sodium concentration minus the chloride plus the bicarbonate concentration. Other causes of bicarbonate loss with normal anion gap include proximal RTA and primary hyperparathyroidism. *(Fauci, Chapter 48)*

43. **(C)** Causes of acute respiratory acidosis include narcotic overdose, myasthenia gravis, airway obstruction, and trauma to the chest. Acute increases in $PaCO_2$ result in carbon dioxide narcosis. This starts with somnolence and confusion and can lead to coma. Asterixis may be present. Cerebral vasodilation may result in frank papilledema. *(Fauci, Chapter 48)*

44. **(B)** Diuretics are a common cause of metabolic alkalosis. The disorder can occur in volume expanded patients in whom the alkalosis is unresponsive to sodium chloride loading, as in primary hyperaldosteronism or volume contraction with secondary hyperaldosteronism, as in this case. *(Fauci, Chapter 48)*

45. **(A)** INH can result in impaired oxygen utilization, leading to lactic acidosis (type B), accumulation of lactate, and increased anion gap. *(Fauci, Chapter 48)*

46. **(D)** Chronic salicylate use can cause respiratory alkalosis. Severe salicylate toxicity results in an anion gap metabolic acidosis such as during an overdose. During acute hyperventilation, plasma bicarbonate concentrations fall by approximately 3 mEq/L when the arterial pressure of CO_2 falls to about 25 mm Hg. Acute respiratory alkalosis can be caused by anxiety, central nervous system (CNS) disorders, drugs, or fever. Chronic respiratory alkalosis occurs in pregnancy and liver disease as well. *(Fauci, Chapter 48)*

47. **(E)** During the recovery phase of ATN there can be a large diuretic response characterized by large losses of sodium and water due to delayed recovery of tubular cell function. *(Fauci, Chapter 273)*

48. **(C)** Primary polydipsia can cause greater medullary washout than either nephrogenic or central DI because primary polydipsia tends to cause expansion of the ECF volume. This tends to increase total delivery of sodium chloride and water to the inner medulla. It also increases renal blood flow, and increased flow through the vasa recta reduces ability to trap solutes in the medulla. *(Fauci, Chapter 334)*

49. **(A)** Nephrogenic DI can be caused by hypokalemia as well as hypercalcemia. *(Fauci, Chapter 334)*

50. **(C)** Both thioridazine and chlorpromazine have been associated with primary polydipsia. *(Fauci, Chapter 334)*

51. **(A)** There is little or no response to vasopressin after fluid deprivation in complete nephrogenic DI. Incomplete nephrogenic DI will show some response. *(Fauci, Chapter 334)*

52. **(D)** High protein tube feeds may cause a solute diuresis because of excessive excretion of urea. Other causes of solute diuresis include glucosuria, mannitol, radiographic contrast media, and chronic renal failure. *(Fauci, Chapter 45)*

53. **(H)** The combination of ECF volume contraction with high urinary sodium (20 mmol/L)

suggests renal fluid loss. This is commonly caused by diuretics or glucosuria. *(Fauci, Chapter 46)*

54. **(C)** SIADH is associated with many CNS diseases including meningitis, encephalitis, tumors, trauma, stroke, and acute porphyria. It is assumed that antidiuretic hormone (ADH) in these patients is secreted in response to direct stimulation of the hypothalamic osmoreceptors. *(Fauci, Chapter 46)*

55. **(C)** Amitriptyline is one of the psychoactive drugs that cause SIADH. Others include phenothiazines, serotonin reuptake inhibitors, and monoamine oxidase inhibitors (MAOIs). Antineoplastic drugs such as vincristine and cyclophosphamide also cause SIADH, as does the hypoglycemic agent chlorpropamide. *(Fauci, Chapter 46)*

56. **(B)** The combination of ECF volume contraction and low urinary sodium (<10 mmol/L) suggests extrarenal sodium loss. Common causes are vomiting, diarrhea, or excessive sweating. *(Fauci, Chapter 46)*

57. **(A)** Hyponatremia associated with nephrotic syndrome, cirrhosis, or CHF is characterized by edema. It is believed that the hyponatremia is caused by a decrease in "effective" circulating volume secondary to decreased cardiac output or sequestration of fluid. *(Fauci, Chapter 46)*

58. **(J)** This man has osmotic diuresis and associated hyponatremia. The clue to the extra osmoles in the serum is the increased serum osmolality in the setting of hyponatremia. This situation is frequently seen in Type 2 diabetes. *(Fauci, Chapter 46)*

59. **(B)** In patients who have prior diuretic use, resulting in hypokalemia at the time of evaluation, the bicarbonate tends to be elevated and the urine potassium low (<25 mmol/L). *(Fauci, Chapter 46)*

60. **(G)** Glucocorticoid and licorice ingestion can result in hypertension with low plasma renin and aldosterone levels. *(Fauci, Chapter 46)*

61. **(C)** RTA types I and II cause hypokalemia with high potassium excretion (>25 mmol/L) and a low bicarbonate in the absence of hypertension. Diabetic ketoacidosis can also result in this constellation of findings. *(Fauci, Chapter 46)*

62. **(F)** Primary hyperaldosteronism is characterized by hypertension with high plasma aldosterone and low plasma renin. *(Fauci, Chapter 46)*

63. **(A)** In lower GI loss (diarrhea), the blood pressure is normal, the urine potassium is low (<25 mmol/L), and the bicarbonate is either normal or low. *(Fauci, Chapter 46)*

64. **(B)** Metabolic acidosis and respiratory alkalosis are seen in salicylate overdose. *(Fauci, Chapter 48)*

65. **(B)** Sepsis can cause cardiovascular insufficiency with lactic acidosis, whereas fever and endotoxemia stimulate the respiratory center, causing respiratory alkalosis. *(Fauci, Chapter 48)*

66. **(C)** Chronic pulmonary disease often causes respiratory acidosis, whereas the steroids frequently used in therapy may cause a metabolic alkalosis. *(Fauci, Chapter 48)*

67. **(E)** Renal failure causes metabolic acidosis, whereas the loss of H+ ions in vomiting causes a metabolic alkalosis. *(Fauci, Chapter 48)*

68. **(B)** Hepatic cirrhosis frequently results in chronic respiratory alkalosis. AKI with metabolic acidosis is common in patients with cirrhosis. *(Fauci, Chapter 48)*

69. **(A)** This is a case of Henoch–Schönlein purpura (HSP). Diffuse proliferative GN is characterized by acute nephritic syndrome: AKI over days to weeks, with hypertension, edema, oliguria, and active urine sediment. Less severe clinical presentation correlates with a more benign biopsy. The pattern of glomerular involvement is similar to IgA nephropathy. *(Fauci, Chapter 277)*

70. **(A)** Systemic lupus erythematosus (SLE) can cause a wide variety of renal disorders, and can progress to ESRF. Because of the active urine sediment this individual has a proliferative GN. It is difficult to diagnose the type of glomerular involvement in SLE without a biopsy. Based on the biopsy results lupus nephritis (LN) is divided into 6 classes (WHO classification). Class I, minimal mesangial LN; Class II, mesangial proliferative LN; Class III, focal LN; Class IV, diffuse segmental LN; Class V, membranous LN; and Class VI, advanced sclerosing LN. *(Fauci, Chapter 277)*

71. **(G)** Gold is one of the drugs causing nephrotic syndrome secondary to membranous GN. It is not commonly used in the treatment of RA anymore as other disease modifying agents are more common like methotrexate. Captopril and penicillamine have also been implicated. Signs and symptoms of nephrotic syndrome (low albumin, edema, hyperlipidemia) are common, and membranous GN is also associated with a thrombotic diathesis. *(Fauci, Chapter 277)*

72. **(I)** This presentation is typical for an inherited disorder of basement membranes such as Alport syndrome. It is inherited as an X-linked dominant disorder. It is relatively benign in women but frequently progresses to ESRF in men. It is often associated with sensorineural hearing loss. *(Fauci, Chapter 277)*

73. **(E)** Rifampin can cause minimal change disease as well as more severe renal damage. The described case is typical for minimal change GN with nephrotic syndrome. Drug-induced minimal change GN frequently has an associated interstitial nephritis. INH is not usually associated with renal disease. *(Fauci, Chapter 277)*

74. **(G)** Rickets and osteomalacia can be secondary to a variety of renal tubular defects. Fanconi syndrome is a rare disorder of tubule function that results in excess amounts of glucose, bicarbonate, phosphates, uric acid, potassium, sodium, and certain amino acids being excreted in the urine. There are genetic defects that result in hereditary Fanconi syndrome and acquired causes usually due to tubular toxins such as heavy metals, certain drugs and myeloma. There are also two variants of vitamin D-dependent rickets caused by renal tubular defects. In one variant, there is impaired production of 1,25(OH)2 D3, and in the other, there is renal resistance to the action of the hormone. *(Fauci, Chapter 279)*

75. **(A)** The autosomal dominant form of polycystic kidney disease is often associated with hepatic cysts, intracranial aneurysms, and colonic diverticula. The occurrence of renal failure is usually in the third decade or later. Complications include infection, obstruction by stone or clot, and gross hematuria. *(Fauci, Chapter 278)*

76. **(D)** Bartter syndrome and Liddle syndrome can be inherited in an autosomal dominant fashion. Patients with Liddle syndrome have hypertension, whereas those with Bartter syndrome do not. In both syndromes, hypokalemia is prominent. *(Fauci, Chapter 278)*

77. **(F)** Many of the listed disorders can cause nephrolithiasis, but cystinuria is the most common cause of stones in childhood. It is a common inborn error of amino acid transport and is inherited as an autosomal recessive trait. The disorder affects transport of all dibasic amino acids (lysine, arginine, ornithine, and cystine) in the kidney and the gut, but symptoms arise from the overexcretion of cystine because it is the least soluble. *(Fauci, Chapter 281)*

78. **(C)** In prerenal AKI (ie, no histologic damage), the urinalysis reveals only hyaline casts. The urine sodium is low (<20), the urinary osmolality is high (>500), and the fractional excretion of sodium is <1. *(Fauci, Chapter 273)*

79. **(F)** In renal failure from ATN, the urinalysis can reveal heme-granular casts, and tubular cells. The fractional excretion of sodium is >1, and the urinary sodium is generally >40. *(Fauci, Chapter 273)*

CHAPTER 9

Rheumatology
Questions

DIRECTIONS (Questions 1 through 25): For each of the questions in this section select the one lettered answer that is the best response in each case.

1. A 42-year-old man of Eastern European Jewish descent develops aseptic necrosis of the femoral head. The other femur shows evidence of osteopenia, and there is diffuse osteopenia of the spine with some collapse. Review of medical records reveals he has had splenomegaly and mild pancytopenia for years. A bone marrow examination is abnormal for infiltration with lipid-laden macrophages called "Gaucher cells." **Which of the following is the most likely mechanism for this condition?**

   (A) insulin deficiency
   (B) abnormal elastic tissue
   (C) excess iron in tissue
   (D) homocystinuria
   (E) abnormal lysosomal enzymes

2. A 26-year-old woman presents to the clinic for evaluation of a red rash over her cheeks and pain, and swelling in both wrists, as well as several small joints in her hands. She notes that the rash gets worse on sun exposure and involves her cheeks, nose, ears, and chin. Medical evaluation reveals a facial rash with nasal fold sparing, oral ulcers, and 3+ proteinuria. **Which of the following is the most specific test for diagnosis of this condition?**

   (A) lupus erythematosus (LE) cells
   (B) antinuclear antibody (ANA)
   (C) anti-Sm antibody
   (D) anti-Ro antibody
   (E) antiphospholipid antibody

3. An 18-year-old man presents to the clinic for assessment of fever symptoms for the past several weeks. The fever occurs on an almost daily basis and is associated with an evanescent salmon-colored truncal rash. He also complains of diffuse arthralgias, and an extensive investigation for infections causes and malignancy is negative. A tentative clinical diagnosis of adult onset Still disease is made. **Which of the following is diagnostic of this condition?**

   (A) high-titer rheumatoid factor (RF)
   (B) positive ANA
   (C) response to steroid therapy
   (D) response to nonsteroidal anti-inflammatory drug (NSAID) therapy
   (E) lymph node biopsy

4. A 32-year-old woman presents to the clinic complaining of symptoms of a dry mouth and dry eyes. She otherwise feels well and reports no joint or systemic symptoms. On physical examination, the only findings are enlarged salivary glands. Studies for autoantibodies to Ro (SS-A) are positive. A salivary gland biopsy reveals lymphocytic infiltration. **Which of the following is the most likely diagnosis?**

   (A) sarcoidosis
   (B) primary Sjögren syndrome
   (C) human immunodeficiency virus (HIV) infection
   (D) lymphoma
   (E) amyloidosis

5. A young woman presents to the clinic for evaluation of a facial rash, as well as symptoms of arthralgias and fatigue. The symptoms started a few months ago and are not resolving. On physical examination, the rash on her face is erythematous and raised, the heart and lungs are normal, and the wrists are swollen and tender on palpation. Laboratory evaluation is only significant for mild thrombocytopenia (90,000/mL). **Which of the following is the most appropriate initial autoantibody test?**

(A) anti-double-stranded (ds) deoxyribonucleic acid (DNA)

(B) anti-Sm

(C) anti-Ro or La

(D) ANA

(E) antiphospholipid antibodies (lupus anticoagulant)

6. A 39-year-old woman complains of developing painful pale fingers on cold exposure for the past 5 years. Recently, she has noticed swollen fingers and tight skin, which limit flexion and extension. She also has new abdominal symptoms that are bothersome. On examination, the skin on the fingers is smooth and shiny with associated edema. The rest of the examination is normal. **Which part of the gastrointestinal (GI) tract is most frequently involved in this condition?**

(A) esophagus

(B) stomach

(C) duodenum

(D) ileum

(E) colon

7. A 67-year-old woman presents to the clinic complaining of frequent headaches and scalp tenderness. She has also noticed symptoms of arthralgias, fatigue, and discomfort in her jaw when she chews her food. On physical examination, her head and neck is normal, but the right temporal artery is tender on palpation. Laboratory investigations reveal an erythrocyte sedimentation rate (ESR) of 50 mm/h and a hemoglobin of 10.5 g/dL. A temporal artery biopsy is obtained for diagnostic confirmation.

Which of the following is the most appropriate next step in management?

(A) intravenous high-dose steroids

(B) acetylsalicylic acid

(C) indomethacin

(D) prednisone 60 mg/day

(E) topical steroid creams

8. A 57-year-old man comes to the clinic complaining of pain in his left hand and right knee, which is interfering with his work. The pain came on gradually, first in his hand 6 months ago and now in his knee. It is usually fine when he wakes up, but gets worse as the day progresses. There is no history of any trauma, and he is otherwise well. Taking over-the-counter NSAIDs usually relieves the pain. On examination, there is bony soft tissue swelling of his second and third distal inter-phalangeal (DIP) joints in the left hand and crepitus over the right knee with flexion. There is no erythema or joint effusion. **Which of the following is the initial change noticed in the pathogenesis of osteoarthritis?**

(A) abnormal chondrocyte function

(B) a defect in the extracellular matrix of cartilage

(C) inflammatory changes in subchondral bone

(D) ligament inflammation

(E) synovial inflammation

9. A 22-year-old woman develops color change in her fingers with cold exposure. The fingers turn white, then blue, and finally red. **Which of the following statements regarding this condition is incorrect?**

(A) may lead to gangrene of the fingers

(B) may precede the onset of scleroderma

(C) symptoms can be brought on by vibration or stress

(D) pallor (white color) associated with coldness and numbness while rubor (red color) associated with pain and tingling

(E) affects the sexes equally

10. A 63-year-old man presents to the emergency room with severe pain and swelling in his right knee. The pain started suddenly, and there is no history of injury to the knee. On physical examination, the knee is warm, red, and swollen with decreased range of movement. A diagnostic aspiration of the knee is performed. **Which of the following will most likely distinguish pseudo-gout from gout?**

(A) positive birefringent crystals
(B) acute onset
(C) involvement of single joints
(D) involvement of large joints
(E) association with diabetes

11. A 54-year-old woman with rheumatoid arthritis (RA) presents to the clinic for evaluation of symptoms of progressive fatigue. She has no active joint symptoms and her RA is controlled by low-dose methotrexate and NSAIDs. On examination, she has chronic joint deformities of her hands and a palpable spleen, which is a new finding. Routine laboratory investigations are significant for a low white count (white blood cells [WBC] 2500/mL). **Which of the following is the most likely diagnosis for her low white count?**

(A) methotrexate therapy
(B) rheumatoid nodules disrupting bone marrow architecture
(C) Felty syndrome
(D) normal variation
(E) myelofibrosis

12. A 74-year-old woman has pain in her right hand and lower back, which started months ago, and is now interfering with her activities of daily living. The pain gets worse as the day progresses. There is no history of any trauma, and she is otherwise well. Taking over-the-counter acetaminophen usually relieves the pain. On examination, there is bony soft tissue swelling of her second and third DIP joints in the right hand and pain in her lower back on forward flexion. There is no erythema or joint effusion in any of the other joints. **Which of the following is the most likely explanation for the joint pain of osteoarthritis?**

(A) synovial inflammation is not the cause
(B) ligament inflammation is a common cause
(C) clinically visible (via plain x-ray) fractures are a common cause of pain
(D) osteophytes can cause pain
(E) muscles are not involved

13. A 10-year-old child has recurrent signs and symptoms of palpable purpura on the buttocks, arthralgias, colicky abdominal pain, diarrhea, and microscopic hematuria. **Which of the following is the most likely diagnosis?**

(A) influenza
(B) immune complex vasculitis
(C) juvenile RA
(D) systemic lupus erythematosus (SLE)
(E) Wegener granulomatosis

14. A 75-year-old woman presents to the emergency room for assessment of abrupt onset of soreness, and stiffness of the shoulders, upper thighs, and hips with a low-grade fever. She was previously well, has no significant past medical history, and is not taking any prescription medications. Her physical examination is entirely normal, but the ESR is over 100 mm/h. **Which of the following is the most likely diagnosis?**

(A) dermatomyositis (DM)
(B) osteoarthritis
(C) polymyalgia rheumatica (PMR)
(D) midline granuloma
(E) sarcoidosis

15. A 63-year-old man presents to the clinic for assessment of muscle weakness symptoms. He also mentions intermittent episodes of hemoptysis, but no fever, cough, or sputum production. He has a 60-pack-per-year history of smoking. On physical examination, there is a blue purple discoloration of the upper eyelids and erythema on his knuckles. He also has proximal muscle weakness rated 4+/5, normal reflexes, and sensation. A chest x-ray (CXR) reveals a lung mass with mediastinal widening. **Which of the following is the most likely diagnosis for his muscle weakness?**

   (A) SLE
   (B) scleroderma
   (C) dermatomyositis (DM)
   (D) polyarteritis
   (E) Weber–Christian disease

16. A 26-year-old man presents to the clinic complaining of intermittent joint pain and swelling in both knees over the past year. The symptoms last weeks at a time and then improve. His past medical history is negative and he is not taking any medications. About 2 years ago he recalls having a round, pruritic skin lesion in his left groin, which appeared shortly after a camping trip. The lesion expanded slowly over a week and then resolved on its own. **Which of the following is the most appropriate initial diagnostic test?**

   (A) positive serologic studies only
   (B) synovial fluid analysis
   (C) skin biopsy
   (D) positive serology and clinical symptoms
   (E) synovial biopsy

17. A 27-year-old man has a history of low back pain and stiffness. After several months of mild symptoms, he notes more severe stiffness at night and hip pain. On physical examination, there is paravertebral muscle tenderness and limited forward flexion of the lumbar spine. X-ray of the lumbar spine shows sacroiliitis. **In addition to recommending physiotherapy and exercise, which of the following is the most appropriate next step in management?**

   (A) NSAID therapy
   (B) methotrexate
   (C) azathioprine
   (D) acetaminophen
   (E) prednisone

18. A 24-year-old woman notices pain in her left arm, made worse with use. She also has fatigue, fever, night sweats, and arthralgias. On examination, there are no palpable lymph nodes, and the joints and muscle strength are normal. The left radial pulse is absent, and there is a bruit over the left subclavian and common carotid arteries. Preliminary laboratory investigations reveal an elevated ESR and mild anemia. **Which of the following vascular findings is most likely to be found in her?**

   (A) high pressure in the legs and low pressure in the arms
   (B) low pressure in the legs and high pressure in the arms
   (C) high-pitched diastolic murmur
   (D) a relentless course to death
   (E) hypotension

19. A 54-year-old man presents to the clinic complaining of headache symptoms. On clinical examination, there is maxillary sinus tenderness on palpation suggesting a diagnosis of sinusitis. A skull x-ray of the sinuses is shown in Figure 9–1. The sinuses are normal but there is another incidental finding seen on the x-ray. **Which of the following is the most likely diagnosis?**

   (A) normal variant
   (B) osteomyelitis
   (C) Paget disease
   (D) hemangioma
   (E) metastatic disease

Figure 9–1.

(A) D-penicillamine

(B) an antimalarial

(C) methotrexate

(D) NSAID or aspirin

(E) gold

20. A 34-year-old woman presents to the clinic for evaluation of new symptoms of a red rash over her cheeks, frequent oral ulcers, and pain and swelling in both wrists, as well as in several small joints in her hands. Medical evaluation confirms the above clinical symptoms and laboratory investigations reveal a positive ANA, and 3+ proteinuria. **Which of the following organ involvement will cause the most symptoms during the course of this disease?**

(A) renal pathology

(B) cardiopulmonary pathology

(C) musculoskeletal pathology

(D) thrombotic events

(E) skin changes

21. A 29-year-old woman presents to the clinic complaining of painful swelling of both hands. She also notes being very stiff in the morning and takes much longer to get ready for work than previously. The physical examination reveals redness, swelling, and tenderness of the proximal interphalangeal joints and metacarpophalangeal (MCP) joints. Laboratory investigations are significant for a positive rheumatoid factor (RF) and negative ANA. **Which of the following medications is most likely to improve her joint pain symptoms?**

22. A 55-year-old woman presents to the clinic for evaluation of several weeks of fever, abdominal pain, weight loss, and lack of energy. Three days prior to the assessment, she developed a left foot drop. Her blood pressure is 160/90 mm Hg, pulse 80/min, and the physical examination confirms left peroneal nerve damage and a bilateral sensory neuropathy in both legs. There are no skin rashes. Laboratory evaluation reveals an ESR of 105 mm/h, WBC of 14,000/mL, and negative serologic tests for antineutrophil cytoplasmic antibody (ANCA) and ANA. The eosinophil count is normal, and urinalysis is negative for casts, protein, and red cells. A clinical diagnosis of polyarteritis nodosa is made. **Which of the following is the most likely mechanism for renal injury in this condition?**

(A) nephrotic syndrome

(B) diffuse glomerulonephritis

(C) granuloma formation

(D) necrotizing vasculitis of vessels

(E) exclusively small vessel involvement

23. A 20-year-old man presents to the clinic with symptoms of back pain. The pain is dull, and intermittent. There is no history of injury and he reports no fever, chills, or weight loss. His past medical history is significant for Marfan syndrome. On physical examination, he has characteristic features of Marfan, as well as a curvature of his thoracic spine to the left. **Which of the following is the most appropriate next step in management?**

(A) a vigorous exercise program

(B) bisphosphate therapy

(C) mechanical back bracing

(D) a prophylactic surgical procedure

(E) appropriate footwear

24. A 27-year-old man presents to the clinic for evaluation of low back pain and stiffness. The discomfort started many months ago, but recently he has noticed more severe stiffness at night and new symptoms of hip pain. The pain improves in the morning after doing some "stretching" exercises. On physical examination, there is paravertebral muscle and sacroiliac joint tenderness on palpation with limited forward flexion of the lumbar spine. A 2/6 diastolic murmur is also heard at the left sternal border radiating to the apex. Plain x-rays of the spine are suggestive of sacroiliitis. **Which of the following is the most likely diagnosis for the diastolic murmur?**

    (A) mitral stenosis
    (B) tricuspid stenosis
    (C) aortic insufficiency
    (D) pulmonic insufficiency
    (E) tetralogy of Fallot

25. A 35-year-old woman notices a red rash over her cheeks, and pain and swelling in both knees, as well as several small joints in her hands. She has difficult-to-control hypertension and 2 months ago was started on a new medication to control her blood pressure. On physical examination, the blood pressure is 167/89 mm Hg, heart rate 76/min, there is a raised erythematous rash on her cheeks, and numerous small joints (MCP and DIP) in both hands that are swollen and tender on palpation. Her ANA and antihistone antibodies are positive. **Which of the following medications is most likely to cause her condition?**

    (A) hydralazine
    (B) hydrochlorothiazide
    (C) ramipril
    (D) nifedipine
    (E) methyldopa

DIRECTIONS (Questions 26 and 27): The following group of numbered items is preceded by a list of lettered options. For each question, select the one lettered option that is most closely associated with it. Each lettered option may be used once, multiple times, or not at all.

Questions 26 and 27: For each patient with monoarthritis, select the most likely interpretation of the synovial fluid analysis.

    (A) normal synovial fluid
    (B) noninflammatory effusion
    (C) inflammatory effusion
    (D) septic arthritis
    (E) hemorrhagic effusion

26. A 57-year-old man presents with a swollen, painful left knee. He fell on the knee 3 days ago while hurrying up the stairs. On examination, there is a swollen knee with palpable effusion and decreased range of motion. A diagnostic tap is preformed and 5 cc of transparent fluid is removed. The WBC count is 1000/mL (20% polymorphonuclear neutrophils [PMNs]), glucose is equal to plasma, viscosity is high, and lactate dehydrogenase (LDH) is low.

27. A 77-year-old woman presents with a swollen, painful right knee. She fell on the knee 3 days ago while hurrying up the stairs. On examination, there is a swollen knee with palpable effusion and decreased range of motion. A diagnostic tap is preformed and 5 cc of opaque fluid is removed. The WBC count is 20,000/mL (50% PMNs), glucose is lower than plasma, viscosity is low, and the LDH is high.

DIRECTIONS (Questions 28 through 59): For each of the questions in this section select the one lettered answer that is the best response in each case.

28. A 27-year-old woman presents to the clinic because she is concerned about a red rash over her cheeks. The rash is more intense on sun exposure, and a recent trial of a mild topical steroid did not make any difference. She also reports new symptoms of joint discomfort in her hands and knees that seem to be worse in the morning. Her past medical history is negative and she is not taking any medications. On physical examination, the vital signs are normal, there are some oral ulcers on the buccal mucosa, a small patch of hair loss, and a raised nontender rash over her cheeks. Laboratory

investigations are significant for a positive ANA, low complements, and 3+ proteinuria. **Which of the following is the most likely mechanism for the renal damage in this condition?**

(A) vasculitis

(B) microemboli

(C) antibasement membrane antibodies

(D) deposition of circulating immune complexes

(E) primary tubular atrophy

29. A 50-year-old man presents to the clinic complaining of fatigue and painful swelling of both hands. He also describes being very "stiff" in the morning and requires much longer time to get ready for work. On physical examination, there is erythema, swelling, and tenderness on palpation of the proximal interphalangeal joints and MCP joints. The pattern of joint swelling is symmetric. Plain x-rays of the hand are ordered. **Which of the following x-ray findings is characteristic of this condition?**

(A) loss of articular cartilage and bone erosion

(B) normal

(C) osteolytic changes

(D) osteosclerotic changes

(E) osteolytic and osteosclerotic changes together

30. A 23-year-old man presents to the clinic for evaluation of new symptoms of low back pain, stiffness, and left eye discomfort. Sunlight also bothers his eyes. The back pain is worse at night and described as a dull ache in the back and buttock area. On physical examination, there is paravertebral muscle, iliac crest, and ischial tuberosity tenderness on palpation. Active range of motion reveals limited forward flexion of the lumbar spine. His eye is also inflamed and the pupil is constricted. Lumbar and pelvic x-rays show sacroiliitis. **Which of the following is the most likely diagnosis for his eye symptoms (it is the most common extra-articular manifestation of this condition)?**

(A) glaucoma

(B) acute anterior uveitis

(C) keratitis

(D) conjunctivitis

(E) episcleritis

31. A 24-year-old man presents to the clinic for assessment of shortness of breath on exertion. On physical examination, he is tall and thin (Figure 9–2), the visual acuity is poor with his glasses off, the jugular venous pressure (JVP) is 4 cm, first heart sound is normal, second sound is soft, a 3/6 early diastolic murmur is heard at the right second intercostal space radiating to the apex. The pulses are bounding, lungs are clear, and his arms are quite long in comparison to his total length. **Which of the following is the most likely diagnosis for his cardiac murmur?**

Figure 9–2.

(A) aortic root dilatation and aortic stenosis

(B) left ventricular dilatation and mitral valve prolapse

(C) aortic root dilatation and aortic regurgitation

(D) aortic dissection

(E) mitral stenosis

32. A 40-year-old woman presents to the clinic complaining of being very "stiff" in the morning, in addition to having sore hands and wrists. The symptoms have come on very gradually and she cannot recall when they started. Her only other complaint is feeling fatigued all the time. Physical examination reveals active inflammation of the proximal interphalangeal joints, MCP joints, and wrist joints in a symmetrical fashion. She also has nodules over both elbows. **Which of the following is predictive of developing extra-articular features of her condition?**

(A) her knees are involved early
(B) there is a poor articular response to disease-suppressing medication
(C) humoral immunity is suppressed
(D) cellular immunity is suppressed
(E) she develops high titers of rheumatoid factor (RF)

33. A 24-year-old woman is referred to the clinic for assessment of a low white-cell count. She has no past medical history and is not on any medications. Her only symptoms are of joint discomfort in her hands, and occasional sharp chest pains that change with breathing. On physical examination, there is inflammation of some MCP and DIP joints in both hands, and the rest of the examination is normal. Her WBC is 3500/mL and on the differential the lymphocytes are low (15%) and PMNs are normal. **Which of the following is the most likely diagnosis?**

(A) periarteritis nodosa
(B) SLE
(C) scleroderma
(D) DM
(E) osteoarthritis

34. A 69-year-old man presents to the clinic for routine assessment. His past medical history includes hypertension, COPD, and dyslipidemia. His current medications are amlodipine, tiotropium, salbutamol and simvastatin. He quit smoking 2 years ago, and has stable symptoms of shortness of breath on exertion. On physical examination, air entry in both lungs is normal, expiration is prolonged and there are no wheezes. On peripheral examination, the pertinent findings are clubbing of his fingers. **Which of the following is most likely associated with this condition?**

(A) RF
(B) aortic stenosis
(C) periosteal inflammation
(D) crystal-induced arthritis
(E) diffuse osteoarthritis

35. A 30-year-old woman presents to the emergency department with symptoms of pleuritic chest pain, shortness of breath on exertion, and painful swelling of her hands. She is also very stiff in the morning. On physical examination, there is inflammation of the proximal interphalangeal joints and MCP joints, air entry is decreased to the right lower lobe and the area is dull on percussion. Investigations reveal an elevated RF level, and a large right pleural effusion on the CXR. A diagnostic thoracentesis is performed, and 500 cc of a straw-colored fluid is removed. **Which of the following biochemical patterns is consistent with a pleural effusion due to her primary condition?**

(A) exudate protein and LDH ratios with low glucose
(B) exudate protein and LDH ratios with high glucose
(C) transudate protein and LDH ratios with high glucose
(D) transudate protein and LDH ratios with low glucose
(E) normal pleural fluid

36. A 67-year-old man has a long history of symmetrical small joint arthritis with deformities due to rheumatoid arthritis. He now develops shortness of breath on exertion with a dry cough, but no sputum or chest discomfort. His heart sounds have a loud P_2, and the lungs have fine bibasilar crackles. **Which of the following is the most likely diagnosis of the pulmonary condition associated with his arthritis?**

(A) pleuritis
(B) cavitating lesions
(C) intrapulmonary nodules

(D) interstitial fibrosis

(E) diffuse pneumonitis

37. A 71-year-old woman comes to the office with a history of headaches, fatigue, and weight loss for 3 months. The headaches are new for her, and usually not very severe. Her jaw also hurts when she is chewing food. Two days prior, she had briefly lost partial vision in her left eye. There were no other neurologic symptoms at the time. On physical examination, her neck is supple to flexion, fundi, and neurologic examinations are normal. She is started on prednisone 60 mg/day and a biopsy is performed to confirm the diagnosis. **Which of the following is the most likely change seen on the biopsy to confirm the diagnosis?**

(A) immune complex deposition

(B) arteritis with giant cells

(C) lymphocytic infiltration

(D) type II muscle fiber atrophy

(E) atherosclerosis

38. A 30-year-old woman presents to the clinic for assessment of a new rash over her cheeks, nose, and ears. She also complains of pain and swelling in her wrists, as well as several small joints in her hands. Her past medical history is negative and she is not taking any medications. Physical examination reveals a raised facial rash on her cheeks and chin, oral ulcerations, a patch of hair loss, and swelling and tenderness of the MCP joints. Her investigations are abnormal for 3+ proteinuria, a positive ANA titer, low serum complement levels, and normal plain x-rays of the hands. **Which of the following is the most likely cardiac manifestation of her disease?**

(A) pericarditis

(B) myocarditis

(C) aortic regurgitation

(D) nonbacterial endocarditis

(E) myocardial vasculitis with infarction

39. A 32-year-old woman presents to the clinic for assessment of shoulder and knee discomfort. Her past medical history is significant for intermittent bloody diarrhea and crampy abdominal pain. Recently, her bowel symptoms have increased and she is having 4–6 bowel movements a day with mucus and blood in the stool. She now has a low-grade fever, loss of appetite, 10 lb weight loss, and new musculoskeletal symptoms. **Which of the following is the best description of this patient's accompanying arthritis?**

(A) asymmetric migratory polyarthritis involving the large joints of the arms and legs

(B) not usually associated with disease flares

(C) a progressive, crippling course

(D) symmetrical small joint involvement

(E) seropositive

40. A 42-year-old woman presents to the clinic for evaluation of symptoms consisting of several weeks of fever, abdominal pain, weight loss, and low energy. Three days prior to assessment, she developed a left foot drop and rash on her legs. Her blood pressure is 164/92 mm Hg, pulse 88/min, and physical examination confirms left peroneal nerve damage. The rash looks like livedo reticularis. Laboratory investigations reveal an ESR of 105 mm/h, WBC of 14,000/mL, and negative serologic tests for ANCA and ANA. Eosinophil count is normal, and urinalysis is negative for casts, protein, and red cells. Biopsy of the skin rash shows inflammation of the small blood vessels. **Which of the following is the most appropriate next step in management?**

(A) plasmapheresis

(B) steroid therapy alone

(C) combination therapy with steroids and cyclophosphamide

(D) cyclophosphamide therapy alone

(E) combination therapy with steroids and methotrexate

41. A 67-year-old man presents to the clinic complaining of frequent headaches that are new for him. They are not very severe, and relieve with acetaminophen. He is also experiencing some back, shoulder, and hip discomfort, which is worse in the morning. He feels quite fatigued and does not have his usual energy level. On physical examination, his neck is supple to flexion, and fundi and thyroid examination are normal. Range of motion in the shoulders and hips is reduced because of discomfort but there is no active inflammation or crepitus. There are no focal deficits on screening neurologic examination. **Which of the following is the most appropriate initial diagnostic test?**

    (A) immunoelectrophoresis
    (B) c-ANCA levels
    (C) ESR
    (D) creatine kinase (CK)
    (E) hemoglobin and red cell indices

42. A 45-year-old man presents to the emergency room complaining of fever, abdominal pain, weight loss, and fatigue. One week ago he fell while walking and thinks that his left foot now drags a little while walking. On physical examination, there is weakness of the left foot on dorsiflexion suggestive of peroneal nerve damage. Reflexes in the legs are normal, strength in the other muscle groups is 5/5, and sensory testing reveals symmetric loss of sensation in the feet. There are no skin rashes. Laboratory investigations reveal an ESR of 115 mm/h, WBC of 16,000/mL, and negative serologic tests for ANCA and ANA. Eosinophil count is normal. A presumptive diagnosis of polyarteritis nodosa is made. **Which of the following chronic viral infections is sometimes associated with this condition?**

    (A) high cytomegalovirus (CMV) titers
    (B) herpesvirus material in circulating immune complexes
    (C) hepatitis B material in circulating immune complexes
    (D) epidemiologic relationship to Coxsackie B virus
    (E) triggering of symptoms following viral gastroenteritis secondary to rotavirus infection

43. A 19-year-old man presents to the clinic for evaluation of low back pain. The discomfort is dull in quality and associated with morning stiffness. He reports no fever, chills, night sweats, or weight loss. His past medical history is significant for a chronic papulosquamous skin disorder involving his knees and elbows. On physical examination, forward flexion at the lumbar spine is reduced but neck movements are normal. There is stress tenderness of both sacroiliac joints. On serologic testing the RF and ANA are negative. **Which of the following is the most likely diagnosis?**

    (A) RA
    (B) ankylosing spondylitis (AS)
    (C) psoriatic arthritis
    (D) reactive arthritis
    (E) PMR

44. A 68-year-old man is worried that he has RA because his RF serology is positive in a low titer (1:32). He has pain in his left hand and right knee, which usually bother him in the evening. He has not noticed any inflammation or swelling and there is no history of morning stiffness. On examination, there are no active joints. **Which of the following statements regarding the presence of RF is correct?**

    (A) is positive in 10%–20% of people over age 65
    (B) is positive in almost 100% of "classical" RA
    (C) is seen only in RA
    (D) is always abnormal
    (E) is frequently present in osteoarthritis

45. A 45-year-old man presents to the clinic complaining of intermittent swelling and pain in the superior part of his auricles for several years. He also notes that mild joint discomfort usually accompanies these episodes. Last year he also had redness, pain, and swelling over the bridge of his nose. On physical examination, there is erythema and swelling of both ears, as well as tenderness on palpation. **Which of the following is the most likely diagnosis?**

    (A) psoriatic arthritis
    (B) Behçet syndrome

(C) Wegener granulomatosis

(D) relapsing polychondritis

(E) rheumatoid arthritis

46. A 72-year-old man is brought to the emergency room after injuring his right knee in a car accident. The pain started soon after the accident. Later that same day he developed swelling and more intense pain making walking difficult. On physical examination, the knee is warm, swollen, and extremely painful to bend. There are clinical signs of an effusion. X-rays of the knee rule out a fracture, and joint fluid aspiration reveals an opaque-colored fluid containing rhomboid crystals with weak-positive birefringence. **Which of the following is the most appropriate next step in management?**

(A) oral prednisone

(B) intravenous antibiotics

(C) oral NSAIDs

(D) acetaminophen

(E) allopurinol

47. A 64-year-old man presents to the clinic because he is experiencing generalized weakness. He notes difficulty getting out of a chair, and lifting objects above his head as examples of the muscle weakness. He has lost 15 lb and feels unwell. On physical examination, there is a blue purple rash on his eyelids and knuckles, and muscle strength in his proximal muscles is rated 4 out of 5. His laboratory investigations are abnormal for an elevated creatinine kinase (CK) level. He is started on prednisone therapy. **Which of the following is the most important in monitoring response to therapy?**

(A) testing of muscle strength

(B) sedimentation rates

(C) urine transaminase enzymes

(D) EMG

(E) alkaline phosphatase

48. A 25-year-old woman with SLE presents to the clinic for assessment of increasing fatigue and shortness of breath on exertion. She denies her usual SLE symptoms of joint discomfort, chest pain, and fevers. On physical examination, there are no active joints, but she is jaundiced. Laboratory studies reveal a hemoglobin 9 g/dL, WBC 5000/mL, platelets 150,000/mL, reticulocyte count 4%, direct antiglobulin test: positive, total bilirubin 4 g/dL, direct 0.5 mg/dL, aspartate amino transferase (AST) 20 U/L, alanine amino transferase (ALT) 15 U/L, LDH 300 U/L. **Which of the following is the most likely diagnosis?**

(A) autoimmune hepatitis

(B) hemolytic anemia

(C) viral hepatitis

(D) acute blood loss

(E) Gilbert syndrome

49. A 38-year-old man presents to the clinic with 3 months of intermittent joint pain and swelling in both knees. The symptoms last weeks at a time and then improve spontaneously. His only past medical history is that of an oval-shaped, red pruritic skin lesion in his right axilla 4 months earlier, which appeared shortly after a camping trip. His immunoglobulin G (IgG) serology for *Borrelia burgdorferi* is positive. **Which of the following is the most appropriate next step in management?**

(A) high-dose glucocorticoids

(B) low-dose glucocorticoids

(C) high-dose NSAID therapy

(D) long-term penicillin

(E) long-term doxycycline

50. A 56-year-old man presents to the clinic complaining of joint symptoms that are progressively getting worse and interfering with his work and activities of daily living. His hands are particularly bad and mentions there is swelling and redness in his knuckle joints. **Which of the following statements concerning the articular manifestations of RA is correct?**

(A) wrists are rarely involved

(B) involvement of hands is characteristically asymmetric

(C) fever up to 104°F is common with joint involvement

(D) ulnar deviation at the wrist is common

(E) absence of morning stiffness makes RA an unlikely cause of articular symptoms

51. A 22-year-old man presents to the clinic complaining of low back pain and stiffness. The discomfort started several months ago as a mild dull ache in his back. The pain is more intense now, and it involves his back and hips. The symptoms seem worse at night and prevent him from sleeping. On physical examination, there is paravertebral muscle tenderness and limited flexion of the lumbar spine. Chest expansion as measured with a tape measure at the nipple line is also reduced. Figure 9–3 shows an x-ray of the lumbar spine. **Which of the following is the most likely diagnosis?**

Figure 9–3.

(A) osteoarthritis
(B) Marfan syndrome
(C) ankylosing spondylitis (AS)
(D) RA
(E) pseudogout

52. A 64-year-old woman presents to the clinic for evaluation of fatigue, and musculoskeletal symptoms. The joint pain is most noticeable in her hips and shoulders. Prior to the onset of these symptoms she has no prior history of joint discomfort. She reports of no headache, jaw discomfort, or visual disturbance. Her physical examination is normal, and laboratory testing reveals an elevated ESR of 75 mm/h. She is started on prednisone 10 mg/day and notices a dramatic improvement in her symptoms after 1 week. **Which of the following are the most typical symptoms of this disorder?**

(A) heliotrope rash
(B) proximal muscle weakness
(C) painful peripheral neuropathies
(D) stiffness and pain of proximal muscles
(E) hematuria

53. A 69-year-old man presents to the office complaining of fatigue and weight loss of 3 months in duration. He also reports having frequent headaches, which are new for him. There are no other constitutional symptoms of fever, chills, or night sweats. He does have chronic lower back pain but lately he has noticed pain in his shoulder, and hip as well. The muscle and joint symptoms are worse in the morning, and the stiffness lasts for 1 hour. His jaw also hurts when he is chewing food. Head and neck examination is normal, there is no lymphadenopathy and funduscopy is normal. Range of motion in the shoulders and hips is reduced because of discomfort but there is no active inflammation. **Which of the following is the most feared complication in patients with this condition?**

(A) blindness
(B) cortical stroke
(C) limb claudication
(D) renal infarction
(E) aortic aneurysm

54. A 67-year-old woman has pain in her left hand and right knee, which is interfering with her activities. The pain came on gradually, first in her hand 6 months ago and now in her knee. It is usually fine when she wakes up, but gets worse as the day progresses. There is no history of any trauma, and she is otherwise well. Taking over-the-counter NSAIDs usually relieves the pain. On examination, there is bony soft tissue swelling of his second and third DIP joints in the left hand and crepitus over the right knee with flexion. There is no erythema or joint effusion. **Which of the following best describes this disease condition?**

(A) disease of the synovial membrane
(B) disease of the articular cartilage
(C) disease of the entire joint
(D) disease of the subchondral bone
(E) disease of the ligaments

55. A very tall, slender 16-year-old boy is referred for evaluation of an abnormal CXR. He reports no pulmonary or cardiac symptoms, and feels well. On physical examination, he has long fingers, pectus excavatum, and a high arched palate. **Which of the following is most likely to be seen on his CXR?**

(A) dextrocardia
(B) aortic dilatation
(C) pneumothorax
(D) apical interstitial fibrosis
(E) rib notching

56. A 29-year-old woman develops symptoms of painful swelling, and stiffness of both hands. She notes that the symptoms are worse in the morning and it takes her half an hour to "loosen up" her fingers. Physical examination reveals erythema, swelling, and joint line tenderness of the proximal interphalangeal, MCP, and wrist joints. Her RF is positive, ANA is negative, and x-rays of the hands do show erosive joint changes. A clinical diagnosis of rheumatoid arthritis is made. **Which of the following is the most likely cause of the inflammation in her joints?**

(A) activated T cells
(B) antineutrophil antibodies
(C) microvascular injury
(D) interleukin-4 (IL-4)
(E) precipitated RF

57. For the above case **which of the following medications is most likely to prevent progression of disease?**

(A) D-penicillamine
(B) antimalarial
(C) methotrexate
(D) NSAID or aspirin
(E) gold

58. A 22-year-old woman develops a red rash over her cheeks, and pain and swelling in both knees, as well as several small joints in her hands. The rash gets worse on sun exposure but is not painful or itchy. On examination, the rash involves the cheeks, chin, and tips of the ears but not the nasolabial folds. It is raised, faint in color and non-scaly. Medical investigations reveal a mild normocytic anemia and 3+ proteinuria. **Which of the following is the most sensitive test for the diagnosis of this condition?**

(A) LE cells
(B) ANAs
(C) anti-Sm
(D) anti-Ro
(E) antiphospholipid

59. A 74-year-old man presents with a history of increasing frequency of headaches, fatigue, and weight loss for 3 months. He has had migraine headaches in the past, but these are different from them. He is also experiencing back, shoulder, and hip discomfort, which is worse in the morning. His head and neck examination is normal. Range of motion in the shoulders and hips is reduced because of discomfort but there is no active inflammation. **Which of the following signs or symptoms is most helpful in the diagnosis?**

(A) throat pain on swallowing
(B) pain in the jaw when chewing
(C) malaise
(D) fatigue
(E) sweating

DIRECTIONS (Questions 60 through 69): The following group of numbered items is preceded by a list of lettered options. For each question, select the one lettered option that is most closely associated with it. Each lettered option may be used once, multiple times, or not at all.

Questions 60 through 64: For each autoantibody, select the most likely clinical manifestation.

- (A) associated with hemolysis
- (B) seen in mixed connective tissue disease
- (C) most sensitive test for SLE
- (D) most sensitive test for drug-induced lupus
- (E) causes false-positive VDRL (Venereal Disease Research Laboratory)
- (F) relatively disease specific

60. ANA.

61. Anti-dsDNA.

62. Antiphospholipid.

63. Antihistone.

64. Anti-ribosomal nuclear protein (RNP).

Questions 65 through 69: For each extra-articular manifestation of RA, select the most likely diagnosis.

- (A) Felty syndrome
- (B) rheumatoid vasculitis
- (C) episcleritis
- (D) Sjögren syndrome
- (E) rheumatoid nodules
- (F) rheumatoid pleural involvement
- (G) Caplan syndrome
- (H) pericardial disease
- (I) Conjunctivitis

65. May present as small brown spots in the nail folds.

66. Most common form of eye involvement.

67. Associated with increased frequency of infections.

68. Found in association with occupational lung disease.

69. Commonly involves Achillis tendon.

DIRECTIONS (Questions 70 through 78): For each of the questions in this section select the one lettered answer that is the best response in each case.

70. A 67-year-old woman develops symptoms of cough and sputum production after an upper respiratory tract infection. A CXR does not show any signs of pneumonia but the report mentions a "pseudofracture" sign (Looser zones) seen in the left scapula compatible with osteomalacia. She has no pain in the scapula. **Which of the following best differentiates rickets and osteomalacia?**

- (A) the mineralization defect is less severe in osteomalacia
- (B) osteomalacia is only produced by vitamin D deficiency, unlike rickets
- (C) the skeleton is at a different stage when affected
- (D) parathyroid hormone levels are only routinely elevated in rickets
- (E) rickets always is characterized by hypocalcemia

71. A 72-year-old man is recently found to have hypocalcemia and osteomalacia is suspected based on the decrease in the cortical bone thickness and osteopenia seen on x-rays. **Which of the following is the most likely mechanism of the resistance to the effects of vitamin D?**

- (A) excess parathyroid hormone secretion
- (B) insufficient parathyroid hormone secretion
- (C) defective receptors for 25(OH) vitamin D
- (D) defective receptors for 1,25(OH)2 vitamin D
- (E) mineralocorticoid excess

72. A 66-year-old woman presents to the clinic complaining of pain in her left hip when walking. Three days ago, she tripped and fell in her apartment. On physical examination, there is decreased range of motion in the hip, and no leg length discrepancy. X-rays of the hip reveal osteopenia, but no fracture. **Which of the following is the primary defect in vitamin D metabolism that causes osteopenia associated with aging?**

    (A) impaired intestinal absorption of vitamin D
    (B) impaired liver hydroxylation of vitamin D
    (C) impaired renal hydroxylation of 1(OH) vitamin D
    (D) low parathyroid hormone levels
    (E) low phosphate levels

73. **Which of the following clinical findings is characteristic of both osteomalacia and rickets?**

    (A) frontal bossing in the skull
    (B) muscle weakness
    (C) prominent costochondral junctions
    (D) defects in tooth enamel
    (E) knock-knees

74. An 84-year-old man presents to the clinic for evaluation of a painful left knee. The pain is so severe that walking is difficult. He feels well otherwise and reports no other symptoms. His only past medical history is osteoarthritis which is treated with acetaminophen. On physical examination, there is an exquisitely tender, red, and swollen left knee with reduced active range of motion. **Which of the following is the most likely finding on synovial fluid analysis?**

    (A) staphylococcal infection
    (B) gonococcal infection
    (C) calcium hydroxyapatite crystals
    (D) calcium pyrophosphate crystal deposition
    (E) calcium oxalate

75. For the above case, **which of the following methods is the most effective prophylaxis for this condition?**

    (A) allopurinol
    (B) continuous NSAIDs
    (C) low-dose glucocorticoids
    (D) continuous antibiotic therapy
    (E) colchicine

76. A 69-year-old woman presents to the clinic for assessment of sudden onset severe left knee pain. She denies any falls and her past medical history is significant for chronic kidney disease due to type 2 DM for which she is on hemodialysis three times a week. On physical examination, the knee is warm, swollen, and painful to move. Diagnostic joint aspiration is performed. **Which of the following is the most likely finding in her joint fluid?**

    (A) uric acid crystals
    (B) calcium pyrophosphate crystals (CPPD)
    (C) calcium hydroxyapatite crystals
    (D) calcium oxalate crystals
    (E) crystallized urea

77. An 81-year-old woman develops progressive pain and immobility of her right shoulder. A series of x-rays over 8 months reveals destruction of the shoulder joint and an aspiration reveals blood in the effusion. Her only other articular manifestations are mild episodes of pain in her knees. **Which of the following is the most likely diagnosis?**

    (A) a chronic bacterial infection
    (B) uric acid deposition
    (C) CPPD disease
    (D) calcium oxalate deposition
    (E) calcium hydroxyapatite deposition

78. A 59-year-old woman with RA, under reasonable control with methotrexate, develops a hot, swollen, red knee. Joint aspiration removes 10 cc of an opaque yellow-colored fluid with a white count of 100,000/μL, predominantly neutrophils. The joint fluid protein is high and glucose is much lower than in the blood. **Which of the following is the most likely diagnosis?**

    (A) uric acid deposition
    (B) CPPD deposition
    (C) septic arthritis
    (D) reactivation of RA
    (E) calcium hydroxyapatite deposition

DIRECTIONS (Questions 79 through 83): The following group of numbered items is preceded by a list of lettered options. For each question, select the one lettered option that is most closely associated with it. Each lettered option may be used once, multiple times, or not at all.

For each patient with vasculitis syndrome, select the most likely diagnosis.

(A) polyarteritis nodosa (PAN)
(B) Churg–Strauss disease
(C) Henoch–Schönlein purpura
(D) vasculitis associated with infectious diseases
(E) vasculitis associated with connective tissue diseases
(F) Wegener granulomatosis
(G) giant cell arteritis
(H) Kawasaki disease
(I) Behçet syndrome

79. A 48-year-old man presents with 3 weeks of fever, fatigue, and shortness of breath. He has a history of "nasal allergies" and asthma, which have been poorly controlled in the past month. Two days prior to presentation, he developed weakness in his left foot and it now "drags" when he walks. On examination, his blood pressure is 165/90 mm Hg, pulse 100/min, respirations 20/min, and lungs have bilateral expiratory wheezes. There is left foot drop, and the rest of the neurologic examination is normal. Laboratory evaluation reveals ESR of 90 mm/h, WBC of 14,000/mL with 10% eosinophils, and 1+ proteinuria. A CXR shows bilateral pulmonary infiltrates.

80. A 39-year-old man has had several weeks of fever, weight loss, and lack of energy. Three days prior to the assessment, he developed a left foot drop. Physical examination confirms left peroneal nerve damage and a bilateral sensory peripheral neuropathy in both legs. Laboratory evaluation reveals ESR of 105 mm/h, neutrophilia of 14,000, and a negative serologic test for ANCA. Eosinophil count is normal. Angiography reveals small aneurysms of the celiac and renal arteries.

81. A 40-year old man complains of cough, shortness of breath, and nasal ulcers. He was previously well until 1 month ago. He noticed some blood in his sputum on the day of presentation. On examination, his blood pressure is 170/90 mm Hg, pulse 90/min, respirations 22/min, and there are bilateral inspiratory crackles. The oral cavity is normal, but there is a 1-cm nasal septal ulcer. Investigations reveal a positive c-ANCA, 3+ proteinuria with red cell casts, and pulmonary infiltrates on the CXR. His ESR is 110 mm/h and WBC 12,000/mL with normal eosinophils.

82. A 24-year-old woman presents with abdominal pain, joint discomfort, and lower limb rash. She was well until 1 week before presentation. On examination, she has a palpable purpuric rash on her legs, nonspecific abdominal discomfort, and no active joints. She has 3+ proteinuria, normal WBC, no eosinophils, and elevated creatinine of 1.6 mg/dL. Biopsy of the rash confirms vasculitis with immunoglobulin A (IgA) and C3 (complement 3) deposition on immunofluorescence.

83. A 34-year-old man has recurrent painful oral and genital ulcers. Recently, he has noticed multiple painful joints and a decrease in his vision. Last year he had deep vein thrombosis that required treatment. On examination, he has multiple small shallow oral ulcers and similar lesions on his scrotum. The left eye is red and tearing, while his left wrist and right knee are warm and inflamed. Laboratory investigations including complete blood count (CBC), biochemistry, and ANCA are all normal. His ESR and C-reactive protein are elevated.

Answers and Explanations

1. **(E)** Each syndrome in the lysosomal storage diseases is caused by a mutation-produced deficiency in the activity of a lysosomal enzyme. For example, Tay–Sachs disease is caused by a deficiency of hexosaminidase A, resulting in accumulation of GM2 ganglioside. Gaucher disease is caused by a deficiency of beta-glucocerebrosidase, resulting in an accumulation of glucosylceramide. It has several forms and, as in this case, is most common in Ashkenazi (Eastern European) Jews. Type I Gaucher disease, as described in this case, is the most common type. Severe bone disease and hepatosplenomegaly is characteristic. Lipid-laden macrophages (Gaucher cells) are found in the bone marrow. *(Fauci, Chapter 355)*

2. **(C)** Anti-Sm detects a protein complexed to six species of small nuclear ribonucleic acid (RNA). It is believed to be very specific for SLE. However, only 30% of patients have a positive test. In the case presented, there are enough clinical criteria (four) to confirm the diagnosis of SLE with 98% specificity and 97% sensitivity. ANA is a sensitive marker for SLE but not specific. Anti-Ro is usually found in Sjögren syndrome and antiphospholipid antibody can be found in some patients with SLE but is not diagnostic of the disorder. *(Fauci, Chapter 313)*

3. **(D)** Still disease (juvenile RA) in an adult may present as fever of unknown origin. Serology including ANA and RF is negative, and a response to NSAIDs along with exclusion of other diseases confirms the diagnosis. *(Fauci, Chapter 18)*

4. **(B)** The sicca syndrome is a recognized feature of Sjögren syndrome. It can be primary or secondary to other autoimmune disorders such as RA, SLE, scleroderma, or vasculitis. Primary Sjögren syndrome is most common in middle-aged women; sicca symptoms can also occur as a complication of HIV infection or in sarcoidosis. Sjögren syndrome is more likely to have positive serology, while the serology in sarcoid or HIV is negative. Both HIV and Sjögren can have lymphocytic infiltration, but in HIV it is predominantly by $CD8^+$ lymphocytes, whereas in Sjögren syndrome, the infiltration is by $CD4^+$ lymphocytes. In sarcoidosis, biopsy reveals granulomas. *(Fauci, Chapter 317)*

5. **(D)** ANA is the most important diagnostic autoantibodies in patients being evaluated for SLE. It is rare to have ANA negative SLE. The other antibodies can occur in SLE but not as sensitive for the diagnosis as ANA. Anti-dsDNA and anti-SM are specific for SLE but not sensitive. *(Fauci, Chapter 313)*

6. **(A)** This patient has scleroderma and esophageal symptoms are present in more than 50% of patients. They are due to the reduced tone of the gastroesophageal sphincter and dilation of the distal esophagus. Gastric and small intestinal motility problems can also occur. Vascular ectasia in the GI tract can result in bleeding. *(Fauci, Chapter 316)*

7. **(D)** The response of pain, stiffness, and headaches to 40–60 mg of prednisone is dramatic in giant cell arteritis (GSA). Intravenous

steroids are not required for the treatment of GSA unless the patient cannot take oral steroids. Anti-inflammatory treatment such as ASA or NSAIDs are not appropriate for GSA. The duration of treatment is not known but most patients require treatment for more than 2 years. ESR is used to monitor response to therapy. Patients need treatment and evaluation for the complications of long-term steroid use such as osteoporosis and diabetes. *(Fauci, Chapter 319)*

8. **(B)** It is most likely that the primary change in osteoarthritis occurs in the cartilage. It is possible that there is a disruption of the collagen network of the cartilage, specifically a disruption of the "glue" holding together adjacent fibers. *(Fauci, Chapter 326)*

9. **(E)** Raynaud phenomenon may lead to gangrene of the fingers. It can be primary (Raynaud disease) or secondary to other diseases, especially scleroderma, in which it can be the presenting symptom. In women, the primary form is common (over 50%), and the phenomenon is generally much more frequent in women. Digital infarction is much more common in relationship to scleroderma than it is in primary Raynaud disease. *(Fauci, Chapter 243)*

10. **(A)** Pseudogout (calcium pyrophosphate crystals—CPPD) is distinguishable from gout by positive birefringent crystals. CPPD are short, blunt rhomboids, and urate crystals (seen in gout) are needle-shaped with negative birefringence. *(Fauci, Chapter 327)*

11. **(C)** The triad of chronic RA, splenomegaly, and neutropenia is called Felty syndrome. It is associated with high titers of RF and extra-articular disease. The increased susceptibility to infections is secondary to both decreased neutrophil number and function. Felty syndrome is rare in African Americans. *(Fauci, Chapter 61)*

12. **(D)** Osteophytes can cause pain by stretching periosteal nerve endings. Synovial inflammation is frequently seen in osteoarthritis, but not in ligament inflammation. Microfractures, but not macrofractures, commonly cause pain.

Muscle spasm can be an important factor in the joint pain. *(Fauci, Chapter 326)*

13. **(B)** The child most likely has Henoch–Schönlein purpura, an immune complex vasculitis affecting the skin, GI tract, and renal glomeruli. Inciting antigens include upper respiratory tract infections, drugs, foods, and insect bites. *(Fauci, Chapter 319)*

14. **(C)** This patient has PMR. Proximal arm and hip muscle/joint discomfort is the hallmark of this disorder. Difficulty in getting out of bed or rising from a chair may suggest polymyositis, but the muscles are normal when muscle strength is assessed. In general, PMR causes painful muscles, not weak muscles. However, pain may lead to profound disuse atrophy and apparent muscle weakness. In these cases, normal CK and nonspecific muscle biopsy still allow accurate differentiation from polymyositis. In dermatomyositis there is a characteristic rash, as well as muscle inflammation (increased CK) and weakness which this patient did not have. The pain and onset of osteoarthritis is more gradual than this patient's. *(Fauci, Chapter 319)*

15. **(C)** This man has dermatomyositis, a paraneoplastic phenomenon of many cancers. The most common tumors associated with DM have been bronchogenic carcinomas, ovarian cancers, breast cancers, and melanoma but many others have occurred. The malignancy may antedate or post-date the myositis. Older age makes malignancy more likely. The extent of the workup for malignancy, if DM is the presentation, depends on clinical circumstances, but history and physical examination, and focused investigations (age appropriate cancer screening) are the cornerstones of evaluation. This patient's characteristic rash and muscle weakness are diagnostic of DM, and rule out the other disorders listed such as scleroderma, SLE, or polyarteritis. *(Fauci, Chapter 383)*

16. **(D)** This story is typical of Lyme disease. The spirochete involved *(B burgdorferi)* is transmitted by ixodic ticks and is most common in the Northeastern and Midwestern parts of the

United States. The host animal varies depending on the exact type of tick. Because antibody studies cannot differentiate between active and inactive disease, the appropriate constellation of symptoms is also required for diagnosis. *(Fauci, Chapter 166)*

17. **(A)** All NSAIDs are probably equally effective in the treatment of this man's ankylosing spondylitis (AS). Options include indomethacin or naproxen, but not phenylbutazone since it can cause aplastic anemia. Exercise and maintaining proper posture are very important. In patients who continue to have symptoms despite NSAID therapy, anti-TNF-α (infliximab, etanercept, or adalimumab) treatment is considered. Prednisone, methotrexate, and azathioprine are not treatment options for AS. *(Fauci, Chapter 318)*

18. **(A)** High pressure in the legs and low pressure in the arms characterize Takayasu syndrome. Clinical manifestations include easy fatigability of the arms and atrophy of the soft tissues of the face. The course is variable, and spontaneous remissions can occur. The disease predominantly affects young women. *(Fauci, Chapter 319)*

19. **(C)** There are typical "cotton wool" changes involving the frontal and parietal bones, and it is typical of Paget disease in which there is calvarial thickening and radiopacity. At this stage of the disease, a cross section through the margin of the lesion reveals a compact inner and outer table in the normal portion, whereas the dipole widens and extends to the outer and inner surfaces of the calvarium without a change in the calvarial thickness in the lesion. *(Fauci, Chapter 349)*

20. **(C)** About 95% of patients will develop musculoskeletal symptoms during the course of SLE. Arthralgias and myalgias predominate, but arthritis, hand deformities, myopathy, and avascular necrosis of bone also occur. About 85% of patients will have hematologic disease and 80% will have skin manifestations. *(Fauci, Chapter 313)*

21. **(D)** This patient has RA and aspirin or other nonsteroidal agents are effective medications for relieving the signs and symptoms of disease. However, they do little to modify the course of the disease. The new generation of NSAIDs that are more specific inhibitors of cyclooxygenase 2 cause less GI toxicity. Glucocorticoids are very powerful at suppressing signs and symptoms of disease and may alter disease progression. Methotrexate is an important disease modifying drug (DMRD) used to prevent joint destruction. Gold and antimaterials were important DMRDs in the past before the use of methotrexate and newer "biological" agents. *(Fauci, Chapter 314)*

22. **(D)** This patient has polyarteritis nodosa (PAN) and in classic PAN, unlike microscopic polyangiitis, both small and medium vessels are involved. The renal lesions are ischemic secondary to fibrinoid necrosis of the vessels. In microscopic polyangiitis, a diffuse glomerulonephritis is frequently present. The most common organ systems involved are the kidneys, musculoskeletal system, and peripheral nervous system. *(Fauci, Chapter 319)*

23. **(C)** The major musculoskeletal issue is progressive scoliosis, which is usually treated with physiotherapy and mechanical bracing. Only severe scoliosis (>45°) is treated with surgery. Vigorous exercise and pregnancy are felt by some experts to increase the rate of aortic root dilatation and not advised. *(Fauci, Chapter 357)*

24. **(C)** The frequency of aortic insufficiency has been about 4% in ankylosing spondylitis (AS). Other cardiac valve anomalies are not increased in incidence. Rarely, congestive heart failure or third degree heart block can occur as well. *(Fauci, Chapter 318)*

25. **(A)** Hydralazine can cause drug-induced lupus (defined by positive ANA and antihistone antibodies). About 25%–30 % of patients treated chronically with hydralazine will develop ANA positivity and about 10%–20% of patients with ANA positivity will develop systemic symptoms compatible with lupus, particularly arthralgias. Genetic variation in drug acetylation rates might be a predisposing factor. *(Fauci, Chapter 313)*

26. **(B)** This man has a noninflammatory effusion likely from the trauma caused by the fall. In the noninflammatory category, the fluid is transparent, WBC 200–2000/mL (<25% PMNs), glucose is normal, and LDH is low. Another cause for a noninflammatory effusion is osteoarthritis. *(Fauci, Chapter 325)*

27. **(C)** This woman has an inflammatory category of effusion in view of the opaque color, high WBC 2000–10,000 (>50% PMNs), low glucose, and high LDH. Common causes for this include crystal-induced arthritis, SLE, and RA. In septic arthritis, WBC is usually 50,000/mL or more and often >100,000/mL with >75% PMNs. Other important tests on synovial fluid include Gram stain and culture when an inflammatory effusion is suspected clinically. *(Fauci, Chapter 325)*

28. **(D)** Renal disease is usually secondary to deposition of circulating immune complex. Although most patients with SLE have such deposits, only half have clinical nephritis as defined by proteinuria. Renal biopsy can provide both prognostic and therapeutic information. *(Fauci, Chapter 313)*

29. **(A)** This patient has features of rheumatoid arthritis, and early in RA there may not be any bony changes seen on x-ray, except nonspecific findings of soft tissue swelling and joint effusions. With longer active inflammation of the joints, loss of cartilage, and bony erosions can be seen. The value of x-rays is to determine the extent of bone and cartilage damage. *(Fauci, Chapter 314)*

30. **(B)** Acute anterior uveitis is the most common extra-articular manifestation of ankylosing spondylitis (AS). Pain, photophobia, and increased lacrimation are the usual symptoms. Attacks are unilateral and tend to recur, often in the other eye. Cataracts and secondary glaucoma are not uncommon sequelae. The iritis is usually managed with local glucocorticoid administration in association with a mydriatic agent. *(Fauci, Chapter 318)*

31. **(C)** The patient has Marfan syndrome (triad of long thin extremities, lens dislocation, and aortic aneurysms). Aortic involvement occurs in about 80%, with degenerative changes predominating. Aortic root dilatation can cause aortic regurgitation or aortic aneurysm and rupture. *(Fauci, Chapter 357)*

32. **(E)** Extra-articular manifestations of RA generally develop in patients with high titers of autoantibody to the Fc component of IgG (also known as rheumatoid factor [RF]). *(Fauci, Chapter 314)*

33. **(B)** Leukopenia occurs in almost two-thirds of the SLE patients, and the differential count is usually normal. Lymphocytes and platelets can also be reduced. *(Fauci, Chapter 313)*

34. **(C)** Clubbing is a hyper-trophic osteoarthropathy (HOA), and not a finding associated with COPD, so its presence should raise the possibility of under lying lung cancer. Secondary (HOA) (eg, lung cancer) is more common than primary HOA. HOA is due to mononuclear cell infiltration and edema in the periosteum, synovial membrane, and joint capsule. *(Fauci, Chapter 330)*

35. **(A)** Pleuritis is common at autopsy in patients with RA but is not usually symptomatic. Typically, the pleural fluid shows increased pleural fluid: serum protein and LDH ratios (exudate pattern), and low glucose and low complement levels. Pleuropulmonary manifestations are more common in men with RA. *(Fauci, Chapter 314)*

36. **(D)** In RA, pleural involvement is very common at autopsy but infrequently causes symptoms. Interstitial lung disease (ILD) is the most common manifestation of rheumatoid lung disease. RA associated interstitial lung disease (RA-ILD) is usually similar to idiopathic pulmonary fibrosis (IPF) in terms of its clinical presentation, pathology, disease spectrum, and pathogenesis. Presentation is more common at age 50–60 years, in men (M:F = 2–3:1), and in association with seropositive and erosive joint disease. If pleural fluid is

present, glucose levels are very low. *(Fauci, Chapter 314)*

37. **(B)** Temporal artery biopsy is required for definitive diagnosis of giant cell arteritis, because of the relatively nonspecific nature of the presenting symptoms, signs, and routine laboratory tests. The arteritis can be segmental, however, and great care must be taken in the pathologic assessment. *(Fauci, Chapter 319)*

38. **(A)** Pericarditis is the most common manifestation of cardiac disease in patients with SLE. It can sometimes present with tamponade and acute cardiac decompensation. Myocarditis does occur and can cause arrhythmias, sudden death, or heart failure. Libman–Sacks endocarditis is associated with thrombotic events or, less commonly, valvular regurgitation. Myocardial infarction is more commonly a result of atherosclerotic disease than vasculitis. *(Fauci, Chapter 313)*

39. **(A)** In inflammatory bowel disease, there are two common types of arthritis involvement. The first is an asymmetric, migratory polyarthritis that affects the large joints of the lower and upper extremities and is closely related to the activity of bowel disease. Spondylitis is also common (though not always symptomatic) and is not always related to activity of bowel disease. *(Fauci, Chapter 318)*

40. **(C)** Current treatment for polyarteritis nodosa (PAN) mimics that of Wegener granulomatosis in the initial treatment with combination steroid and cyclophosphamide therapy. This will result in up to a 90% long-term remission rate even after discontinuation of therapy. In cases associated with hepatitis B infection, plasmapheresis is sometimes used as initial therapy. *(Fauci, Chapter 319)*

41. **(C)** Almost all patients with temporal arteritis will have an elevated ESR. Although a high ESR cannot make the diagnosis, a normal ESR helps in excluding the diagnosis. C-ANCA is a diagnostic tool for Wegener granulomatosis. Elevated CK is not seen in temporal arteritis, even with associated PMR. Normochromic, or slightly hypochromic, anemia often seen in temporal arteritis is too nonspecific to be of much diagnostic help. *(Fauci, Chapter 319)*

42. **(C)** About 20%–30% of patients with PAN have hepatitis B antigenemia. Circulating immune complexes containing hepatitis B antigen and immunoglobulin have been detected, and immunofluorescence of blood vessel walls have also demonstrated hepatitis B antigen. Antiviral therapy has been used in these cases. *(Fauci, Chapter 319)*

43. **(C)** This patient has a sacroiliac form of arthritis seen in patients with psoriasis. Patients with psoriasis can develop 5 different patterns of musculoskeletal symptoms. These include arthritis of the DIP joints; asymmetric oligoarthritis; symmetric polyarthritis similar to RA; spine and sacroiliac type; and arthritis mutilans, a highly destructive form. Most patients with psoriatic arthritis also have nail involvement. Only about a quarter actually develop a progressive, destructive disease. Uric acid may be elevated because of high tissue turnover but is not part of the pathogenesis of joint disease. AS and reactive arthritis are also seronegative arthropathies with sacroiliac involvement but they do not have the rash on the extensor surfaces described in this patient. RA is usually RF positive and involves symmetric joints. *(Fauci, Chapter 318)*

44. **(A)** The presence of RF has little predictive power in determining the diagnosis of RA with out consideration of the clinical history and physical findings. However, it is useful in determining prognosis, as high titers of RF are associated with more severe and progressive disease, as well as with extra-articular manifestations. *(Fauci, Chapter 314)*

45. **(D)** The disease is relapsing polychondritis and is characterized by frequent remissions and exacerbations of lesions and is rarely fatal. Auricular chondritis and nasal chondritis are the most common manifestations. It can also be secondary to SLE, RA, Sjögren syndrome, and vasculitis. *(Fauci, Chapter 321)*

46. **(C)** In traumatic arthritis, swellings, ecchymoses, muscular spasms, and tenderness tend to be present, but fractures must be excluded. This man has calcium pyrophosphate (CPPD) crystal-induced monoarthritis, so called "pseudogout." It is most common in the elderly and can be precipitated by minor trauma. The crystals have a rhomboid shape, and the clinical presentation can mimic that of gout. It can be associated with metabolic abnormalities such as hyper-parathyroidism or hemochromatosis. Treatment is with an NSAID for 7–10 days. If there are multiple joints involved, then steroids can be considered. An alternative to oral NSAIDs is intra-articular steroids for single joint disease. Allopurinol is not effective in CPPD. *(Fauci, Chapter 327)*

47. **(A)** The goal of therapy is to increase muscle strength and function, so following muscle strength is the key clinical assessment of response to therapy. The course of muscle necrosis in dermatomyositis can also be followed by repeated CK determinations. Repeated muscle biopsies or EMGs are rarely required. *(Fauci, Chapter 383)*

48. **(B)** This patient with SLE has developed autoimmune hemolytic anemia. Treatment consists of high-dose oral steroids. The positive Coombs test (direct antiglobulin test), high indirect bilirubin, high LDH, and high retic count are all supportive of hemolytic anemia. A normal AST and ALT rule out hepatitis of any type. There is no history of acute blood loss and the biochemical profile of increased bilirubin, low haptoglobin, and increased LDH is not consistent with blood loss. *(Fauci, Chapter 101)*

49. **(E)** This story is typical of Lyme disease. The spirochete involved (*B burgdorferi*) is transmitted by ixodic ticks and is most common in the Northeastern and Midwestern parts of the United States. The host animal varies depending on the exact type of tick. Treatment is shorter and more effective earlier in the course of the disease. The treatment of choice is doxycycline 100 mg bid for 1–2 months. Amoxicillin is a second choice drug. Steroids or high dose NSAIDs are not part of the recommendations for the treatment of Lyme disease. *(Fauci, Chapter 166)*

50. **(E)** As in most inflammatory arthritides, the patient with RA generally has morning stiffness for more than 1 hour. Wrist involvement is nearly universal and is associated with radial deviation (unlike the ulnar deviation of the digits) and carpal tunnel syndrome. Hand involvement characteristically involves the proximal interphalangeal and MCP joints in a symmetric involvement. High fever (>100.4°F), even with active synovitis, should suggest an intercurrent problem such as infection. *(Fauci, Chapter 314)*

51. **(C)** This man's symptoms are characteristic of AS, and it occurs in 1%–6% of adults inheriting human lymphocyte antigen B27 (HLA-B27). However, the prevalence in B27-positive relatives of patients with AS is up to 30%. Men are 3 times more likely to be affected. The distribution of the joints (back pain) and no hand or wrist involvement rule out RA, and osteoarthritis would be unusual in a man his age. *(Fauci, Chapter 318)*

52. **(D)** This patient has PMR. It is characterized by stiffness, aching, and pain in proximal muscle groups in the neck, shoulders, back, hips, and thighs. It is considerably more common than temporal arteritis. Both diseases are almost exclusively seen in the over 50 age group. Proximal muscle weakness, peripheral neuropathies, and hematuria are not features of PMR. If there is objective muscle weakness then the diagnosis is more likely to an inflammatory myopathy. *(Fauci, Chapter 319)*

53. **(A)** Although all these complications have been reported in giant cell arteritis, the only one with a significant likelihood is blindness secondary to ischemic optic neuropathy. Thus, if the disease is suspected, urgent diagnosis and treatment with high dose prednisone (usually 60 mg/day) is required. *(Fauci, Chapter 319)*

54. **(C)** Although the hallmark of osteoarthritis is the progressive loss of articular cartilage, it is

best considered as a disease of the entire organ, the synovial joint, rather than of any of its component tissues. In fact, all areas of the joint, bone, cartilage, synovium, meniscus, and ligaments are involved. *(Fauci, Chapter 326)*

55. **(B)** In Marfan syndrome, inheritance is autosomal dominant, and the aortic lesion is a cystic medial necrosis with loss of elastic tissue, resulting in aneurysm formation. Pneumothorax can occur but is not as characteristic. Mitral valve prolapse can also be part of the syndrome. Dislocation of the lens is the most apparent eye abnormality. Severe chest deformities and long limbs are characteristic. High, arched palate; high pedal arches; and pes planus are common. *(Fauci, Chapter 357)*

56. **(A)** Numerous mediators of inflammation are found in the synovium of patients with rheumatoid arthritis (RA). The evidence favoring activated T cells as the initiators of the inflammation include the predominance of CD4+ T cells in the synovium, the increase in soluble interleukin-2 (IL-2) receptors (a product of T-cell activation), and amelioration of symptoms by T-cell removal. *(Fauci, Chapter 314)*

57. **(C)** Methotrexate, 7.5–20 mg once weekly, is the most commonly recommended disease-modifying drug, because its effect is more rapid and patients are able to tolerate it for longer periods of time. Maximum improvement with methotrexate occurs after 6 months of therapy. Toxicity includes GI upset, oral ulceration, and liver function abnormalities. GI upset in particular may be ameliorated by concurrent folic acid administration. Pneumonitis has also been reported. *(Fauci, Chapter 314)*

58. **(B)** ANAs are present in 98% of patients with SLE. Repeatedly negative tests make the diagnosis of SLE very unlikely. Unfortunately, the test is not specific and may be positive in normal people (especially in older individuals), or secondary to infections, drugs, or other autoimmune disorders. *(Fauci, Chapter 313)*

59. **(B)** Although malaise, fatigue, and sweating are common in temporal arteritis, they are too nonspecific to help in making the diagnosis. Claudication of the jaw and tongue, while not very sensitive for temporal arteritis, are more specific than the constitutional symptoms. Odynophagia is not a characteristic of this disease. *(Fauci, Chapter 319)*

60. **(C)** Although not specific, ANA is positive in 95% of patients with SLE. A repeatedly negative test makes SLE unlikely. *(Fauci, Chapter 313)*

61. **(F)** Anti-dsDNA is relatively disease-specific and associated with nephritis and clinical activity. Anti-single-stranded (ss) DNA is not very specific. *(Fauci, Chapter 313)*

62. **(E)** The presence of anticardiolipin antibodies is associated with false-positive VDRL, vascular thrombosis, and spontaneous abortion. *(Fauci, Chapter 313)*

63. **(D)** Antihistone antibodies are seen in 95% of patients with drug-induced LE and in 70% of those with SLE. *(Fauci, Chapter 313)*

64. **(B)** Anti-RNP is found in high titer in syndromes with features of polymyositis, scleroderma, lupus, and mixed connective tissue disease. *(Fauci, Chapter 313)*

65. **(B)** Although widespread vasculitis is rare, limited forms of vasculitis are not, particularly in White patients with high titers of RF. Cutaneous vasculitis usually presents as crops of small brown spots in the nail beds, nail folds, and digital pulp. *(Fauci, Chapter 314)*

66. **(D)** Direct eye involvement with the rheumatoid process (episcleritis or scleritis) occurs in less than 1% of patients. However, 15%–20% may develop Sjögren syndrome with attendant keratoconjunctivitis sicca. *(Fauci, Chapter 314)*

67. **(A)** Felty syndrome consists of chronic RA, splenomegaly, and neutropenia. The increased frequency of infections is due to both decreased number and function of neutrophils. *(Fauci, Chapter 314)*

68. **(G)** Caplan syndrome is a diffuse, nodular fibrotic process that may result when rheumatoid nodules occur in the lungs of patients with pneumoconiosis. *(Fauci, Chapter 314)*

69. **(E)** Rheumatoid nodules occur in 20%–30% of patients with RA. Common locations include the olecranon bursa, the proximal ulna, the Achillis tendon, and the occiput. *(Fauci, Chapter 314)*

70. **(C)** Both rickets and osteomalacia are disorders in which mineralization of the organic matrix of the skeleton is defective. Rickets is the name when this disorder occurs in a growing skeleton, whereas osteomalacia occurs after the epiphyseal plates are closed. *(Fauci, Chapter 346)*

71. **(D)** Deficient or defective 1,25(OH)2 vitamin D receptors will result in vitamin D resistance. Parathyroid hormone levels increase secondary to decreased vitamin D effect. The 1(OH) vitamin D is an intermediate metabolite. *(Fauci, Chapter 346)*

72. **(C)** Aging decreases the responsiveness of the renal 25(OH) D-1-hydroxylase to parathyroid hormone (PTH), thus decreasing circulatory levels of the active metabolite 1,25(OH)2 vitamin D. This results in decreased calcium absorption from the gut. There is not a close relationship of 1(OH) vitamin D levels and osteopenia. *(Fauci, Chapter 346)*

73. **(B)** Muscle weakness is common in both rickets and osteomalacia, and proximal leg muscles are particularly involved. The combination of leg deformity and muscle weakness in rickets can result in an inability to walk. The presentation of osteomalacia is more insidious in the elderly, but proximal myopathy may be severe enough to cause a waddling gait and mimic a primary muscle disorder. The other clinical findings listed are found only in rickets. *(Fauci, Chapter 346)*

74. **(D)** The term *pseudogout* refers to crystal deposition disease not due to uric acid (gout). By far the most common cause of pseudogout is calcium pyrophosphate deposition (CPPD). The major predisposing factors are advanced age and preexisting joint disease. The knee is the most common joint involved, and presentation can mimic acute gout. However, in the majority of cases, the deposition of calcium pyrophosphate seems to be asymptomatic. *(Fauci, Chapter 327)*

75. **(E)** Unfortunately, there is no medical means to remove the deposits of CPPD. Colchicine does seem to decrease the rate of recurrence. NSAIDs, steroids (systemic or intra-articular), and colchicine are all helpful in acute attacks. *(Fauci, Chapter 327)*

76. **(C)** Although gout and CPPD disease are found in chronic renal failure, hydroxyapatite deposition is characteristic of end-stage renal failure. The crystals are very small, nonbirefringent, and only seen on electron microscopy. Treatment is symptomatic, and similar to the treatment of gout or CPPD disease. *(Fauci, Chapter 327)*

77. **(E)** "Milwaukee shoulder" represents an unusual manifestation of calcium hydroxyapatite deposition disease. Once destruction changes start occurring, medical management is relatively unsuccessful. The exact reason why destructive arthritis occurs is not understood. The knee is the other joint affected in this manner. *(Fauci, Chapter 327)*

78. **(C)** The high white cell count suggests infection. In RA and crystal-induced arthritis, the white cell count is usually less than 50,000/μL. *Staphylococcus aureus* infection is the most common type in RA. *(Fauci, Chapter 314)*

79. **(B)** Churg–Strauss is a granulomatous vasculitis. Pulmonary involvement often dominates the clinical presentation with severe asthma attacks and pulmonary infiltrates. Peripheral eosinophilia is present in virtually all cases. *(Fauci, Chapter 319)*

80. **(A)** PAN is a multisystem, necrotizing vasculitis of small- and medium-sized muscular arteries. Aneurysmal dilations of the arteries are characteristic. Nonspecific signs and symptoms are the usual method of presentation. Renal

involvement is clinically present in 60% of cases and is the most common cause of death in untreated cases. *(Fauci, Chapter 319)*

81. **(F)** A high percentage of patients with Wegener develop ANCAs. In particular, cytoplasmic or c-ANCAs are both sensitive and specific for Wegener. However, tissue diagnosis is still required. *(Fauci, Chapter 319)*

82. **(C)** Henoch–Schönlein purpura, characterized by palpable purpura, arthralgias, GI symptoms, and glomerulonephritis, can be seen in any age group but is most common in children. It can resolve and recur several times over a period of weeks or months and can resolve spontaneously. *(Fauci, Chapter 319)*

83. **(I)** Behçet syndrome is a leukocytoclastic venulitis characterized by episodes of oral ulcers, genital ulcers, iritis, and cutaneous lesions. Eye involvement can rapidly progress to blindness. *(Fauci, Chapter 319)*

CHAPTER 10

Infectious Diseases
Questions

DIRECTIONS (Questions 1 through 53): For each of the questions in this section select the one lettered answer that is the best response in each case.

1. A 22-year-old man presents to the emergency room after sustaining a work related injury. He is a recent immigrant to the United States and does not recall receiving vaccination for tetanus. On physical examination, there is a small laceration on his leg requiring stitches, but there is dirt and soil contamination of the wound. **Which of the following statements is correct?**

    (A) tetanus usually develops within 2 weeks following exposure
    (B) tetanus always develops within 4 hours following exposure in patients who have not been previously immunized
    (C) tetanus may develop many months or years following exposure in susceptible individuals
    (D) the usual incubation period for tetanus is 48 hours
    (E) tetanus may be prevented with penicillin

2. A 19-year-old man is donating blood for the first time. Despite having no risk factors for human immunodeficiency virus (HIV) infection, his blood tests positive for HIV by enzyme immunoassay (EIA). **Which of the following statements is correct?**

    (A) EIA is currently the most specific test for HIV
    (B) he might have a false-positive secondary to an unsuspected collagen-vascular disease
    (C) he has a 75% chance of truly being infected with HIV
    (D) EIA is an excellent screening test
    (E) a Western blot test would be more sensitive

3. A 27-year-old man presents to the clinic for assessment of symptoms of fever, chills, malaise, and joint discomfort in his hands and knees. He looks unwell, his temperature is 39.4°C, blood pressure 115/70 mm Hg, pulse 110/min, head and neck is normal, and his jugular venous pressure (JVP) has a prominent c-v wave. There is also a 3/6 pansystolic murmur heard at the right sternal border that increases with respiration. His lungs are clear, abdomen is soft, and hand joints are normal. He has multiple puncture sites on his forearms from injection drug use. **Which of the following is the most likely causative organism?**

    (A) *Staphylococcus aureus*
    (B) *Staphylococcus epidermidis*
    (C) *Streptococcus viridans*
    (D) enterococci
    (E) *Candida*

4. A 23-year-old woman presents to the clinic for evaluation of a new skin rash in her genital area. The lesions are painful and itchy, and she is experiencing discomfort with urination. On physical examination, there are multiple vesicular lesions on an erythematous base on her vulvar area. There is also bilateral inguinal lymphadenopathy that is tender on palpation. **Which of the following is the most likely causative organism?**

(A) cytomegalovirus (CMV)
(B) gonococcus
(C) herpes simplex virus type 2 (HSV-2)
(D) *Treponema pallidum*
(E) varicella zoster

5. A 17-year-old man presents to the clinic with new symptoms of fatigue, malaise, fever, and a sore throat. He has no significant past medical history and is not on any medications. Physical examination is entirely normal except for enlarged, palpable cervical lymph nodes. He reports no weight loss or night sweats. Laboratory investigations include a normal chest x-ray, negative throat swab, but abnormal blood film with atypical lymphocytes. The hemoglobin is 15.5 g/dL; hematocrit 42%; platelets 290,000/mL; WBC 10500/mL, with 45% segmented neutrophils, 1% eosinophils, and 54% lymphocytes, of which 36% were atypical. **Which of the following is the most appropriate initial diagnostic test?**

(A) lymph node biopsy
(B) bone marrow
(C) erythrocyte sedimentation rate (ESR)
(D) heterophil antibody (Monospot) test
(E) hepatic biopsy

6. A 34-year-old man is traveling in Southeast Asia on business. He is staying in Western-style hotels and eating food in large restaurants. He does not eat from street vendors. One week after arrival, he develops symptoms of anorexia, nausea, and abdominal cramps followed by the sudden onset of watery diarrhea. He has no fever or chills and there is no blood or pus in the stools. **Which of the following is the most appropriate therapy for his condition?**

(A) amoxicillin
(B) symptomatic therapy with loperamide
(C) doxycycline
(D) oral rehydration only
(E) specific antitoxin

7. An 18-year-old woman presents with headache, anorexia, chilly sensations, and discomfort on both sides of her jaw. She has also noticed discomfort in both lower abdominal quadrants. Physical examination reveals bilateral enlarged parotid glands that are doughy, elastic, and slightly tender; with a reddened orifice of Stensen duct. Her abdomen is soft with bilateral lower quadrant abdominal tenderness; a temperature of 38.5°C; and a pulse rate of 92/min. Laboratory data show hemoglobin 13 g/dL; hematocrit 40%; white blood cells (WBC) 9000/mL, with 35% segmented neutrophils, 7% monocytes, and 58% lymphocytes. **Which of the following is the most likely cause for her abdominal pain and tenderness?**

(A) mesenteric lymphadenitis
(B) oophoritis
(C) gonorrhea
(D) peritoneal metastases
(E) intestinal hyperperistalsis

8. A 32-year-old man, who is previously well, presents to the clinic for evaluation of a fever and dry cough. On physical examination, his chest is clear and the heart sounds are normal. A chest x-ray (CXR) reveals a diffuse interstitial infiltrate in both lower lobes. **Which of the following is the most likely causative organism?**

(A) bacterium
(B) mycoplasma
(C) fungus
(D) rickettsia
(E) spirochete

9. A 25-year-old man presents to the hospital with symptoms of fever and rust-colored sputum. The symptoms started 2 days ago and are getting worse. On physical examination, he looks unwell; the temperature is 38.7°C, pulse 100/min,

and blood pressure 115/80 mm Hg. On auscultation, there are bronchial breath sounds and inspiratory crackles in the right axilla. The CXR is shown in Figure 10–1. **Which of the following is the most likely diagnosis?**

Figure 10–1.

(A) right middle lobe pneumonia
(B) loculated pleural effusion
(C) aspergilloma
(D) aspiration pneumonia
(E) right lower lobe pneumonia

10. A 30-year-old man comes to the clinic complaining of malaise and fever. One week ago he noticed a pustular lesion on his right forearm that developed at the site of a scratch from his cat. Prior to this he was feeling well, and reports no significant past medical history. On physical examination, the pustule is healed but there are multiple tender lymph nodes in the right axilla. **Which of the following is the most likely causative organism?**

(A) *Bartonella henselae*
(B) *Bartonella bacilliformis*
(C) *Bartonella quintana*
(D) *Coxiella burnetii*
(E) *Borrelia burgdorferi*

11. A 7-year-old child develops malaise, cough, coryza, and conjunctivitis with a high fever. Prior to this illness he was completely healthy. Further questioning reveals that he has not received any childhood vaccinations because of his parents' religious beliefs. Examination of his mouth reveals blue white spots on a red base beside his second molars. The next day he develops an erythematous, nonpruritic, maculopapular rash at his hairline and behind his ears, which spreads over his body. **Which of the following is the most likely diagnosis?**

(A) hand-foot-and-mouth disease (coxsackievirus)
(B) measles (rubeola)
(C) rubella (German measles)
(D) mumps
(E) pertussis

12. A 60-year-old man presents to the hospital with symptoms of fever and malaise 6 weeks after mitral valve replacement. On physical examination, his temperature is 38.5°C, blood pressure 130/80 mm Hg, pulse 80/min, and there is a loud pansystolic murmur at the apex, which radiates to the axilla. The skin and neurologic examination is normal. **Which of the following is the most likely causative organism?**

(A) *Staphylococcus aureus*
(B) a fungus
(C) *Staphylococcus saprophyticus*
(D) pneumococcus
(E) *Staphylococcus epidermidis*

13. A 73-year-old man from a nursing home develops headache, fever, cough, sore throat, malaise, and severe myalgia during a community outbreak affecting numerous other residents at the home. The symptoms gradually resolve after 3 days, and he starts feeling better but then there is a reappearance of his fever, with cough and yellow sputum production. On examination, his temperature is 38.5°C, pulse 100/min, respiration 24/min, oxygen saturation 88% and crackles in the right lower lung base, bronchial breath sounds and dullness on percussion. CXR reveals a new infiltrate in the right lower lobe. **Which of the following is the most likely causative organism?**

    (A) primary viral pneumonia
    (B) an autoimmune reaction
    (C) *Mycoplasma pneumoniae*
    (D) *Streptococcus pneumoniae*
    (E) *Neisseria catarrhalis*

14. Two students from a university dormitory building have contracted meningitis due to *Neisseria meningitides*. **Which of the following students in the dormitory are most likely to benefit from chemoprophylaxis?**

    (A) everybody in the dormitory, with oral amoxicillin
    (B) close contacts only, with oral amoxicillin
    (C) everybody in the dormitory, with oral rifampin
    (D) close contacts only, with oral rifampin
    (E) everybody in the dormitory, with meningococcal vaccine

15. A 21-year-old woman visits her physician because of 3 weeks of a "flu-like" illness. She reports symptoms of malaise, fever, fatigue, and a sore throat. There is no weight loss or night sweats, and she has not traveled out of country. Her past medical history is not significant and she is not taking any medications. Physical examination is normal except for enlarged cervical lymph nodes. Laboratory data show hemoglobin 13.2 g/dL; hematocrit 42%; platelets 380,000/mL; WBC 8500/mL, with 35% segmented neutrophils, 1% eosinophils, and 64% lymphocytes, of which 36% were

atypical. A heterophil antibody (Monospot) test is negative. **Which of the following is the most likely causative organism?**

    (A) herpes simplex
    (B) echovirus
    (C) CMV
    (D) coxsackievirus
    (E) reovirus

16. A 23-year-old woman visits your office because of headache, malaise, anorexia, pain in both sides of her jaw, and discomfort in both lower abdominal quadrants. Physical examination reveals enlarged parotid glands; bilateral lower quadrant abdominal tenderness; a temperature of 38.7°C; and a pulse rate of 92/min. Serologic testing (IgM) confirms the diagnosis of mumps. **Which of the following is the most appropriate treatment for this condition?**

    (A) symptomatic
    (B) immunization
    (C) broad-spectrum antibiotics
    (D) sulfonamides
    (E) steroids

17. A 10-year-old boy is brought to the emergency room with symptoms of fever, headache, photophobia, and neck discomfort in the middle of summer. He is alert and oriented, but describes neck pain with flexion and extension of the head. His fundi are normal, and there are no focal neurologic findings or skin changes. A lumbar puncture reveals normal protein and glucose with a cell count of 240/mL (90% lymphocytes). **Which of the following is the most likely causative organism?**

    (A) enterovirus (coxsackievirus or echovirus)
    (B) *Streptococcus pneumoniae*
    (C) *Neisseria meningitides*
    (D) *Listeria monocytogenes*
    (E) HSV-1

18. An 18-year-old woman has eaten homemade preserves. Eighteen hours later, she develops diplopia, dysarthria, and dysphagia. She presents to the emergency room for assessment and

on examination her blood pressure is 112/74 mm Hg, heart rate 110/min, and respirations 20/min. The pertinent findings are abnormal extraocular movements due to cranial nerve palsies, difficulty swallowing and a change in her voice. The strength in her arms is 4/5 and 5/5 in her legs, and the reflexes are normal. **Which of the following is the most likely causative organism?**

(A) *Clostridium botulinum* toxin
(B) staphylococcal toxin
(C) salmonellosis
(D) brucellosis
(E) shigellosis

19. A previously healthy 19-year-old female university student develops myalgia, headache, fever, and malaise. Blood tests reveal lymphocytosis, with 20% of the lymphocytes being atypical. She remains tired and unwell for 6 weeks, but repeated tests for heterophil antibody are negative. **Which of the following is the most likely diagnosis?**

(A) Epstein–Barr virus (EBV) infection
(B) primary HIV infection
(C) human herpes virus type 7 (HHV-7)
(D) CMV infection
(E) toxoplasmosis

20. A 43-year-old man develops a cough shortly after returning from a 1-month hiking trip in California. He was previously healthy and not taking any medications. While there, he was hiking in the central California valleys. During his trip, he reports developing a "flu-like" illness consisting of fever, cough, and muscle pains, which resolved spontaneously. A CXR shows a thin-walled cavity in the right upper lobe, and his sputum reveals fungal elements. **Which of the following is the most likely causative organism?**

(A) ringworm
(B) *Cryptococcus neoformans*
(C) *Candida albicans*
(D) mycobacteria
(E) coccidioidomycosis

21. An 8-year-old boy from an impoverished inner-city area has never been vaccinated appropriately. He develops fever, cough, and coryza. The next day, blue-white spots develop on the buccal mucosa. On the third day, an erythematous, nonpruritic maculopapular rash develops on the face and spreads over the entire body. **Which of the following is the most likely complication?**

(A) pneumonia
(B) encephalitis
(C) otitis media
(D) bronchitis
(E) mastoiditis

22. A 27-year-old man presents to the clinic with symptoms of diarrhea and abdominal pain. He returned from a trip to rural South America 3 weeks ago. Over the past few days, he has gradually developed lower abdominal pain and diarrhea. Now the symptoms are much worse with 8 stools a day consisting mostly of mucus and blood. On physical examination, he is afebrile, the abdomen is tender in the left lower quadrant, and the remaining examination is normal. His stool is mostly comprised of blood and mucus. **Which of the following is the most appropriate initial diagnostic test?**

(A) stool culture
(B) Clostridium difficile toxin assay
(C) examination of a dried stool specimen
(D) immunofluorescence of stool specimen
(E) stool samples for culture and ova and parasites

23. A 4-year-old boy is sent to the emergency room because he is suspected of having meningitis. He has been ill for 2 days with fever and lethargy. On physical examination, he is febrile (38.4°C), the neck is stiff on flexion and causes discomfort, and on funduscopy papilledema is present. There is no skin rash, the lungs are clear, and the heart sounds normal. **Which of the following is the most likely causative organism?**

   (A) *Neisseria meningitidis*
   (B) *Streptococcus pneumoniae*
   (C) *Haemophilus influenzae*
   (D) *Staphylococcus*
   (E) *Listeria* species

24. **Which of the following is a contraindication to receiving the live rubella vaccine?**

   (A) children between 1 year old and puberty
   (B) infants <1 year old
   (C) all adults
   (D) pregnant women
   (E) all exposed patients

25. A 24-year-old woman presents to the emergency department with symptoms of fever, chills and rigors. On physical examination, she looks unwell; the temperature is 39.4°C, blood pressure 100/60 mm Hg, pulse 110/min, and oxygen saturation 95%. There is a 3/6 pansystolic murmur at the right sternal border, which increases with inspiration. Her arms have multiple tattoos and needle marks from injection drug use. Blood cultures (2/2 sets) are positive for *S aureus*, and she is started on appropriate antibiotics. Her renal function is mildly impaired and her urinalysis is positive for protein, and microscopy reveals red cell casts. **Which of the following mechanisms is the most likely explanation for her renal abnormalities?**

   (A) septic emboli
   (B) cardiac failure with prerenal azotemia
   (C) a high level of circulating immune complexes
   (D) fungal disease
   (E) inevitable progression to renal failure

26. A 22-year-old university student complains of fatigue and malaise for the past 2 weeks. She also reports feeling feverish, and recently had a sore throat. Physical examination reveals enlarged tonsils and palpable cervical lymph nodes. There is also tenderness in the right upper quadrant on deep palpation, and minimal splenomegaly. Laboratory data show hemoglobin 13 g/dL; hematocrit 40%; platelets 340,000/mL; WBC 9400/mL, with 35% segmented neutrophils, 1% eosinophils, and 64% lymphocytes, of which 36% were atypical. A heterophil antibody (Monospot) test is positive. **Which of the following is the most appropriate initial treatment for this condition?**

   (A) intravenous gamma-globulin
   (B) adequate rest and supportive treatment
   (C) ciprofloxacin
   (D) moxifloxacin
   (E) ampicillin

27. A 26-year-old woman presents to the clinic for assessment of a painless chronic genital ulcer on her vulva. She recently arrived to study in the United States from Southern India. The lesion began as a papule and then ulcerated. It has persisted for several months. Physical examination reveals a painless elevated area of beefy red, friable granulation tissue. She has been sexually active for several years. **Which of the following is the most likely causative organism?**

   (A) spirochete
   (B) Gram-positive coccus
   (C) intracellular Gram-negative bacteria
   (D) chronic viral infection
   (E) fungus

28. A 20-year-old woman presents to the emergency department with symptoms of headache, fever, and neck stiffness. On physical examination, her blood pressure is 100/70 mm Hg, pulse 100/min, temperature 38.6°C, and the neck is stiff and painful on flexion and extension. The ears, throat, and sinuses are normal, there are no focal neurologic signs, and the remaining examination is normal. There are no reported similar cases in the community.

Which of the following is the most likely source of her infection?

(A) an infected heart valve

(B) nasopharynx

(C) skin

(D) oral ingestion

(E) bowel

29. A 44-year-old man with a prior renal transplant presents to the clinic for evaluation of symptoms consisting of a cough and shortness of breath on exertion. There is no sputum production and he has no prior respiratory or cardiac illnesses. On physical examination, he appears dyspneic, respirations 24/min, pulse 110/min, and oxygen saturation 88%. His lungs are clear on auscultation and heart sounds are normal. CXR shows bilateral diffuse perihilar infiltrates. Bronchoscopy and bronchial brushings show clusters of cysts that stain with methenamine silver. **Which of the following is the most appropriate next step in management?**

(A) amphotericin B

(B) cephalosporins

(C) trimethoprim-sulfamethoxazole

(D) aminoglycosides

(E) penicillins

30. A 34-year-old man presents to the clinic for assessment of new symptoms of diarrhea. He returned recently from a trip to Southeast Asia 3 weeks ago. He now complains of lower abdominal pain associated with the diarrhea. He is having 8 stools a day consisting mostly of mucus and blood. On physical examination he is afebrile, the abdomen is tender in left lower quadrant, and the remaining examination is normal. Stool tests show trophozoites of *Entamoeba histolytica*. **Which of the following is the most likely site of extraintestinal involvement?**

(A) genitals

(B) pleura

(C) pericardium

(D) liver

(E) cerebral cortex

31. A 20-year-old woman complains of headache and discomfort in both sides of her jaw. Physical examination reveals enlarged parotid glands that are slightly tender on palpation. There is reddening of the orifice of Stensen duct on intra oral examination; her temperature is 38.3°C, and the pulse rate is 80/min. Laboratory data show hemoglobin 14 g/dL; hematocrit 40%; WBC 11000/mL, with 33% segmented neutrophils, 7% monocytes, and 60% lymphocytes. **Which of the following diagnostic tests will help to confirm the diagnosis of epidemic parotitis?**

(A) single blood sample for a specific immunoglobulin G (IgG)

(B) blood cell count

(C) blood culture

(D) single blood test for a specific immunoglobulin M (IgM)

(E) serum amylase

32. Three hours after a church social, 8 people develop severe diarrhea. Other symptoms included nausea, vomiting, and abdominal cramps. Food served included chicken salad and cream-filled pastries. All affected individuals had the chicken salad. **Which of the following is the most likely causative organism?**

(A) staphylococcal enterotoxin

(B) *C botulinum*

(C) *Clostridium perfringens*

(D) *Salmonella* species

(E) ptomaine poisoning

33. A 22-year-old woman presents to the clinic complaining of hair loss, loss of hair luster, and intense scalp irritation. The symptoms started a few weeks ago, and seem to be getting worse. Physical examination of the hair reveals patches of hair loss with tiny little black dots where the hair shaft has broken off. There are also annular scaly patches with raised erythematous borders and central clearing. A Wood light examination is positive. **Which of the following is the most likely diagnosis?**

(A) seborrheic dermatitis

(B) *Aspergillus* infection

(C) *Trichophyton* infection

(D) neurosis

(E) excess androgen levels

34. A 9-year-old boy is brought to the emergency department because of a severe sore throat with fever and dysphagia. On physical examination, there are grayish-white papulovesicular lesions on an erythematous base that ulcerate. They are located on the soft palate, anterior pillars of the tonsils and uvula. There are no lesions on the gingiva, tongue, or lips. A clinical diagnosis of herpangina is made. **Which of the following is the most likely causative organism?**

(A) measles (Morbillivirus)

(B) rubella (Rubivirus)

(C) coxsackievirus A

(D) HSV-1

(E) HSV-2

35. A 19-year-man presents to the emergency department because he is bitten by a stray dog. On physical examination, there is a penetrating wound to the right forearm. The dog is nowhere to be found. The wound is cleaned with water and povidone-iodine solution. **Which of the following is the most appropriate next step in management?**

(A) start postexposure prophylaxis

(B) contact the local public health professional for further advice

(C) treat with oral doxycycline

(D) treat with IV ceftriaxone

(E) start IV acyclovir

36. **Which of the following malignancies in the United States is most likely to contain EBV deoxyribonucleic acid (DNA) in a non-HIV patient?**

(A) gastric cancer

(B) well-differentiated thyroid cancer

(C) anaplastic nasopharyngeal carcinoma

(D) Burkitt lymphoma

(E) Hodgkin disease

37. A 24-year-old man presents to the clinic complaining of fatigue, malaise, fever, and a sore throat. He was previously well, but now feels tired all the time and has to rest multiple times a day. Physical examination shows enlarged tonsils and there are palpable anterior and posterior cervical, axillary, and inguinal lymph nodes. There is also tenderness in the right upper quadrant with a liver span of 10 cm. Laboratory data is significant for a heterophil antibody (Monospot) test that is positive. **Which of the following rare complications is associated with this condition?**

(A) retinitis

(B) esophagitis

(C) splenic rupture

(D) Kaposi sarcoma

(E) hemorrhage

38. A 40-year-old man develops erythema nodosum, conjunctivitis, and a pleural effusion. Over several weeks, pulmonary lesions lead to cavitation and a large, thin-walled cavity. He was traveling in Arizona before becoming ill. Sputum samples reveal mature spherules. **Which of the following is the most likely diagnosis?**

(A) *Streptococcus*

(B) coccidioidomycosis

(C) candidiasis

(D) *Staphylococcus*

(E) *Pneumocystis carinii*

39. A patient undergoing emergency surgery for trauma receives 20 blood transfusions during the operation. Four weeks later, she develops a syndrome resembling infectious mononucleosis. **Which of the following is the most likely causative organism?**

(A) EBV

(B) hepatitis C virus

(C) delayed hemolysis

(D) CMV

(E) serum sickness

40. A 32-year-old woman presents to the emergency department after acutely developing a high fever, lightheadedness on standing, and a rash. At the hospital she develops vomiting, diarrhea, confusion, and abdominal pain. She goes on to develop evidence of multiorgan failure and is transferred to the intensive care unit. One week after the acute illness she develops desquamation of the skin. On further history, the illness started 3 days after the onset of menstruation. **Which of the following is the most likely diagnosis?**

(A) *S aureus* toxic shock syndrome (TSS)

(B) streptococcal infection (scarlet fever)

(C) clostridial infection

(D) Rocky mountain spotted fever (RMSF)

(E) staphylococcal scaled skin syndrome

41. An 18-year-old man develops fever, neck stiffness, and headache. On examination, his blood pressure is 105/80 mm Hg, pulse 100/min, temperature 38.7°C, and neck flexion is very painful. The ears, throat, and sinuses are normal; there are no focal neurologic signs, and the remaining examination is normal. His is the second case of meningitis in his university dormitory building. **Which of the following is the most likely causative organism?**

(A) *Neisseria meningitidis*

(B) *Streptococcus pneumoniae*

(C) *Haemophilus influenzae*

(D) *Staphylococcus*

(E) *Listeria* species

42. A 45-year-old woman is undergoing chemotherapy for breast cancer. She presents 10 days after her last chemotherapy dose with fever (temperature >38.5°C), but no other symptoms except a sore throat and mouth. On examination, she looks well, there is oral mucositis, ears are normal, lungs are clear, and the central line site is clean. The CXR, urinalysis, and biochemistry are normal. Her WBC is 800/mL and the absolute neutrophil count is low (<500). **Which of the following is the most appropriate next step in management?**

(A) start empiric bacterial antibiotics

(B) start empiric antifungal and bacterial antibiotics

(C) acetaminophen alone until culture results are available

(D) start antiviral medications for HSV-1

(E) start antiviral and bacterial antibiotics

43. An 84-year-old bedridden patient in the hospital develops cough, fever, and shortness of breath. On physical examination, the JVP is at 4 cm, heart sounds are normal, and there are crackles on inspiration in the right lower lobe. A CXR reveals a new right lower lobe infiltrate and his WBC is 15,000/mL. He was admitted to the hospital 7 days ago for the treatment of congestive heart failure. **Which of the following is the most likely diagnosis?**

(A) hospital-acquired pneumonia

(B) atelectasis

(C) pulmonary embolism

(D) community-acquired pneumonia

(E) asymmetric congestive heart failure

44. A 74-year-old man residing in a nursing home develops symptoms of high fever, diarrhea, chest pain, and nonproductive cough. His temperature is 40°C, blood pressure 120/80 mm Hg, respiration 24/min, and oxygen saturation 90%. He has bibasilar crackles, normal heart sounds, and a soft nontender abdomen. His CXR reveals bilateral lower lobe infiltrates. He is not able to provide any sputum, and the urine is positive for legionella antigen. **Which of the following is the most appropriate antibiotic choice?**

(A) trimethoprim-sulfamethoxazole

(B) azithromycin

(C) ceftriaxone

(D) cefuroxime

(E) gentamicin

45. A businesswoman needs to make frequent trips to South America, but every time she is there, she develops traveler's diarrhea, which requires her to change her business schedule. To prevent future episodes during business trips, she is inquiring about prophylaxis methods. **Which of the following is the most helpful advice for her?**

(A) take loperamide for symptoms

(B) take trimethoprim-sulfamethoxazole every day

(C) take azithromycin every day

(D) take doxycycline every day

(E) take ciprofloxacin only if moderate or severe symptoms develop

46. The dental condition illustrated in Figure 10–2 is usually associated with a congenital infectious disease. The teeth are characterized by centrally notched, widely spaced, peg-shaped upper central incisors and molars that have poorly developed cusps. **Which of the following is the most likely diagnosis?**

Figure 10–2.

(A) congenital rubella

(B) congenital syphilis

(C) congenital toxoplasmosis

(D) congenital HIV

(E) congenital measles

47. A 53-year-old man with alcoholic cirrhosis presents to the emergency room with increasing jaundice and abdominal discomfort. He reports no fevers or chills. On physical examination, his blood pressure is 100/60 mm Hg, pulse 100/min, and temperature 38.1°C. The abdomen is distended; there is 2+ peripheral edema, and shifting dullness. It is tender on palpation and bowel sounds are present. A diagnostic paracentesis is performed; the total cell count is 940/mL with polymorphonuclear neutrophils (PMNs) equal to 550/mL, Gram stain is negative, and cultures are pending. **Which of the following is the most likely diagnosis?**

(A) pancreatic ascites

(B) malignant ascites

(C) spontaneous bacterial peritonitis (SBP)

(D) secondary peritonitis

(E) tuberculous ascites

48. A 45-year-old man presents to the clinic complaining of diffuse joint discomfort which started 1 week ago. He reports no other symptoms. He recently came back from a camping trip to Maine and is concerned that he might have Lyme disease. He does not recall any tick bites, or characteristic skin lesions. His physical examination is completely normal. **Which of the following statements concerning Lyme disease is correct?**

(A) the incubation period is 3 months

(B) after an initial brisk immune response, immunity wanes with continuous infection

(C) the disease is caused by a spirochete

(D) the disease is caused by a tick

(E) the characteristic skin lesion of erythema migrans is found in over 95% of cases

49. An 18-year-old woman presents to the clinic complaining of malaise for the past 3 weeks, fever for 2 weeks, and a sore throat. Physical examination shows pharyngeal infection with enlarged tonsils and a patchy, white exudate; enlarged, palpable anterior and posterior cervical, axillary, and inguinal lymph nodes; tenderness in the right upper quadrant; and minimal splenomegaly. Laboratory data show hemoglobin 14 g/dL; hematocrit 42%; platelets 380,000/mL; WBC 8500/mL, with 35% segmented neutrophils, 1% eosinophils, and 64% lymphocytes, of which 36% were atypical. **Which of the following is the most likely diagnosis?**

    (A) infectious hepatitis
    (B) lymphocytic leukemia
    (C) infectious mononucleosis
    (D) Hodgkin disease
    (E) cat-scratch fever

50. An 18-year-old man develops fever, neck stiffness, and headache. On examination, his blood pressure is 110/80 mm Hg, pulse 100/min, temperature 38.7°C, and neck flexion is very painful. The ears, throat, and sinuses are normal; there are no focal neurologic signs; and the remaining examination is normal. There are no reported similar cases in the community. **Which of the following is the most likely causative organism?**

    (A) *Neisseria meningitides*
    (B) *Streptococcus pneumoniae*
    (C) *Haemophilus influenzae*
    (D) *Staphylococcus*
    (E) *Listeria* species

51. A 43-year-old businessman is developing a new enterprise in Mexico. On his most recent trip, he developed diffuse watery diarrhea with severe cramps 1 week after arriving. The illness resolved after about 2 days with no further complications. **Which of the following is the most likely causative organism?**

    (A) *Campylobacter*
    (B) *E coli*

    (C) *Salmonella*
    (D) *Shigella*
    (E) rotavirus

52. A 22-year-old man is an avid spelunker (cave explorer) and has recently been exploring several caves. A routine CXR taken for a new job reveals hilar adenopathy and two patches of pneumonitis. His physical examination is completely normal. Careful questioning reveals he has just gotten over a "cold" with mild fever, cough, and malaise. **Which of the following is the most likely diagnosis?**

    (A) tuberculosis (TB)
    (B) sarcoidosis
    (C) candidiasis
    (D) histoplasmosis
    (E) coccidioidomycosis

53. A previously well 28-year-old female presents to the clinic for evaluation of fever and generalized malaise over 2–3 weeks. She also complains of arthralgias and myalgias. Repeated measurement of her temperature reveals a low-grade fever between 38°C and 39°C. On physical examination, the pertinent findings are oval retinal hemorrhages with a clear, pale center; a pansystolic cardiac murmur heard best at the apex; and small, tender nodules on her fingertips. **Which of the following is the most likely causative organism?**

    (A) *Staphylococcus aureus*
    (B) *S epidermidis*
    (C) *Viridans streptococci*
    (D) *enterococcus*
    (E) *Candida*

DIRECTIONS (Questions 54 through 63): The following group of numbered items is preceded by a list of lettered options. For each question, select the one lettered option that is most closely associated with it. Each lettered option may be used once, multiple times, or not at all.

Questions 54 through 58: For each patient with impaired immunity, select the most likely pathogen causing infection.

- (A) *Staphylococcus aureus*
- (B) *Candida*
- (C) *P carinii*
- (D) *Streptococcus pneumoniae*
- (E) Gram-negative enteric bacilli
- (F) *Haemophilus influenzae*
- (G) *Neisseria* species
- (H) *Nocardia* species
- (I) *Salmonella*
- (J) rubella virus

54. A 55-year-old man is receiving chemotherapy for colon cancer. His last dose was 2 weeks ago, and he now has symptoms of fevers and chills but no other localizing symptoms. His examination is normal except that he is pale. Investigations reveal that he is neutropenic (absolute neutrophil count <500/mL), and his CXR is normal.

55. An 18-year-old man of European decent with selective immunoglobulin A (IgA) deficiency presents with another respiratory tract infection. He has had two episodes of pneumonia in the past year requiring antibiotic therapy. He now has symptoms of fever, cough, and sputum production. His CXR reveals a right lower lobe infiltrate.

56. A 4-year-old boy is diagnosed with an inherited disorder of the complement system after having recurrent sinopulmonary infections.

57. A 24-year-old woman complains of pain in the upper chest every time she eats or drinks anything. She is HIV positive, but currently not on any antiretroviral therapy. Her last CD4 count was 400/mL.

58. A 67-year-old man has back pain and newly discovered hypercalcemia. Further investigations determine that he has multiple lytic lesions, anemia, and a monoclonal protein in his serum. A bone-marrow aspirate confirms the diagnosis of multiple myeloma.

Questions 59 through 63: For each patient with foodborne illness, select the most likely pathogen.

- (A) *Staphylococcus aureus*
- (B) *C perfringens*
- (C) *Vibrio cholerae*
- (D) enterotoxigenic *E coli*
- (E) *Salmonella*
- (F) *Shigella*
- (G) *Vibrio parahaemolyticus*
- (H) *Bacillus cereus*

59. A 34-year-old woman is at a family picnic where she has a ham sandwich and potato salad. Three hours after the meal, she feels nauseous and throws up.

60. A 22-year-old university student is backpacking in South America. Ten days after arriving, she develops symptoms of anorexia, malaise, and abdominal cramps followed by a sudden onset of watery diarrhea. There are no symptoms of fever or chills, and the stools are nonbloody.

61. A 24-year-old man is traveling in Southeast Asia. He is eating at local restaurants and from street vendors. He now develops high fevers, anorexia, and frequent passage of small-volume stools containing blood, pus, and mucus. This is associated with severe abdominal cramps and painful straining when having bowel movements.

62. A 27-year-old woman is on holiday on the East coast of the United States. She is at a seafood restaurant and has fresh shellfish for dinner. Twenty-four hours later, she develops symptoms of nausea, vomiting, abdominal cramps, and watery diarrhea.

63. A family of four has dinner at a local Asian restaurant, where multiple dishes are ordered and shared amongst the group. Three hours after the meal, all members develop stomach symptoms consisting of nausea and vomiting.

DIRECTIONS (Questions 64 through 79): For each of the questions in this section select the one lettered answer that is the best response in each case.

64. A 19-year-old man is seen in the office 9 days after a hiking trip in Colorado. Five days ago, he developed a fever, headache, myalgia, and nausea. Two days later, he noticed the start of a nonitchy rash on his wrists and ankles. He presents today because of light-headedness while standing and progression of the rash on to his body. He reports that he had numerous insect bites during his hike. On examination, his blood pressure is 90/60 mm Hg, pulse 100/min, and respirations 20/min. There are multiple 1–5 mm macules on his body and some of them have a hemorrhagic center consistent with petechia. His heart sounds are normal, lungs clear, and legs are edematous. **Which of the following is the most likely diagnosis?**

(A) circulating immune complex disease
(B) a drug reaction
(C) infective endocarditis
(D) Rocky mountain spotted fever (RMSF)
(E) *S aureus* sepsis

65. A 22-year-old sexually active man presents to the clinic with symptoms of painful urination. He reports no joint discomfort, rash, fever, or penile discharge. Examination of the prostate, testes, and penis are normal, and there is no visible discharge that can be expressed from the urethra. **Which of the following is the most appropriate initial diagnostic test?**

(A) Urine sample for nucleic acid amplification tests (NAATs)
(B) anterior urethral swab
(C) routine urinalysis
(D) Gram stain of a midstream urine specimen
(E) urine culture

66. A 21-year-old man presents to the clinic for evaluation of cough, headache, malaise, and fever. He reports minimal whitish sputum production and now has chest soreness from coughing so much. He has no other past medical history and no risk factors for HIV. On physical examination, his temperature is 38.3°C, pharynx is normal, and lungs are clear. A CXR reveals diffuse bilateral infiltrates.

Mycoplasma pneumonia is considered in the possible differential diagnosis of his pneumonia. **Which of the following skin manifestations is most likely seen in mycoplasma pneumonia?**

(A) erythema nodosum
(B) erythema multiforme
(C) maculopapular rash
(D) vesicular rash
(E) urticaria

67. A 6-year-old boy develops symptoms of cough, fever, and malaise followed by a generalized maculopapular rash that has spread from the head downward. A clinical diagnosis of measles is made. A few days after the onset of the rash he is drowsy, lethargic, and complaining of headache. A lumbar puncture, electroencephalogram (EEG), and computerized tomography (CT) of the brain exclude other etiologies and confirm the diagnosis of encephalitis. **Which of the following is the most likely delayed neurologic complication of measles virus encephalitis?**

(A) meningitis
(B) pure motor paralysis
(C) autonomic neuropathy
(D) mental retardation or epilepsy
(E) "stocking-glove" peripheral neuropathy

68. A 23-year-old university student presents to the clinic for evaluation of symptoms consisting of painful urination and a penile discharge. The symptoms started 3 days ago and are not improving. He reports no joint symptoms, rash, back pain or fever. Examination of the prostate, testes, and penis are normal, but there is a visible discharge that can be expressed from the urethra. **Which of the following is the most likely causative organism?**

(A) *Neisseria gonorrhoeae*
(B) *Chlamydia trachomatis*
(C) herpes simplex virus (HSV)
(D) *Ureaplasma urealyticum*
(E) *Mycoplasma genitalium*

69. A 56-year-old man presents to the clinic for assessment of intermittent fevers and malaise for the past 2 weeks. He has no other localizing symptoms. Two months ago, he had valve replacement surgery for a bicuspid aortic valve. A mechanical valve was inserted and his postoperative course was uncomplicated. On examination, his temperature is 38°C, blood pressure 124/80 mm Hg, pulse 72/min, and head and neck are normal. There is a 3/6 systolic ejection murmur, the second heart sound is mechanical in quality, and a 2/6 early diastolic murmur is heard. The lungs are clear and the skin examination is normal. Three sets of blood cultures are drawn and an urgent echocardiogram is ordered. **Which of the following is the most likely causative organism?**

(A) *Staphylococcus aureus*
(B) *S epidermidis*
(C) *S viridans*
(D) enterococci
(E) *Candida*

70. A 22-year-old woman presents to the clinic for assessment of symptoms consisting of vulvar itching, burning, and pain when voiding urine. She reports no other symptoms of fever, vaginal discharge, or urinary frequency. On physical examination, there is some vulvar ulceration but no vaginal discharge. The ulcers are small 2–3-mm lesions with an erythematous base. **Which of the following is the most likely diagnosis?**

(A) HSV infection
(B) *Trichomonas vaginalis* infection
(C) *N gonorrhoeae* infection
(D) *C trachomatis* infection
(E) *M genitalium* infection

71. A 29-year-old sexually active man presents to the clinic complaining of painful urination and penile discharge. He reports no other symptoms and is otherwise well with no significant past medical history. He recalls having similar symptoms 8 years ago that were treated successfully with antibiotics. On physical examination, he is afebrile, the penis, testes, and prostate are normal on palpation. There is a visible discharge that can be expressed from the urethra. Microscopic examination of the appropriate specimens is not possible in this clinic. **Which of the following is the most appropriate next step in management?**

(A) send the patient to another clinic for cultures
(B) treat for *C trachomatis* with azithromycin
(C) treat for *N gonorrhoeae* infection with ceftriaxone
(D) treat for *N gonorrhoeae* infection with penicillin
(E) treat for *C trachomatis* and *N gonorrhoeae* with azithromycin and ceftriaxone

72. A 56-year-old previously healthy man is admitted to the hospital for community-acquired pneumonia. He is started on empiric antibiotics. Two days later, his blood cultures are positive of *S pneumoniae*. **Which of the following statements concerning the epidemiology of *S pneumoniae* is correct?**

(A) most children are nasopharyngeal carriers
(B) most adults are nasopharyngeal carriers
(C) bacteremia is not common in people over 55
(D) in adults, bacteremia is most common in midwinter
(E) bacteremia always occurs with pneumonia

73. A 62-year-old woman presents with fever, cough, sputum production, and pleuritic chest pain. CXR reveals a right middle lobe infiltrate, and she is started on antibiotics for the treatment of pneumonia. Her sputum Gram stain is positive for *S pneumoniae*. **Which of the following immunologic mechanisms is the most specific host defense against pneumococcal infection?**

(A) intact splenic function
(B) intact complement function
(C) IgG antibody directed against capsular antigens

(D) alveolar macrophages

(E) liver macrophages

74. A 5-year-old boy presents to the clinic for evaluation of symptoms of left ear pain and associated fever. On physical examination, the left eardrum is inflamed with a small perforation in it and pus is seen in the external canal. A swab of the fluid grows *S pneumoniae*. **Which of the following is the most likely mechanism for *S pneumoniae* to cause otitis media?**

(A) hematogenous spread

(B) direct extension from the nasopharynx

(C) direct inoculation on the ear

(D) spread through lymphatic tissue

(E) associated dental disease

75. A 31-year-old woman presents with symptoms of vulvar itching and burning made worse by urinating. She has no fever or frequency, but has noticed a recent whitish vaginal discharge. Clinical examination reveals vulvar erythema, edema, and fissures. On speculum examination, there is a white discharge with small white plaques loosely adherent to the vaginal wall. **Which of the following treatments is appropriate for her asymptomatic male sexual partner?**

(A) azole cream to the penis

(B) oral fluconazole

(C) standard urethritis investigation

(D) no investigation or treatment

(E) azithromycin plus cefixime

76. A 29-year-old man is seen in the office after returning from a hiking trip in Colorado. He complains of feeling unwell and reports symptoms of fever, myalgia, headache, and nausea. Two days ago, he noticed a rash on his wrists and ankles that has now spread to his body. He recalls having had numerous insect bites during his trip. On examination, his blood pressure is 90/60 mm Hg, pulse 100/min, and respirations 20/min. There are multiple 1–5 mm macules on his body and some of them have a hemorrhagic center consistent with a petechia. His neck is supple and fundi are normal. The heart sounds are normal, lungs clear, and legs are edematous. Cranial nerve, motor, and sensory examination is normal. A clinical diagnosis of Rocky Mountain Spotted Fever (RMSF) is made and he is started on appropriate therapy. **Which of the following is the most common type of central nervous system (CNS) presentation in this condition?**

(A) hemiplegia

(B) cranial nerve abnormalities

(C) paraplegia

(D) encephalitis

(E) ataxia

77. Three individuals living on the same floor in a university dormitory residence develop symptoms and signs of pneumonia. The diagnosis is confirmed by CXR, and sputum samples are positive for *S pneumoniae*. **In an outbreak, which of the following conditions most likely predisposed these 3 individuals to developing pneumococcal pneumonia?**

(A) immotile cilia syndrome

(B) previous viral infection

(C) asthma

(D) cigarette-induced chronic lung disease

(E) allergies

78. A 78-year-old woman with a prior stroke is not feeling well. Her appetite is poor, and today her family noticed that she is confused so they send her to the emergency room for an assessment. She reports no cough, fever, or sputum production but her CXR reveals a left lower lobe infiltrate. Blood cultures are drawn, and she is started on antibiotics. The next day the cultures are positive for *S pneumoniae* sensitive to penicillin. **Which of the following is the most likely complication of pneumococcal pneumonia?**

(A) peritonitis

(B) empyema

(C) pericarditis

(D) endocarditis

(E) osteomyelitis

79. A 19-year-old man presents with cough, malaise, and fever. He reports minimal whitish sputum production and now has chest soreness from coughing so much. His past medical history is negative and there are no risk factors for HIV. On examination, he looks well, the temperature is 38.3°C, pharynx is normal, and the lungs are clear. A CXR reveals diffuse bilateral infiltrates. Mycoplasma pneumonia is considered in the possible differential diagnosis of his pneumonia. **Which other symptom besides cough is also prominent in patients with mycoplasma pneumonia?**

(A) sputum

(B) shortness of breath

(C) headache

(D) shaking chills

(E) pleuritic chest pain

DIRECTIONS (Questions 80 through 99): The following group of numbered items is preceded by a list of lettered options. For each question, select the one lettered option that is most closely associated with it. Each lettered option may be used once, multiple times, or not at all.

Questions 80 through 84: For each mechanism of antibiotic action, select the most likely drug.

(A) beta-lactams (penicillins and cephalosporins)

(B) vancomycin

(C) erythromycin

(D) sulfonamides and trimethoprim

(E) ciprofloxacin

80. Major cellular target is interference with cell metabolism.

81. Work by inhibiting DNA synthesis.

82. Resistance can be caused by drug inactivation.

83. Work by inhibiting protein synthesis.

84. Decreased intracellular accumulation can result in resistance.

Questions 85 through 89: For each antibiotic side effect, select the most likely drug.

(A) erythromycin

(B) ciprofloxacin

(C) tetracycline

(D) sulfonamides

(E) metronidazole

(F) rifampin

85. Can cause unwanted pregnancy.

86. Can contribute to hypoglycemia in non-insulin-dependent diabetes mellitus (NIDDM).

87. Can cause severe reaction to alcohol.

88. Drug interaction can result in rejection for transplant recipients.

89. Can result in phenytoin toxicity.

Questions 90 through 94: For each of the following patients, select the most likely diagnosis.

(A) brucellosis

(B) coccidioidomycosis

(C) histoplasmosis

(D) leprosy

(E) leptospirosis

(F) infectious mononucleosis

(G) TB

(H) tularemia

90. A previously healthy 43-year-old man presents with symptoms of cough, fever, weight loss, and lymphadenopathy for the past 2 months. His physical examination reveals multiple axillary and cervical lymph nodes and oropharyngeal ulcerations. His CXR reveals fibronodular pulmonary infiltrates in the apex, his sputum is negative for TB, and the HIV test is negative. A bronchoalveolar lavage (BAL) confirms the diagnosis.

91. A 34-year-old man presents with fever, cough, and sputum production. The CXR reveals a thin-walled pulmonary cavity. His tests for TB

and HIV are negative. Four weeks ago, he was traveling in southern California, including visiting the San Joaquin valley. While there he did experience a "flu-like" illness, which slowly improved but then his symptoms of cough and sputum started. A BAL confirmed the diagnosis.

92. A 42-year-old man presents with symptoms of cough, sputum, fever, and weight loss. His CXR reveals upper lobe pulmonary infiltrates and his Mantoux test (purified protein derivative [PPD]) is positive. He emigrated from Southeast Asia 3 years ago.

93. A 25-year-old woman presents with fever, night sweats, and muscles aches for the past 1 month. She was previously well. On examination, she has axillary and cervical lymph nodes, but no active joints or hepatosplenomegaly. She currently works on a hog farm. Her investigations are negative for EBV, CMV, and HIV. Serologic tests for the infecting agent confirm the diagnosis in her.

94. A 42-year-old man presents with sudden-onset fever, chills, headaches, myalgias, and arthralgias. He has no prior medical history, but noticed a new ulcer on his hand 1 week ago. On examination, there is a small "punched out" ulcer, which is erythematous and indurated on his hand, as well as epitrochlear and axillary lymph nodes that are tender. As a hobby, he keeps rabbits in a large pen outside his house and recalls being bitten by one 2 weeks ago. Serologic testing for the organism confirms the diagnosis.

Questions 95 through 99: For each of the following patients, select the most likely infecting organism.

   (A) toxoplasmosis
   (B) tetanus

   (C) syphilis
   (D) *Streptococcus*
   (E) *Staphylococcus*
   (F) smallpox
   (G) salmonellosis

95. A 28-year-old man presents with a new genital ulcer on his penis that is painless. He is sexually active and noticed the lesion 1 week ago. The ulcer is 1 cm in size, has an eroded base, and an indurated margin. Dark-field examination of the ulcer fluid confirmed the diagnosis.

96. Infection with this organism during pregnancy can cause congenital hydrocephalus.

97. A 35-year-old woman develops nausea, vomiting, abdominal pain, and diarrhea 1 day after attending an outdoor picnic. Other people who attended the picnic have similar gastrointestinal symptoms. Most symptomatic individuals recall having egg salad sandwiches.

98. For this infectious disease, preventive measures are no longer used since it has been effectively eradicated.

99. A 34-year-old man who works as a carpenter presents with symptoms of jaw discomfort, dysphagia, and pain as well as stiffness in his neck, back, and shoulders. On examination, he is unable to open his jaw, his proximal limb muscles are stiff as is his abdomen and back, but the hands and feet are relatively spared. He occasionally has violent generalized muscles spasms that cause him to stop breathing, but there is no loss of consciousness. A clinical diagnosis is made and he is treated with antibiotics, antitoxin, and diazepam as well as muscle relaxants for the spasms.

Answers and Explanations

1. **(A)** In tetanus, an acute onset is usual. The median onset is 7 days, and 90% present within 14 days of injury. The organism is an anaerobic, motile Gram-positive rod. It has the ability to survive for years in the form of spores, which are resistant to disinfectants and heat. Tetanus can occur in nonimmunized individuals, or those who have neglected their booster shots. Penicillin, or metronidazole, is used in treatment, but their efficacy is not clear. *(Fauci, Chapter 133)*

2. **(D)** EIA is an excellent screening test for HIV infection as it is positive in over 99.5% of cases. However, it lacks specificity, and in low risk populations, only about 10% of EIA positive results are true positives. Recent influenza vaccination, acute viral infections, and liver disease are common causes for false positives. The Western blot test is more specific and is the usual confirmatory test, although even more specific tests are now available. *(Fauci, Chapter 182)*

3. **(A)** *S aureus* causes more than 50% of cases of native valve endocarditis in drug abusers. The onset is usually acute, and the tricuspid valve is the most commonly affected. In staphylococcal tricuspid endocarditis, septic pulmonary emboli are common. Frequently, no murmur is heard. *(Fauci, Chapter 118)*

4. **(C)** HSV-2 genital infections may be associated with fever, malaise, and anorexia. Vesicular lesions usually ulcerate rapidly and become covered with exudate. There is a 90% chance of recurrent symptoms in the first year following a primary infection. HSV-1 genital infections are similar, but the chance of recurrence is less. *(Fauci, Chapter 172)*

5. **(D)** Heterophil antibodies are present in 50% of children and 90%–95% of adolescents and adults with infectious mononucleosis. Monospot tests are the best diagnostic tools but may not turn positive until the second or third week of the illness. The presence of IgG antibodies by the indirect immunofluorescence test indicates recent or prior EBV infection. IgM antibodies indicate recent infection only. Specific EBV antibodies and cultures are rarely used. *(Fauci, Chapter 174)*

6. **(B)** Current recommendations for the treatment of traveler's diarrhea suggest that mild diarrhea be treated with oral rehydration alone, but when enteric symptoms such as cramps are bothersome, treatment with loperamide or bismuth subsalicylate is warranted. More severe infections with severe diarrhea, severe pain, or fever should be treated with antibiotics such as fluoroquinolones or trimethoprim-sulfamethoxazole. *(Fauci, Chapter 117)*

7. **(B)** This patient's clinical presentation suggests a diagnosis of mumps. Pain referring to either or both lower quadrants is common when oophoritis is present. Fever usually accompanies oophoritis. Sterility is not a consequence of mumps oophoritis. Other causes for abdominal pain in mumps can be due to pancreatitis. *(Fauci, Chapter 187)*

8. **(B)** Mycoplasmas have no cell walls and have filtration characteristics of viruses, but morphologically are closer to bacteria. The typical *M pneumoniae* infection produces an influenza-like respiratory illness characterized by headache, malaise, fever, and cough.

If pneumonia occurs, physical examination can be relatively benign despite a grossly abnormal CXR. *(Fauci, Chapter 168)*

9. **(A)** The x-ray shows a silhouette sign with loss of the right heart border indicating right middle lobe pneumonia. The organism is most likely to be pneumococcus, but care must be taken to consider blockage of the right middle lobe bronchus and post obstruction pneumonia. *(Fauci, Chapter 128)*

10. **(A)** The cause of cat-scratch fever (CSD) is a tiny Gram-negative bacillus, *B henselae*. The other Bartonella species listed do not cause CSD. Cats acquire the organism from the soil and inoculate humans via scratches or bites. The disease is generally self-limited, and is treated with analgesics and antipyretics. Encephalitis, seizures, coma, meningitis, and transverse myelitis can occasionally occur even in immunocompetent patients. Azithromycin is recommended for treatment of severe disease and in patients that are immunosuppressed. *(Fauci, Chapter 153)*

11. **(B)** This is a typical case of measles. The Koplik spots in the mouth are easily missed with poor illumination. They are white-blue spots of 1 mm on a red background and are not seen in any other infectious disease. The rash of measles becomes confluent while that of rubella does not. Pneumonia is an infrequent complication but accounts for many measles deaths. Giant cell pneumonia is also seen, most commonly in children suffering with a severe disease such as leukemia or immunodeficiency. Treatment for most patients is supportive care. The other potentially lethal complication of measles is encephalitis. The Koplick spots help differentiate this illness from rubella, and the distribution of the rash rules out infection from coxsackievirus. *(Fauci, Chapter 185)*

12. **(E)** About half of all early-onset (<60 days after surgery) prosthetic endocarditis is caused by staphylococcal infection, with *S epidermidis* predominating. Early-onset prosthetic endocarditis is generally the result of intraoperative contamination of the prosthesis or a bacteremic postoperative complication. *(Fauci, Chapter 118)*

13. **(D)** This man has a complication of viral influenza; a secondary bacterial pneumonia has developed. This usually occurs 2–3 days after the initial viral symptoms resolve. Primary viral pneumonia with influenza is not common. *S pneumoniae, Staphylococcus,* and *H influenzae* are the most common bacterial invaders in pulmonary complications of influenza. Pneumonia is the leading cause of death and may also be due to *S pneumoniae* and *H influenzae*. Mixed viral and bacterial pneumonia is common; pure viral pneumonia in influenza is uncommon (but can be very severe). *(Fauci, Chapter 180)*

14. **(D)** Although only close contacts need chemoprophylaxis, it is sometimes given more widely than recommended because of community concern. Meningococcal vaccine is effective against serotype A and C, and will prevent late secondary infection in close contacts. Ciprofloxacin or ofloxacin are alternatives to rifampin. *(Fauci, Chapter 376)*

15. **(C)** The most common cause of non-EBV mononucleosis-type syndrome is CMV. It is the most common presentation of CMV in nonneonates with normal immune function. *(Fauci, Chapter 175)*

16. **(A)** Symptomatic treatment including mouth care, analgesics, and a bland diet are usually recommended for patients with mumps. Antibiotics, steroids, and mumps convalescent sera are of no value. There is no evidence to support the use of glucocorticoids for orchitis. Prevention via vaccination is the preferred strategy for mumps. *(Fauci, Chapter 187)*

17. **(A)** The cerebrospinal fluid (CSF) picture in this individual is consistent with viral meningitis rather than a bacterial process. Enteroviruses are a prominent cause of viral meningitis in the summer and fall months. They received their name because they multiply in the GI tract. Fever, sometimes associated with respiratory symptoms, is the most common sequela of

enterovirus infection. There are about 70 enteroviruses that affect humans. These include polioviruses, coxsackieviruses, echoviruses, and others. The spectrum of disease includes paralytic disease, encephalitis, aseptic meningitis, pleurodynia, exanthems, pericarditis, myocarditis, and nonspecific febrile illnesses. They can, on occasion, cause fulminant disease in a newborn. The most important enteroviruses are the three poliovirus serotypes. *(Fauci, Chapter 376)*

18. **(A)** The incubation period of *C botulinum* toxin is 18–36 hours but ranges from a few hours to days. There are no sensory symptoms. Foodborne botulinum is associated primarily with home-canned food. Severe foodborne botulinum can produce diplopia, dysarthria, and dysphagia; weakness then can progress rapidly to involve the neck, arms, thorax, and legs. There is usually no fever. Nausea, vomiting, and abdominal pain can precede the paralysis or come afterward. *(Fauci, Chapter 134)*

19. **(D)** Heterophil antibody-negative mononucleosis syndrome is the most common manifestation of CMV infection in immunocompetent adults and is more common than the similar syndrome caused by toxoplasmosis. As of yet, no syndromes caused by HHV-7 have been identified in adults. Acute HIV infection seroconversion at 3–6 weeks after exposure can cause an acute mono like syndrome. The atypical lymphocytosis suggests that this illness is either due to EBV or CMV and not HIV. *(Fauci, Chapter 175)*

20. **(E)** Coccidioidomycosis is the usual cause of pulmonary cavitation resulting from fungal infection. A rarefaction may be demonstrable in a pneumonic lesion within 10 days of onset. In the United States, most cases are acquired in California, Arizona, and western Texas. TB and cryptococcus are less likely in this individual given his previously healthy status (and presumed normal immune status) and unlikely exposure to TB during his vacation. *(Fauci, Chapter 193)*

21. **(C)** The most common complication of measles is otitis media, other complications include mastoiditis, pneumonia, bronchitis, encephalitis, and lymphadenitis. Otitis media is usually a bacterial superinfection, and should be treated with antibiotics. *(Fauci, Chapter 185)*

22. **(E)** Examination of stool samples for enteroinvasive bacteria and ova and parasites is important in establishing the correct diagnosis in this patient. Demonstration of hematophagous trophozoites of *E histolytica* in stool confirms the diagnosis for bloody diarrhea. The trophozoites are rapidly killed by drying, so wet mounts of stool should be examined. Stool toxin assay is not helpful unless there is an antecedent history of antibiotic use. *(Fauci, Chapter 117)*

23. **(B)** Since the introduction of *H influenzae* type B and meningococcal vaccine, *S pneumoniae* has become the most common type of meningitis in infants and toddlers. *(Fauci, Chapter 376)*

24. **(D)** Pregnancy or anticipated pregnancy within 4 weeks of vaccination is a contraindication to receiving the rubella vaccine. There is a theoretical concern that fetus might develop congenital rubella syndrome from the live attenuated virus used for the vaccine. Vaccination is usually given to children combined with measles and mumps vaccine between 12 and 15 months of age, and then repeated during childhood at age 4–6 years. It is given even to children with HIV infection. Infants <1 year old can be given the vaccine but may not develop adequate immunity and should still be given the recommended two doses. *(Fauci, Chapter 185)*

25. **(C)** Glomerulonephritis, arthritis, and many of the mucocutaneous lesions are secondary to circulating immune complexes. The clinical manifestations of infective endocarditis are a result of three factors: (1) direct infection in the heart, (2) septic emboli, and (3) high levels of circulating immune complexes. Renal emboli cause hematuria and flank pain, but rarely impair renal function. *(Fauci, Chapter 118)*

26. **(B)** Adequate rest is the treatment of choice, but forced bed rest is not necessary. Glucocorticoids hasten defervescence and resolution of pharyngitis but are not routinely used. Acyclovir halts oropharyngeal shedding of EBV but has minimal effect on the clinical disease. Similarly alpha-interferon and ganciclovir have antiviral efficacy but have no role to play in uncomplicated infectious mononucleosis. Antibiotics are not helpful, and ampicillin is likely to cause a pruritic maculopapular rash in most patients. *(Fauci, Chapter 174)*

27. **(C)** Donovanosis, or granuloma inguinale, is a mildly contagious, chronic, indolent disease that can be sexually transmitted. *Calymmatobacterium granulomatis*, a Gram-negative intracellular bacterium, is felt to be the cause. It is endemic in many tropical areas. Daily doxycycline or weekly azithromycin until the lesions are healed are the usual treatments. Erythromycin is used in pregnant patients. *(Fauci, Chapter 124)*

28. **(B)** *S pneumoniae* colonizes the nasopharynx of 5%–10% of healthy adults and up to 20%–40% of children. The source of pneumococcal meningitis is either direct extension from middle ear or sinus infections, or via seeding from a bacteremia. In the latter circumstance, bacteremia from pneumonia would be more likely than from infective endocarditis. *(Fauci, Chapter 376)*

29. **(C)** The treatment of choice is trimethoprim-sulfamethoxazole. The patient has *Pneumocystis jiroveci* pneumonia, since he is immunocompromised from antirejection medications for his renal transplant. Alternate therapies include IV pentamidine or IV clindamycin and primaquine. *(Fauci, Chapter 200)*

30. **(D)** All the sites mentioned can be involved by amebiasis, but the liver is the most common. Most travelers who develop an amebic liver abscess will do so within a few months of their return. Pleuropulmonary and pericardial involvement results from extension from the liver. *(Fauci, Chapter 202)*

31. **(D)** A single test revealing a specific IgM antibody can confirm the disease. Acute and convalescent titers of specific IgG antibodies will also confirm the diagnosis of mumps. Urine, saliva, and throat swabs will grow the mumps virus, but blood does not. Salivary amylase is elevated but is relatively nonspecific. Of course, a typical presentation during an epidemic probably does not require any confirmatory tests. Sporadic cases require more active confirmation. Other causes of parotitis requiring specific treatment include calculi, bacterial infections, and drugs. Tumors, sarcoid, TB, leukemia, Hodgkin disease, Sjögren syndrome, and lupus erythematosus can also cause parotid enlargement. *(Fauci, Chapter 187)*

32. **(A)** Staphylococcal enterotoxin food poisoning is characterized by violent GI upset with severe nausea, cramps, vomiting, and diarrhea. It occurs very rapidly after ingestion (1–6 hours) and usually resolves by 12 hours. *(Fauci, Chapter 122)*

33. **(C)** The patient has tinea capitis, which may be caused by *Trichophyton* or *Microsporum* species. It may be successfully treated with topical azole drugs (eg, clotrimazole). More severe infections are usually treated with systemic medications. The scalp lesions are not seborrheic dermatitis because of the description of the lesions and it also does not illuminated with Wood light. Aspergillus does not affect the skin (or scalp) except in immunocompromised individuals and then usually at sites of skin trauma. *(Fauci, Chapter 191)*

34. **(C)** Coxsackie A viruses may cause a number of syndromes, including herpangina, exanthem, aseptic meningitis, common cold, paralysis, pneumonitis, and summer febrile illness. It is distinguished from HSV-1 herpes stomatitis by the fact that most of the lesions are concentrated in the posterior portion of the mouth and that there is no gingivitis. The other viruses do not cause oral lesions. HSV-2 can occasionally cause oral lesions. *(Fauci, Chapter 184)*

35. **(B)** Rabies is transmitted through the saliva of infected animals. Once clinical signs develop, the disease is almost 100% fatal. Symptoms of rabies may include apathy, as well as hyperexcitability. Finding Negri bodies in nerve cells of the brain in infected animals confirms the diagnosis. Polymerase chain reaction for detection of viral material is another method of confirming the diagnosis. In cats and dogs that are not available for observation (lasting 10 days) to determine if they have signs of rabies, public health authorities should be consulted to determine the potential risk of rabies in the animal based on local rates of rabies in wild animals. Alternatively, if there is a high risk the animal is infected, then postexposure prophylaxis should be started with rabies vaccination on days 0, 3, 7, 14, and 28 as well as one dose of rabies immune globulin on day 0. *(Fauci, Chapter 188)*

36. **(C)** EBV genetic material has been found in association with many malignancies. In Africa, about 90% of patients with Burkitt lymphoma have an association with EBV, but in the United States, only 15% of cases are associated with EBV. In contrast, almost all cases of anaplastic nasopharyngeal carcinoma and also HIV-related CNS lymphomas are associated with EBV genetic material. *(Fauci, Chapter 174)*

37. **(C)** Splenic rupture occurs during the second or third week of the illness and can be insidious or abrupt in presentation. Surgery is required. Hemorrhage is not a usual complication of infectious mononucleosis. Over 90% of cases are benign and uncomplicated, but liver involvement is clinical in 5%–10%. Over 85% of EBV-associated neurologic problems resolve spontaneously. Although hemorrhage does not occur, autoimmune hemolytic anemia can occur. It is usually mediated by IgM antibodies with anti-i specificity. *(Fauci, Chapter 174)*

38. **(B)** Coccidioidomycosis may present with a syndrome of erythema nodosum, fever, and conjunctivitis. Serious complications include cavitating lung lesions or meningitis. *(Fauci, Chapter 193)*

39. **(D)** CMV is probably transmitted in the leukocyte component of transfusions. The syndromes include fever and lymphocytosis. Screening donors for this virus reduces the incidence of transmission. HCV transmission can occur with blood transfusions but it does not cause a mono-like syndrome, and EBV transmission does not occur with blood transfusions. *(Fauci, Chapter 175)*

40. **(A)** TSS is most characteristically seen in females using vaginal tampons and is secondary to staphylococcal enterotoxins called TSS toxin 1 (TSST-1). Abrupt onset is characteristic. The clinical criteria for diagnosis include high fever, a diffuse rash that desquamates on the palms and soles over the subsequent 1–2 weeks, hypotension, and involvement in 3 or more organ systems. This involvement can include GI dysfunction (vomiting and diarrhea), renal insufficiency, hepatic insufficiency, thrombocytopenia, myalgias with elevated creatine kinase (CK) levels, and delirium. Staphylococcal-scaled-skin syndrome most often affects newborns and children. It results in localized or quite extensive fluid-filled blisters that easily rupture to expose denuded skin. It is caused by an exfoliative toxin. *(Fauci, Chapter 129)*

41. **(A)** In epidemics, *N meningitidis* is usually the cause, generally serotype A (sub-Saharan Africa) or C (North America). Serotype B is more common in sporadic outbreaks. *(Fauci, Chapter 376)*

42. **(A)** This patient has "febrile neutropenia." Several antibiotic combinations could be used and may vary with the indigenous organisms. Aminoglycoside and cephalosporin are commonly used in combination. The antibiotic combination must cover both Gram-positive and Gram-negative organisms. Antifungal or viral agents are not empirically started unless there is an appropriate clinical fungal or viral infection. In some centers, empiric antifungal agents are started if the patient remains febrile on antibiotics after 5 days. Observation alone is not an option, since these individuals usually have some form of bacteremia causing the fever. *(Fauci, Chapter 82)*

43. (A) Hospital-acquired pneumonia is defined as pneumonia occurring >48 hours after admission and not incubating at the time of admission. It is caused by *S aureus*, *Gram-negative bacilli*, or *Streptococcus pneumoniae*. Mixed aerobic and anaerobic infections are also common. Pulmonary embolism is always a consideration in the diagnosis based on clinical probability. The elevated WBC makes atelectasis unlikely and the normal JVP rules out congestive heart failure. *(Fauci, Chapter 125)*

44. (B) Treatment of choice is either a newer generation macrolide-like azithromycin, or a respiratory quinolone-like levofloxacin or moxifloxacin. Erythromycin is also an option but the newer macrolides are better tolerated. Tetracyclines or TMP/SMX are second line options, and the cephalosporins are not effective for legionella. Legionnaires disease is transmitted via infectious aerosols and may cause severe disease characterized by dry cough and fevers. Mild infections and asymptomatic seroconversion also occur. Natural reservoirs for the organisms include streams, hot springs, and stagnant lakes. Amplifiers are man-made water supplies that favor growth of *legionellae*. Common amplifiers are hot-water systems and heat-exchange units. *(Fauci, Chapter 141)*

45. (E) Prophylactic antibiotics can prevent enteric bacterial infections, but at the cost of drug side effects (rash, *Clostridium difficile* colitis) and the possibility of developing an infection with a drug-resistant organism. Most experts recommend against taking daily prophylaxis unless the consequences of traveler's diarrhea outweigh the risks of the side effects. Such individuals include patients with inflammatory bowel disease (IBD), or immunocompromised states like transplant recipients. Bismuth subsalicylate at a dosage of 2 tablets (525 mg) 4 times a day is safe and effective for up to 3 weeks, but can be difficult to take because of the large quantity required. It is also only 60% effective in preventing symptoms. Improving food and drink selection and appropriate caution are the best advice, and medications are only indicated if moderate or severe symptoms develop, including taking loperamide for severe diarrhea. *(Fauci, Chapter 117)*

46. (B) Figure 10–2 illustrates Hutchinson teeth, which is a manifestation of late congenital syphilis. This may be associated with cardiovascular and neurologic manifestations as well as "saddle nose" and "saber shins." *(Fauci, Chapter 162)*

47. (C) The findings of SBP can be subtle and not as dramatic as that of secondary peritonitis (when bacteria contaminate the peritoneum). As many as 80% of patients with SBP will present with fever. Preexisting ascites is almost always present, but only 10% of cirrhotics at most will develop SBP. The microbiology is characteristically that of a single organism (*E coli* most commonly). Polymicrobial infection should suggest the possibility of peritonitis secondary to a perforation. More than 250 PMNs/μL of ascitic fluid is diagnostic. *(Fauci, Chapter 121)*

48. (C) Lyme disease is caused by the spirochete *B burgdorferi*, a fastidious microaerophilic bacterium. It is a tick-transmitted disease but is not caused by the tick. The incubation period is 3–32 days and is associated, initially, with minimal immune response. Perhaps as many as 25% of patients lack the characteristic skin lesion. *(Fauci, Chapter 166)*

49. (C) Infectious mononucleosis is an acute, self-limited infection of the lymphatic system by the EBV. Typical infectious mononucleosis has an incubation period of 4–8 weeks. The prodrome includes malaise, anorexia, and chills, and then the classic symptoms of pharyngitis, fever, and lymphadenopathy develop. Headache is also common. *(Fauci, Chapter 174)*

50. (B) In adults (age >15 years), *S pneumoniae* is the single most common organism, accounting for one-third to one-half of all cases of bacterial meningitis. This pneumococcal predominance is even more pronounced in sporadic cases. *(Fauci, Chapter 376)*

51. **(B)** The most common cause of traveler's diarrhea worldwide is toxigenic *E coli*. In North Africa and Southeast Asia, *Campylobacter* infections predominate. Other causative organisms include *Salmonella*, *Shigella*, rotavirus, and the Norwalk agent. The most common parasite causing traveler's diarrhea is *Giardia lamblia*. *(Fauci, Chapter 117)*

52. **(D)** *Histoplasma capsulatum* is a dimorphic fungus with worldwide distribution. In the United States, it is particularly common in Southeastern, mid-Atlantic, and Central states. In the US, the endemic areas spread over the Ohio and Mississippi river valleys. It is frequently found in soil enriched by droppings of certain birds and bats. Caves are common sites of infection. Most infections are asymptomatic or mild and require no therapy. Acute disseminated infection usually occurs in patients with HIV infection or other immuno-compromised states, but chronic dissemination can occur in immunocompetent patients. Findings may include hepatosplenomegaly, lymphadenopathy, anemia, and Addison disease. Mediastinal fibrosis can result in superior vena cava compression. Fibrosis can also involve the pulmonary arteries, esophagus, and pulmonary veins. *(Fauci, Chapter 192)*

53. **(C)** This woman likely has native valve endocarditis, probably in the setting of a previous valvular abnormality. Streptococci cause over half the cases of native valve endocarditis in nonintravenous drug abusers. Of these, 75% are viridans streptococci. *Streptococcus bovis* is the most common nonviridans streptococcus causing endocarditis and is usually found in the older population (60 years), particularly if bowel lesions are present. Staphylococcal endocarditis is the next most common type, but it is usually associated with a more acute presentation. Enterococci cause about 6% of cases in native valve endocarditis, but fungi are rare causes. *(Fauci, Chapter 118)*

54. **(E)** Cytotoxic chemotherapy frequently results in neutropenia and subsequently Gram-negative bacillary infection. *Pseudomonas, Staphylococcus, Candida*, and *Aspergillus* infections are also common. *(Fauci, Chapter 82)*

55. **(D or F)** Selective immunoglobulin A (IgA) deficiency predisposes to *S pneumonia, G lamblia*, hepatitis virus, and. *H influenzae* infection. *(Fauci, Chapter 310)*

56. **(D, or F, or G)** Defects in the complement pathway predisposes individuals to recurrent infections with encapsulated organisms such as *H influenzae, Neisseria* species, or *S pneumonia*. *(Fauci, Chapter 308)*

57. **(B)** All forms of T-lymphocyte deficiency/dysfunction are characterized by candidal infections. *Candida* species can cause thrush, skin lesions, esophagitis, and cystitis. Hematogenous spread can occur and disseminate the organism widely in individuals with low CD4 counts. *(Fauci, Chapter 182)*

58. **(D)** Patients with myeloma have defects in humoral immunity and are prone to recurrent pneumonias due to *S pneumoniae*. Lung infections with *S aureus* and *Klebsiella pneumoniae* are also frequent. *E coli* and other Gram-negatives cause recurrent urinary tract infections. *(Fauci, Chapter 108)*

59. **(A)** The preformed toxin of *Staphylococcus* causes nausea within 1–6 hours of ingestion. Ham, poultry, potato and egg salad, mayonnaise, and cream pastries are common food sources. *(Fauci, Chapter 122)*

60. **(D)** Enterotoxigenic *E coli* causes 15%–50% of traveler's diarrhea, depending on geographic location. The incubation period is more than 16 hours, and water and many foods can be the source. *(Fauci, Chapter 117)*

61. **(F)** *Shigella* causes an invasive diarrhea with blood and has an incubation period of more than 16 hours. Potato and egg salad, lettuce, and raw vegetables are common food sources. *(Fauci, Chapter 117)*

62. **(C)** *Vibrio cholerae* causes profuse watery diarrhea with an incubation period of more than 16 hours. Shellfish are a common source. *(Fauci, Chapter 149)*

63. **(H)** *B cereus* causes an early onset of food poisoning when found in fried rice. This occurs within 1–6 hours and, like staphylococcal food poisoning, is characterized by vomiting. The enteric form of *B cereus* food poisoning is characterized by watery diarrhea and occurs 8–16 hours after ingestion of contaminated food such as meat, vegetables, dried beans, or cereals. *(Fauci, Chapter 122)*

64. **(D)** The location of infection, the possibility of tick exposure, and the nonspecific nature of the presentation are consistent with a rickettsial infection, likely RMSF. *(Fauci, Chapter 167)*

65. **(A)** A urine sample for nucleic acid amplification tests (NAATs) are easy, rapid and more comfortable for patients when screening for STIs such as gonorrhoeae or chlamydia. The diagnosis can also be made by proximal to distal "milking of the urethra" and showing evidence of a purulent or mucopurulent discharge and sending it for culture. Other methods include examining a urethral swab or the sediment from the first 20–30 mL of voided urine (after the patient has not voided for several hours). Dysuria without inflammation may represent a functional problem and usually does not benefit from antibiotics. *(Fauci, Chapter 124)*

66. **(B)** Although all the skin problems listed have been described with *M pneumoniae* infection, the only clearly linked entity is erythema multiforme. *(Fauci, Chapter 168)*

67. **(D)** Subacute sclerosing panencephalitis causes involuntary spasmodic movements and progressive mental deterioration, frequently ending in death within a year. It usually occurs in children whose measles occurred at an early age (= 2 years). It occurs 6–8 years after the primary infection. It presents with nonspecific symptoms such as poor school performance or mood and personality changes. It then progresses to intellectual decline, seizures, myoclonus, ataxia, and visual disturbances. Continued deterioration results in inevitable death. *(Fauci, Chapter 185)*

68. **(B)** *C trachomatis* causes 30%–40% of the cases of urethritis in men in the United States. The exact prevalence depends on the effectiveness of *Chlamydial* control programs in the population. The other organisms can all cause urethritis in men. *(Fauci, Chapter 124)*

69. **(B)** *S epidermidis* is still the leading cause of prosthetic valve endocarditis in the early postoperative period (usually defined <2 months). It is usually the consequence of intraoperative contamination or postoperative bacteremia. Endocarditis occurring 12 months after surgery is usually due to the same organisms that cause native valve endocarditis. *(Fauci, Chapter 118)*

70. **(A)** HSV and *C albicans* are the common causes of vulvar infection. Although they can cause dysuria, it is of the "external" variety (ie, secondary to urine passing over the inflamed vulvar area). The other infections cause "internal dysuria" and/or vaginal discharge. *(Fauci, Chapter 172)*

71. **(E)** Empiric treatment should include coverage for both *Chlamydial* infection (with azithromycin) and *N gonorrhoeae* infection (usually with ceftriaxone). There are numerous alternatives for *N gonorrhoeae* infection, such as oral cefixime (not available in the United States), oral ciprofloxacin, or intramuscular (IM) ceftriaxone. However, resistance to penicillin is too common to allow the routine use of this drug. *(Fauci, Chapter 124)*

72. **(D)** There is a definite midwinter spike in bacteremia in adults, but not in children. Invasive disease is highest in children under 2 years of age. Bacteremia is more common in certain groups (eg, Native Americans, Native Alaskans, African Americans), suggesting a genetic predisposition. Up to 40% of healthy

children and 10% of healthy adults are asymptomatic carriers. In adults, the organism can persist in the nasopharynx for up to 6 months. *(Fauci, Chapter 128)*

73. **(C)** The most specific immunologic defense is directed at capsular antigens and is serotype specific. Antibodies are not naturally occurring, but are the result of prior colonization, infection, or vaccination. Intact spleen, complement and macrophage function is important in clearance of pneumococci from sterile areas, but specific immunoglobulin G (IgG) antibody coating of a pneumococcal polysaccharide capsule is essential for macrophages to ingest and kill the bacteria. *(Fauci, Chapter 128)*

74. **(B)** Infections of the middle ear, trachea, sinuses, bronchi, and lungs are caused by direct spread from nasopharyngeal colonization. Disease of the CNS, heart valves, bones, joints, and peritoneal are usually caused by hematogenous dissemination. *(Fauci, Chapter 128)*

75. **(D)** There is no need to investigate or treat an asymptomatic male partner of a patient with vulvovaginal candidiasis. If candidal dermatitis of the penis is present, topical azole therapy would be appropriate. *(Fauci, Chapter 196)*

76. **(D)** Although all these can be manifestations of RMSF, encephalitis as manifested by confusion or lethargy is by far the most common CNS manifestation. It occurs in about one-quarter of cases, and can progress to coma. *(Fauci, Chapter 167)*

77. **(B)** It is possible that such outbreaks can occur in people with no predisposing factors, unlike the vast majority of sporadic cases. However, the only common predisposing factor in a young healthy population such as this would be a previous viral respiratory infection. *(Fauci, Chapter 128)*

78. **(B)** Approximately 2% of cases of pneumococcal pneumonia are complicated by empyema. However, not all pleural effusions in the setting of pneumococcal pneumonia represent pleural infection. Frank pus, a positive Gram stain, or a pH = 7.1 on thoracentesis suggest empyema and the need for aggressive drainage with a chest tube. *(Fauci, Chapter 128)*

79. **(C)** The most common presentation is with cough and headache. Both can be quite severe. Cough becomes more prominent if a lower respiratory tract infection ensues, but sputum production is not usually prominent. Shaking chills and pleuritic chest pain are quite uncommon. *(Fauci, Chapter 168)*

80. **(D)** Sulfonamides and trimethoprim competitively inhibit enzymes involved in folic acid biosynthesis. *(Fauci, Chapter 161)*

81. **(E)** Ciprofloxacin, rifampin, and metronidazole inhibit DNA synthesis, albeit by different mechanisms. *(Fauci, Chapter 161)*

82. **(A)** Beta-lactams can be inactivated by beta-lactamase. *(Fauci, Chapter 161)*

83. **(C)** Macrolides (clarithromycin, azithromycin, erythromycin), lincosamides (clindamycin), and chloramphenicol inhibit protein synthesis by binding to the 50S ribosomal subunit. Tetracyclines and aminoglycosides inhibit protein synthesis by binding to the 30S ribosomal subunit. *(Fauci, Chapter 161)*

84. **(E)** Some Gram-negative bacteria acquire mutations in their outer membrane pori, so they are no longer permeable to ciprofloxacin. Some Gram-positive bacteria develop a mutation that allows them to actively pump the drug out. The most common form of resistance, however, is a mutation in the DNA gyrase, which is the target of ciprofloxacin action. *(Fauci, Chapter 161)*

85. **(F)** Rifampin is an excellent inducer of many cytochrome P450 enzymes and increases the hepatic clearance of a number of drugs, including oral contraceptives. *(Fauci, Chapter 161)*

86. **(D)** Sulfonamides potentiate the effects of oral hypoglycemics through reduction in metabolism or displacement from serum protein. *(Fauci, Chapter 161)*

87. **(E)** Metronidazole can cause a disulfiram-like syndrome when alcohol is ingested. Instructions to avoid alcohol should be given when this drug is prescribed. *(Fauci, Chapter 161)*

88. **(F)** Rifampin enzyme-induction properties can result in increased metabolism of cyclosporine, with resultant organ rejection. In contrast, erythromycin inhibits the enzyme involved in cyclosporine metabolism and can result in enhanced toxicity. *(Fauci, Chapter 161)*

89. **(D)** Sulfonamides may potentiate the effects of phenytoin through reduction in metabolism or displacement from serum protein. *(Fauci, Chapter 161)*

90. **(C)** Disseminated histoplasmosis has many features in common with hematogenously disseminated TB. Common findings include fever, weight loss, cough, lymphadenopathy, anemia, abnormal liver enzymes, and hepatosplenomegaly. The chronic pulmonary disease is characterized by cough, increasing sputum production, and apical infiltrates. One-third improve or stabilize spontaneously while the remainder progress slowly to develop cavitation of the upper lobes and altered pulmonary function. In histoplasmosis, oropharyngeal ulcerations begin as solitary indurated plaques with no pain present at first, although eventually pain becomes deep-seated. These oropharyngeal manifestations are usually part of disseminated infection. *(Fauci, Chapter 192)*

91. **(B)** In coccidioidomycosis, hemoptysis may call attention to cavitations, or patients may complain of pain at the cavity site. However, only half of the patients with a thin-walled pulmonary cavity secondary to coccidioidomycosis will have symptoms. *(Fauci, Chapter 193)*

92. **(G)** The intracutaneous tuberculin test with purified protein derivative (PPD) is read for evidence of delayed hypersensitivity at 48 hours. Although induration >10 mm is felt to be positive, interpretation is really dependent on the population being studied. In an HIV-infected patient, any reaction should be considered significant. When testing household contacts,

>5 mm is probably enough to warrant prophylactic treatment. *(Fauci, Chapter 158)*

93. **(A)** In the United States, brucellosis is rare and found most commonly among farmers, meat-processing workers, and veterinarians. Transmission is by contact of *Brucella* organisms with abraded skin, through the conjunctiva, or by inhalation. Person-to-person transmission is rare or nonexistent. The disease can be acute, localized, or chronic. It requires prolonged antibiotic treatment. A typical treatment course would be doxycycline plus an aminoglycoside for 4 weeks followed by a further 4 weeks of doxycycline and rifampin. *(Fauci, Chapter 150)*

94. **(H)** Tularemia can be acquired through direct contact with an infected rabbit, which may occur in preparation or cooking inadequately. The incubation period is 2–5 days, and the syndrome includes fevers, chills, headaches, myalgias, and tender hepatosplenomegaly. In addition, specific syndromes such as ulceroglandular or oculoglandular tularemia can accompany the nonspecific syndrome. *(Fauci, Chapter 151)*

95. **(C)** On dark-field examination, *T pallidum* (the spirochete that causes syphilis) is a thin, delicate organism with tapering ends and 6–14 spirals. When dark-field examination is not possible, direct fluorescent antibody tests are used. *(Fauci, Chapter 162)*

96. **(A)** Congenital toxoplasmosis is initiated in utero usually as a complication of a primary infection. Infants may be asymptomatic at birth but later can present with a multitude of signs and symptoms, including chorioretinitis, strabismus, epilepsy, and psychomotor retardation. The presence of hydrocephalus is a bad prognostic sign. *(Fauci, Chapter 207)*

97. **(G)** Salmonellosis is an acute infection resulting from ingestion of food containing bacteria and is characterized by abdominal pain and diarrhea. *Salmonella* gastroenteritis is not usually treated with antibiotics because the length of the illness is not shortened, but the length of time the organism is carried is increased.

Antibiotics are used for more serious systemic *Salmonella* infections. *(Fauci, Chapter 146)*

98. **(F)** Preventive measures are not used because smallpox is thought to be eradicated worldwide, and vaccination may be associated with serious side effects. As humans are the only reservoir for smallpox, there is no longer any risk of infection from natural sources. However, smallpox could be used in bioterrorism. *(Fauci, Chapter 214)*

99. **(B)** Patients with tetanus develop hypertonus, seizures, respiratory distress, and asphyxia unless they are treated with diazepam and muscle relaxants. The treatment of tetanus requires diazepam, muscle relaxants, antitoxin, respiratory care, and managing autonomic dysfunction. Antibiotics are given but are probably of little help. *(Fauci, Chapter 133)*

CHAPTER 11

Immunology and Allergy
Questions

DIRECTIONS (Questions 1 through 20): For each of the questions in this section select the one lettered answer that is the best response in each case.

1. A 29-year-old woman presents to the clinic with symptoms of joints discomfort and hives 6 days after starting penicillin for a "strep throat" infection. She has also noticed some lumps in her neck, but no lip or tongue swelling, and no difficulty breathing. On physical examination, she has small mobile cervical lymph nodes, skin changes of urticaria, and no oral lesions. Her urinalysis is positive for protein and red cells. **Which of the following is the most likely mechanism of this drug reaction?**

   (A) immunoglobulin E (IgE) release
   (B) mast cell degranulation
   (C) immediate-type hypersensitivity
   (D) macrophage-endothelial cell interaction
   (E) circulating immune complexes

2. A 24-year-old man is diagnosed with disseminated histoplasmosis after developing symptoms of fever, lymphadenopathy, hepatosplenomegaly, and pancytopenia. **Which of the following is the body's major immunologic defense against histoplasmosis?**

   (A) immunoglobulin G (IgG) antibodies
   (B) mononuclear leukocytes
   (C) complement

   (D) immunoglobulin M (IgM) antibody
   (E) neutrophils

3. **Which of the following are large, granular lymphoid cells that are mediators of antibody-dependent cellular cytotoxicity?**

   (A) macrophages
   (B) natural killer (NK) cells
   (C) T lymphocytes, suppressor subset
   (D) B lymphocytes
   (E) granulocytes

4. A 9-year-old boy presents to the clinic for assessment of sneezing, runny nose, and nasal congestion. His mother reports that the symptoms are seasonal and worse in the spring time. The physical examination is completely normal. A clinical diagnosis of hay fever (allergic rhinitis) is made. **Which of the following statements about hay fever is correct?**

   (A) sufferers may develop asthma
   (B) symptoms are not improved by moving to different locations
   (C) sufferers are less prone to develop upper respiratory infections (URIs)
   (D) sufferers are severely disturbed emotionally
   (E) hay fever can be improved symptomatically only with steroids

5. A 19-year-old man presents to the emergency department with symptoms of recurrent attacks of gastrointestinal colic type discomfort and swelling of his face and legs. He states that there is no relationship of the attacks to any foods or activity. His father has a similar syndrome. **Which of the following is the most likely cause of death in this disease?**

   (A) an unrelated condition
   (B) non-cardiogenic pulmonary edema
   (C) edema of the glottis
   (D) overtreatment
   (E) an arrhythmia

6. A 34-year-old woman is seen in the clinic for her annual assessment and has a routine complete blood count performed. The patient's past health history is significant for human immunodeficiency virus (HIV) which was diagnosed 2 years ago. She is not on any antiretroviral therapy currently, and is doing well with no symptoms. Her physical examination is completely normal. **Which of the following changes is most likely seen on her peripheral blood cell counts?**

   (A) granulocytosis
   (B) lymphopenia
   (C) increased helper T cells
   (D) monocytosis
   (E) decreased NK cells

7. A 30-year-old woman presents to the clinic complaining of fatigue. In addition, she reports that her urine is very dark and "tea color" like, and today her partner commented that her eyes look yellow. Her past medical history is significant for myasthenia gravis for which she is taking azathioprine and pyridostigmine. Laboratory investigations reveal findings in keeping with autoimmune hemolytic anemia. The chest x-ray (CXR) reveals an anterior mediastinal mass. **Which of the following is the most likely diagnosis?**

   (A) thymoma
   (B) nodular sclerosing Hodgkin disease

   (C) small cleaved cell non-Hodgkin lymphoma
   (D) teratoma
   (E) bronchogenic carcinoma, small cell undifferentiated type

8. A 19-year-old man presents to the emergency department complaining of coughing up blood and decreased urine output. On physical examination, there is normal air entry in the lungs, and the heart sounds are normal. There is no skin rash or palpable lymph nodes and his abdomen is normal. CXR reveals patchy infiltrates in both lower lobes and his creatinine is elevated. Urinalysis is positive for red cells and protein. A renal biopsy is performed and it reveals autoantibodies to basement membranes. **Which of the following is the most likely diagnosis?**

   (A) thyroiditis
   (B) myasthenia gravis
   (C) Goodpasture syndrome
   (D) thrombocytopenia
   (E) hemolytic anemia

9. A 25-year-old woman presents to the emergency room with new symptoms of decreased urine output, leg edema, and facial swelling. She was previously well and has no significant past medical history. Laboratory investigations reveal acute kidney injury and a renal biopsy is performed. Immunofluorescence of the biopsy specimen reveals a granular pattern of immune complex-mediated glomerulonephritis. (See Figure 11–1.) **Which of the following conditions is most likely to cause this pattern of renal injury?**

   (A) acute tubular necrosis (ATN)
   (B) Wegener granulomatosis
   (C) postinfectious glomerulonephritis
   (D) hemolytic uremic syndrome (HUS)
   (E) Goodpasture syndrome

Figure 11–1.

10. A 25-year-old woman is receiving desensitization shots for an allergy for the past 1 year. Today she developed diffuse urticaria 5 minutes after the injection. **Which of the following is the most appropriate next step in management?**

(A) discontinuation of subsequent injections for 3 weeks
(B) application of a tourniquet distal to the injection site
(C) administration of steroids prior to the next injection
(D) administration of aminophylline subcutaneously
(E) administration of epinephrine (1:1000) subcutaneously

11. A 23-year-old man is receiving penicillin for the treatment of a group A strep throat infection. He now returns to the clinic with new symptoms of a rash and diffuse joint discomfort. On physical examination, there are areas of urticaria on his arms and back. The joints appear normal and he has no oral lesions. A urinalysis is positive for red cell casts and protein. **Which of the following is most characteristic of the syndrome?**

(A) it usually requires corticosteroids
(B) symptoms last several months
(C) it may recur after apparent recovery
(D) it may be transferred by leukocyte infusions
(E) most patients are children

12. A 22-year-old woman is seen in the clinic for assessment of recurrent fungal infections. Her physical examination is completely normal and she is not on any medications. She is suspected of having immunodeficiency secondary to impaired T-cell function. **Which of the following is the most cost-effective screening test of cellular immunity?**

(A) quantification of serum immunoglobulin A (IgA)
(B) lymphocyte enumeration on a cell sorter
(C) lymphocyte responses to mitogens
(D) nitroblue tetrazolium assay
(E) intradermal skin test with *Candida albicans*

13. A 19-year-old female university student unknowingly eats a noodle dish that has shrimp in it. She is allergic to shrimp. Over the next 20 minutes she develops acute skin lesions consisting of erythematous wheals that are raised on the surface of the skin. (See Figure 11–2.) **Which of the following is most characteristic of these lesions?**

Figure 11–2.

(A) are most common on the palms and soles
(B) are rarely itchy
(C) do not blanch on pressure
(D) are caused by a localized vasculitis
(E) are caused by an ongoing, immediate, hypersensitivity reaction

14. A 27-year-old man presents to the clinic for assessment of an itchy rash that develops when he goes jogging, or while taking a hot shower. There is no rash at present to examine, but he does show you a digital picture of the rash. It appears as small (few millimeters) wheals. His past medical history is negative, he is not on any medications, and reports no known allergies. **Which of the following is most appropriate in the management of this condition?**

(A) discontinuation of all vigorous exercises

(B) counseling regarding recognition and treatment of anaphylactic reactions

(C) treatment with anticholinergic medications

(D) treatment with hydroxyzine

(E) cool baths rather than hot showers

15. A 42-year-old man was seen in the clinic because of pain and redness in his finger. Last week he had injured the finger while working in his garage. On physical examination, there is erythema, swelling, and tenderness of the second digit in the right hand. Flexion and extension of the finger were normal. A clinical diagnose of cellulitis is made and he is prescribed cephalexin. A few days later he presents to the emergency room complaining of difficulty breathing. He has angioedema due to a drug reaction to the cephalexin. **Which of the following physical findings is characteristic of this syndrome?**

(A) invariably severe itching

(B) prolonged nature of the edema

(C) fluid extravasation from subcutaneous and intradermal postcapillary venules

(D) involvement of lips, tongue, eyelids, genitalia, and dorsum of hands or feet

(E) fluid accumulation in the most dependent areas of the body

16. A 47-year-old woman, with Type 1 diabetes of 30 years' duration, is in the hospital for assessment of atypical chest pain. While in the hospital, she develops a true anaphylactic reaction. **Which of the following is the most likely cause for the reaction?**

(A) radiographic contrast media

(B) erythromycin

(C) insulin

(D) folic acid supplement

(E) exposure to nuts

17. A 27-year-old woman presents to the clinic complaining of pain and discomfort on swallowing. This is the third oral thrush infection in the past one year. Her past health history is significant for substance abuse and intravenous (IV) drug use. Physical examination reveals while plaques on her tongue and cheeks. Laboratory investigations reveal a low CD4+ count. **Which factor is true concerning this immunosuppression?**

(A) qualitative defects in T lymphocytes follow quantitative problems

(B) the low CD4 count in advanced disease is secondary to the direct cytotoxic effects of virus infection

(C) B-lymphocyte abnormalities do not occur early in the disease

(D) macrophages are important in viral dissemination

(E) circulating immune complexes are rarely present

18. A 34-year-old man presents to emergency room with headache and left-sided arm and leg weakness. The symptoms started about a week ago and seem to be getting worse. His past medical history is significant for HIV infection, and he has declined antiretroviral therapy in the past. On physical examination, he is alert and oriented; there is left-sided weakness rated 4–/5 in his arm and 4+/5 in his leg. Strength on the right side is normal. A computed tomography (CT) scan with contrast reveals multiple cortical lesions that are spherical and ring enhancing. **Which of the following is the most likely diagnosis?**

(A) glioblastoma multiforme

(B) toxoplasmosis

(C) lymphoma

(D) progressive multifocal leukoencephalopathy

(E) cytomegalovirus (CMV)

19. A 23-year-old woman presents to the clinic for repeat assessment of wheezing symptoms and shortness of breath on exertion. She reports no "triggers" that bring on the symptoms, and they usually only occur in the spring and then resolve spontaneously. She is a lifetime nonsmoker and feels well in between episodes. There is no personal or family history of atopy or asthma. On physical examination, the vital signs and cardiac exam are normal. The lungs are clear on auscultation and there is no wheeze on forced expiration. **Which of the following is the most likely mechanism of wheezing in this woman?**

(A) elevated IgE levels
(B) mast cell instability
(C) nonspecific hyperirritability of the tracheobronchial tree
(D) disordered immediate hypersensitivity
(E) disordered delayed hypersensitivity

20. A 45-year-old man is admitted to the hospital because of increasing shortness of breath and cough due to an asthma exacerbation. He reports having multiple exacerbations in the past year. After treatment with steroids and bronchodilators he is feeling much better. He is interested in avoiding any potential agents that might trigger his asthma in the future. **Which of the following foods is most likely to precipitate an asthmatic reaction in this man?**

(A) red meat
(B) egg whites
(C) green salad
(D) gluten
(E) mayonnaise

DIRECTIONS (Questions 21 through 36): The following group of numbered items is preceded by a list of lettered options. For each question, select the one lettered option that is most closely associated with it. Each lettered option may be used once, multiple times, or not at all.

Questions 21 through 23: For each patient with symptoms after taking a new medication, select the most likely mechanism.

(A) allergic reaction caused by sensitized mast cells
(B) may be mediated by drug effect on kinin system
(C) final mediator of symptoms are leukotrienes

21. A 23-year-old man has a reaction after being given oral penicillin for a sore throat.

22. A 56-year-old woman is given an angiotensin-converting enzyme (ACE) inhibitor for control of hypertension and develops a reaction consisting of urticaria.

23. A 23-year-old man has an exacerbation of asthma when he takes aspirin for a headache.

Questions 24 through 30: Match the following diseases with the appropriate HLA association.

(A) human lymphocyte antigen (HLA) B27
(B) HLA DR4
(C) HLA DR3
(D) HLA B17
(E) HLA B8
(F) multigenic disorder

24. A 29-year-old man presents with severe back pain and a red eye. The pain is located in his lower back and gluteal area, and is associated with morning stiffness that improves after several hours. On examination, he has limited forward flexion and tenderness of the ischial tuberosities.

25. A 24-year-old woman has a facial skin lesion, thrombocytopenia, arthralgia, and pericarditis.

26. A 12-year-old child has severe deforming arthritis of the hands.

27. A 14-year-old girl presents with weight loss, increased thirst, and urination. Her laboratory tests reveal hyperglycemia and a mildly increased anion gap metabolic acidosis.

28. A 22-year-old man with iritis, balanitis, urethritis, and arthritis.

29. A 27-year-old woman has severe symmetrical small joint arthritis. She notices 1 hour of morning stiffness and swelling with redness in her wrists and hand joints. The distal finger joints are spared. X-rays of the hands reveal early bone erosion in some of the joints.

30. A 33-year-old policeman develops acute asymmetric arthritis involving his left knee and ankle and right ankle. The pain in the feet prevents him from walking. He recalls having a diarrheal illness 3 weeks ago.

Questions 31 through 36: For each patient with a medical condition, select the most likely immune dysfunction.

   (A) B-cell deficiency/dysfunction
   (B) mixed T- and B-cell deficiency/dysfunction
   (C) T-lymphocyte deficiency/dysfunction
   (D) neutropenia
   (E) chemotaxis
   (F) C3 (complement 3) deficiency

31. A 73-year-old man has a history of recurrent pneumonias. He now complains of bone discomfort in his back and chest. X-rays reveal multiple lytic lesions and his serum protein electrophoresis has an IgG spike of 12 g/dL.

32. A 22-year-old woman notices multiple lymph nodes in her neck. They are nontender on palpation and mobile. A monospot test is negative and a biopsy of the node reveals Hodgkin disease.

33. A 73-year-old man has 30,000/mL mature lymphocytes on his blood film. This is an incidental finding and he is clinically feeling well.

34. A 24-year-old woman with malar rash, thrombocytopenia, and arthralgia.

35. A 69-year-old man is receiving chemotherapy for acute myeloid leukemia.

36. A young woman with ataxia-telangiectasia syndrome.

Answers and Explanations

1. **(E)** Serum sickness results from circulating immune complexes, and drug hypersensitivity is the most common cause of serum sickness. It is believed that the drug acts as a hapten binding to a plasma protein. The resultant drug–protein complex induces an immune response. Common signs and symptoms include fever, skin rash (urticarial or morbilliform), arthralgias, lymphadenopathy, and albuminuria. Arthritis, nephritis, neuropathy, and vasculitis are less common. Primary sensitization requires 1–3 weeks, but symptoms can occur rapidly on reexposure. Immediate-type hypersensitivity reactions depend on the release of inflammatory mediators from mast cells either directly or through IgE-specific antibodies. These reactions occur with minutes of exposure to the drug, which rules them out in this patient. *(Fauci, Chapter 56)*

2. **(B)** The major reaction to fungal infections such as histoplasmosis is delayed-type hypersensitivity. This is a reaction of T cells, which have been stimulated by antigen to react against infectious agents, grafts, and tumors. A classic example is the response to the tuberculin skin test in a person previously exposed to *Mycobacterium tuberculosis* organisms which occurs between 48 and 72 hours after antigen exposure. *(Fauci, Chapter 158)*

3. **(B)** NK cells may be of T-cell lineage or monocyte-macrophage lineage. They appear to play an important role in surveillance mechanisms. *(Fauci, Chapter 308)*

4. **(A)** Allergic asthma is often associated with a personal and/or family history of allergic diseases. It is dependent on an IgE response controlled by T and B lymphocytes and activated when antigens interact with mast cell-bound IgE molecules. Most provoking allergens are airborne. Allergic asthma can be seasonal. *(Fauci, Chapter 248)*

5. **(C)** Edema of the glottis is the usual cause of death in hereditary angioedema, an autosomal dominant condition. The lesions are tense, rounded, nonpitting, and several centimeters in diameter. The edema, unlike urticaria, involves deeper tissue and is not pruritic. *(Fauci, Chapter 311)*

6. **(B)** Acquired immune deficiency syndrome (AIDS) is characterized by lymphopenia, with a selective diminution of helper T cells. Likely infectious complications and their appropriate prophylaxis can be predicted by the CD4 T lymphocyte count. Lymphocyte dysfunction can occur even when severe lymphopenia is not yet present. *(Fauci, Chapter 182)*

7. **(A)** Thymic tumors may be associated with myasthenia gravis, red cell aplasia, polymyositis, hemolytic anemia, pemphigus, and agranulocytosis. There is also an association with immunodeficiency and thymoma. These patients have B-lymphocyte deficiency and bacterial infections and diarrhea. Erythroid aplasia may develop as well. *(Fauci, Chapter 101)*

8. **(C)** Autoantibodies can be demonstrated by immunofluorescence or electron microscopy on the basement membranes of glomeruli and alveoli in Goodpasture syndrome. The disease is most common in young men but

can strike at any age. The hemoptysis can be minimal or massive. The course of the hemoptysis is variable, but renal involvement is often progressive. Current therapy includes intensive plasma exchange, cytotoxic agents, and glucocorticoids. Other causes of lung–renal syndromes such as various vasculitides, Wegener granulomatosis, mixed essential cryoglobulinemia, Henoch–Schönlein purpura, and systemic lupus erythematosus (SLE) are not characterized by antibodies to basement membranes. (Fauci, Chapter 277)

9. (C) Immune complexes with low complement levels can be seen in idiopathic and postinfectious glomerulonephritis, lupus, cryoglobulinemia, shunt nephritis, and bacterial endocarditis. Immune complexes are not detected in ATN, Wegener's, HUS, or Goodpasture syndrome. Immune complexes with normal complement levels are found in IgA nephropathy and Henoch–Schönlein purpura. (Fauci, Chapter 277)

10. (E) These systemic reactions are uncommon and easily managed in the office if detected with some subcutaneous epinephrine. But if the patient leaves too soon the reaction could be missed. The exact mechanism of benefit for hyposensitization therapy is unclear. No single measurement of immune function correlates well with clinical efficacy, suggesting a complex of effects that likely includes a reduction in T-cell cytokine production. This type of therapy is reserved for clearly seasonal diseases that cannot be adequately managed with drugs. (Fauci, Chapter 311)

11. (C) The symptoms of serum sickness are usually self-limited and may recur after apparent recovery. The natural course is 1–3 weeks. Recurrence can occur rapidly (12–36 hours) if repeat exposure to the offending antigen occurs. (Fauci, Chapter 311)

12. (E) A positive skin test with C albicans extract (erythema and induration of 10 mm or more at 48 hours) excludes virtually all primary T-cell defects. Lymphocyte enumeration and responses to mitogens are much costlier tests. Serum IgA levels are a good screening test

for agammaglobulinemia, and the nitroblue tetrazolium assay is useful to detect killing defects of phagocyte cells. (Fauci, Chapter 311)

13. (E) An ongoing, immediate hypersensitivity reaction in association with degranulation of mast cells is the most common cause of urticaria. Although it can involve any epidermal or mucosal surface, the palms and soles are usually spared. The associated itching indicates stimulation of nociceptive nerves. The increased blood flow results in erythema that blanches on pressure. (Fauci, Chapter 311)

14. (D) Hydroxyzine can be used for the treatment of this man's urticaria. This represents a case of generalized heat urticaria or cholinergic urticaria rather than exercise-induced urticaria. The latter is characterized by larger lesions and possible anaphylactic reactions and is not triggered by hot showers. Although thought to be cholinergically mediated, atropine does not block symptoms in generalized heat urticaria. Because anaphylaxis does not occur and hydroxyzine is so effective, hot showers are not a great danger. (Fauci, Chapter 311)

15. (D) Unlike other causes of edema, angioedema is not dependent and can involve all epidermal and submucosal surfaces, although the lips, tongue, eyelids, genitalia, hands, and feet are the most commonly involved. Angioedema is often not itchy and, like urticaria, is transient; manifestation peaks in minutes to hours and disappears over hours to days. The fluid extravasates from deeper areas such as dermal and subdermal sites. (Fauci, Chapter 311)

16. (E) Nuts, eggs, seafood, and chocolate are among the many foods implicated in anaphylaxis. Anaphylaxis is characterized by an initial exposure followed by the formation of specific IgE antibody. Repeat exposure results in antigen combining with IgE bound to basophils and mast cells and subsequent degranulation. Anaphylactoid reactions, such as those to radiographic contrast media, are generally not immunemediated and do not require prior exposure. Insulin and folic acid rarely cause

anaphylaxis. Similarly, erythromycin is not a common antibiotic to cause anaphylaxis. *(Fauci, Chapter 311)*

17. **(D)** Even in advanced AIDS, only a minority of CD4+ lymphocytes are actually infected. Numerous other factors, including "innocent bystander destruction" and autoimmune phenomena, might be implicated. Impaired soluble antigen recognition by T lymphocytes can occur when absolute counts are still normal. Polyclonal activation of B cells, which occurs early in the disease, is unlikely to be triggered by direct HIV infection of B cells. Macrophages are felt to be particularly important in carrying the virus across the blood–brain barrier. Circulating immune complexes might help explain arthralgias, myalgias, renal disease, and vasculitis that occur in infected individuals. *(Fauci, Chapter 182)*

18. **(B)** The three most common causes of focal brain lesion in HIV disease are toxoplasmosis, primary central nervous system (CNS) lymphoma, and progressive multifocal leukoencephalopathy (PML). Toxoplasmosis lesions are typically multiple, spherical, and ring-enhancing on CT scan. They are most likely located in the basal ganglia and the cortex. The symptoms develop characteristically over days and global brain dysfunction is common. Lymphoma presents with one or relatively few irregular weakly enhancing lesions more commonly in the periventricular area. PML presents with multiple nonenhancing lesions in the white matter. CMV, herpes, and *Cryptococcus* generally cause diffuse brain disease. Glioblastoma multiforme is not characteristic of HIV disease. *(Fauci, Chapter 182)*

19. **(C)** There is a constant state of hyperreactivity of the bronchi, during which exposure to an irritant precipitates an asthmatic attack. A following subacute phase has been described that can lead to late complications. The presence of inflammation in the airways has resulted in increased usage of inhaled corticosteroids for maintenance therapy. Many cases of asthma have no discernible allergic component. *(Fauci, Chapter 248)*

20. **(C)** Sulfites, used to keep salad greens fresh, can cause severe asthmatic reactions. Other sulfite-containing foods include fresh fruits, potatoes, shellfish, and wine. Aspirin, tartrazine (a coloring agent), and beta-adrenergic agonists also commonly provoke asthmatic attacks. *(Fauci, Chapter 248)*

21. **(A)** Penicillin can cause numerous allergic reactions, including anaphylaxis, interstitial nephritis, rashes (the most common manifestation), urticaria, fever, pneumonitis, dermatitis, and even asthma in workers exposed to airborne penicillin. Hemolytic anemia is often IgG-mediated. Skin tests are reliable in predicting low risk (similar to general population) for those claiming previous penicillin reactions, and desensitization is feasible. The frequency of reactions to cephalosporins in penicillin-allergic patients is not definitely known. *(Fauci, Chapter 311)*

22. **(B)** ACE inhibitors can cause angioedema of the face and oropharyngeal structures. This is felt to be a pseudoallergic reaction, possibly due to the drug's effect on the kinin system. It is thought that reactions may be more common in women, Blacks, and those with idiopathic angioedema. If this occurs, therapy with alternate ACE inhibitors should not be attempted. *(Fauci, Chapter 311)*

23. **(C)** Aspirin frequently can precipitate asthma in susceptible individuals. At highest risk are asthmatics with chronic rhinosinusitis and nasal polyps. This is probably a pseudoallergic reaction related to inhibition of cyclooxygenase with a resultant enhancement of leukotriene synthesis or effect. Densensitization regimens have been developed. *(Fauci, Chapter 248)*

24. **(A)** Ankylosing spondylitis and HLA B27. *(Fauci, Chapter 318)*

25. **(F)** SLE is a multigenic disorder. *(Fauci, Chapter 313)*

26. **(B)** Juvenile rheumatoid arthritis (RA) and HLA DR4 *(Fauci, Chapter 314)*

27. **(C)** Type 1 diabetes mellitus and HLA DR3. *(Fauci, Chapter 338)*

28. **(A)** Reiter syndrome and HLA B27. *(Fauci, Chapter 328)*

29. **(B)** RA and HLA DR4. *(Fauci, Chapter 328)*

30. **(A)** Reactive arthritis (eg, *Shigella* or *Yersinia*) and HLA B27. *(Fauci, Chapter 328)*

The relationship between HLA antigens and diseases is not absolute, but rather one of increased relative risk. The presence of HLA B27 increases the relative risk of ankylosing spondylitis by a factor of about 80, of Reiter syndrome by a factor of 40, and also increases the likelihood of reactive arthritis. The presence of HLA DR4 increases the likelihood of juvenile RA by a factor of 7 and RA by a factor of 6. The presence of HLA DR3 increases the likelihood of both SLE and insulin-dependent diabetes mellitus by a factor of approximately 3.

31. **(A)** Multiple myeloma and B-cell deficiency/dysfunction. *(Fauci, Chapter 106)*

32. **(C)** Hodgkin disease and T-cell deficiency/dysfunction. *(Fauci, Chapter 105)*

33. **(A)** Chronic lymphocytic leukemia and B-cell deficiency/dysfunction. *(Fauci, Chapter 105)*

34. **(F)** SLE and complement deficiency. *(Fauci, Chapter 313)*

35. **(D)** Therapy for hematologic malignancy and neutropenia. *(Fauci, Chapter 82)*

36. **(B)** Ataxia-telangiectasia and both T- and B-cell dysfunction. *(Fauci, Chapter 368)*

Multiple myeloma and chronic lymphocytic leukemia are two of the more common causes of B-cell deficiency/dysfunction. Hodgkin disease, AIDS, sarcoidosis, and thymic aplasia or hypoplasia result in T-lymphocyte depletion/dysfunction. SLE has been associated with C3 deficiency, but most severe complement deficiencies result from inherited disorders. Ataxiatelangiectasia, common variable hypogammaglobulinemia, severe combined immunodeficiency, and Wiskott–Aldrich syndrome have mixed T- and B-cell deficiency.

CHAPTER 12

Pulmonology
Questions

DIRECTIONS (Questions 1 through 45): For each of the questions in this section select the one lettered answer that is the best response in each case.

1. A 33-year-old farmer presents to the clinic with symptoms of recurrent wheezing and coughing after working in a barn where hay is stored. He has no prior history of asthma, and is not taking any medications. On physical examination, there are bibasilar crackles on auscultation of the lungs, the heart sounds are normal, JVP is 2 cm above the sternal angle, and there is no peripheral edema.

   His laboratory investigations are normal with no increase in eosinophils on the CBC. The chest x-ray (CXR) reveals patchy lower lobe infiltrates, and a normal cardiac silhouette. **Which of the following is the most likely diagnosis?**

   (A) asthma
   (B) chronic obstructive lung disease
   (C) hypersensitivity pneumonitis
   (D) bronchiectasis
   (E) sarcoidosis

2. A 57-year-old man presents to the clinic for assessment of shortness of breath on exertion. The symptoms started many months ago after a "cold" and seem to be getting worse. There is no associated cough or sputum production, and he reports a 40-pack-per-year history of smoking. He otherwise feels well and his only past health history is hypertension that is well controlled on amlodipine. On physical examination, there are bilateral wheezes on expiration and increased resonance to percussion of the chest. Pulmonary function tests confirm the diagnosis of chronic obstructive lung disease (COPD). **Which of the following is the best definition of this condition?**

   (A) it is caused by bronchial asthma
   (B) it is preceded by chronic bronchitis
   (C) it is airflow limitation that is not fully reversible
   (D) it is due to destruction and dilatation of lung alveoli
   (E) is due to small airways disease only

3. A 24-year-old woman presents to the emergency department with symptoms of severe wheezing and shortness of breath for 2 days. She has asthma that is well controlled but recently acquired a cat and thinks she is allergic to it. She reports using her salbutamol more frequently at home over the past week, and is adherent to inhaled corticosteroids.

   After receiving oxygen, steroids, and salbutamol (Ventolin) in the emergency room, her breathing improves. She is still wheezing and now feels tremulous and anxious with a pulse of 110/min and respirations 30/min. Arterial blood gases on oxygen reveal a pH of 7.40, PO_2 340 mm Hg, PCO_2 40 mm Hg, and bicarbonate of 24 mEq/L. She is hospitalized for further treatment. **Which of the following treatments or medications should be avoided?**

   (A) theophylline
   (B) sedatives
   (C) corticosteroids
   (D) sympathomimetic amines
   (E) intravenous (IV) fluids

4. A 29-year-old woman presents to the clinic for assessment of on-going symptoms of shortness of breath and wheezing. She has a long history of mild asthma that is well controlled on inhaled corticosteroids. She recently experienced a flare that is characterized by recurrent episodes of bronchial obstruction, fever, malaise, and expectoration of brownish mucous plugs.

On physical examination, the heart exam is normal, and there is bilateral wheezing on expiration. A CXR reveals upper lobe pulmonary infiltrates, and on the complete blood count the eosinophil count is 2000/mL. Special testing reveals that the serum precipitating antibodies to *Aspergillus* are positive. **Which of the following is the most appropriate next step in management?**

(A) antihelminthic therapy

(B) a short course of systemic glucocorticoid therapy

(C) desensitization treatment

(D) high-dose glucocorticoids by puffer

(E) long-term systemic glucocorticoid therapy

5. A 31-year-old African-American man presents to the clinic with new symptoms of dyspnea on exertion. He also reports having a fever and a red tender "rash" on his shins that started one week ago. Prior to this he was healthy with no significant health issues or medication use.

Physical examination reveals fine inspiratory crackles in both lower lung lobes and tender erythematous nodules on his legs. There are no other pertinent findings. A CXR shows bilateral hilar adenopathy and reticulonodular changes in both lungs. A transbronchial biopsy reveals noncaseating granulomas. **Which of the following is the most appropriate next step in management?**

(A) aspirin

(B) isoniazid (INH) and streptomycin

(C) steroids

(D) nitrogen mustard

(E) no therapy

6. A 53-year-old man presents to the hospital with increasing symptoms of shortness of breath, increased sputum production, and frequent puffer use. He has a prior history of chronic obstructive pulmonary disease (COPD) as a result of a 44 pack/year history of smoking. He quit smoking 1 year ago but has not noticed any improvement in his breathing. His medications are tiotropium, salmeterol, fluticasone, and prn salbutamol all via the inhaled route.

On physical examination, he appears in moderate respiratory distress, his blood pressure is 145/90 mm Hg, heart rate 110/min, respiratory rate 24/min, O2 saturation of 82%, and temperature 38.5°C. He is admitted to the hospital with a diagnosis of acute exacerbation of COPD and started on oxygen, antibiotics, oral steroids, inhaled bronchodilators, and anticholinergic agents. The next day he is found in his room confused and sleepy. An arterial blood gas reveals a P_{O_2} 110mm Hg, and P_{CO_2} 75 mm Hg. **Which of the following explanations regarding his elevated P_{CO_2} is correct?**

(A) occurs only with CO_2 inhalation

(B) does not occur in obstructive lung disease

(C) does not occur in restrictive lung disease

(D) is due ventilation–perfusion mismatch

(E) occurs with chronic hypocapnia

7. A 63-year-old woman presents to the emergency room with symptoms of sudden onset of shortness of breath. She reports no chest discomfort, cough, sputum, or fever. Her past medical history is negative for any prior heart or lung problems. She was recently diagnosed with breast cancer and is undergoing active treatment. On examination, her blood pressure is 120/80 mm Hg, pulse 100/min, and heart and lungs are normal. There are no clinical signs of deep venous thrombosis (DVT). **Which of the following investigations is most likely to rule out a pulmonary embolism (PE)?**

(A) normal CXR

(B) normal electrocardiogram (ECG)

(C) normal ventilation–perfusion lung scan

(D) normal ventilation scan

(E) normal magnetic resonance image (MRI)

8. A 40-year-old woman is seen in the clinic for follow up assessment of symptoms of shortness of breath and fatigue. The symptoms started 3 years ago and are now progressively getting worse. She has no other significant past medical history. On physical examination, the jugular venous pressure (JVP) is seen at 7 cm above the sternal angle with a prominent *c-v* wave, and a reduced carotid pulse. Precordial examination reveals a left parasternal lift, loud P_2, and right-sided S_3 and S_4. There are no audible murmurs. The lungs are clear on auscultation.

A CXR reveals clear lung fields and an ECG shows evidence of right ventricular hypertrophy. Pulmonary function tests show a slight restrictive pattern. A clinical diagnosis of primary pulmonary hypertension is considered. **Which of the following is the most appropriate test to confirm the diagnosis?**

(A) open lung biopsy

(B) pulmonary angiography

(C) cardiac catheterization

(D) noninvasive exercise testing

(E) electrophysiologic testing

9. A 63-year-old man presents to the clinic for evaluation of symptoms of shortness of breath. The symptoms are worse on exertion, but there is no chest discomfort, cough, or sputum production. His physical examination is completely normal. Investigations include a normal CXR, and on the arterial blood gas the PO2 is 74 mm Hg, and P_{CO_2} is 60 mm Hg. **Which of the following mechanisms is the most likely cause for the elevated P_{CO_2}?**

(A) ventilation–perfusion ratio inequality

(B) right-to-left shunt

(C) impaired diffusion

(D) hypoventilation

(E) carbon monoxide poisoning

10. A 56-year-old man presents to the clinic for assessment of symptoms of chronic cough. It is present most of the time and is progressively getting worse over the past 3 years. With the cough he usually has white to yellow sputum that he has to expectorate. There is no history of wheezing, asthma, heart failure (HF), or acid reflux disease. He currently smokes 1 pack a day for the past 35 years. On examination, his chest is clear. CXR is normal and his forced expiratory volume in 1 second (FEV1) and forced vital capacity (FVC) on spirometry are normal. **Which of the following is the most likely diagnosis?**

(A) chronic obstructive pulmonary disease (COPD)

(B) early cor pulmonale

(C) chronic bronchitis

(D) asthma

(E) emphysema

11. A 58-year-old man is recently diagnosed with bowel cancer. He now complains of vague chest discomfort and shortness of breath. On examination, he is unwell, blood pressure 90/50 mm Hg, pulse 110/min, respirations 26/min, and oxygen saturation 88%. His lungs are normal on auscultation, the JVP is at 8 cm, and P_2 is loud. There is no edema or leg tenderness on palpation.

A quantitative (ELISA) D-dimer assay is positive, ECG reveals sinus tachycardia, and cardiac enzymes are negative. The CT pulmonary angiogram is positive for a large clot in the right pulmonary artery. **Which of the following tests is most likely to help in guiding emergent therapy?**

(A) echocardiogram

(B) CT scan

(C) venous ultrasound of the legs

(D) venography of the legs

(E) pulmonary function tests

12. A 40-year-old man presents to the clinic for assessment of fever, chills, sore throat, and cough. The symptoms started 2 days ago and his sputum is now productive and green-yellow in color. His past medical history is negative, and he reports his son having a similar illness 1 week ago. The physical examination is normal. A CXR is performed, which reveals a posterior mediastinal mass, but no pneumonia. **Which of the following is the most likely diagnosis?**

(A) lipoma
(B) neurogenic tumor
(C) esophageal cyst
(D) fibroma
(E) bronchogenic cyst

13. A 35-year-old man is evaluated in the clinic for symptoms of shortness of breath. He reports no other lung or heart disease. He smokes half pack a day for the past 10 years. On examination, his JVP is at 2 cm, heart sounds normal, and lungs are clear. A CXR shows hyperinflation and increased lucency of the lung fields. A chest CT reveals bullae and emphysematous changes in the lower lobes, while pulmonary function tests show an FEV1/FVC ratio of <70%. Evaluation of his family reveals other affected individuals. **Which of the following is the most likely diagnosis?**

(A) alpha1-antitrypsin deficiency
(B) beta-glycosidase deficiency
(C) glucose-6-phosphatase deficiency
(D) glucocerebrosides deficiency
(E) growth hormone deficiency

14. A 23-year-old man presents to the clinic for assessment of a gradual but progressive increase in breathing difficulty. He mentions a long history of back pain with prolonged morning stiffness. His past medical history is also significant for an episode of iritis in the past.

On physical examination, the pertinent findings are a reduced range of motion in the lumbar spine with forward flexion and pain on palpation of the sacroiliac joint and surrounding soft tissue. X-rays of the pelvis show erosions and sclerosis of the sacroiliac joint.

Which of the following is the most likely pulmonary complication of this condition?

(A) upper lobe fibrosis
(B) airflow obstruction
(C) chronic pulmonary embolism
(D) pleural effusions
(E) hilar adenopathy

15. A 44-year-old woman has been complaining of a 4-year history of increasing dyspnea and fatigue. Physical examination reveals increased JVP and a reduced carotid pulse. Precordial examination reveals a left parasternal lift, loud P_2, and right-sided S_3 and S_4. There are no audible murmurs. CXR reveals clear lung fields and an ECG shows evidence of right ventricular hypertrophy. Pulmonary function tests show a slight restrictive pattern. A diagnosis of primary pulmonary hypertension (PPH) is made. **Which of the following is the most likely cause of death in this condition?**

(A) intractable left ventricular failure
(B) intractable respiratory failure
(C) massive PE
(D) intractable right ventricular failure or sudden death
(E) myocardial infarction

16. A 29-year-old man presents to the clinic because he is concerned about blue fingers. He reports no other symptoms and is otherwise healthy. On physical examination, his vital signs are normal except for an oxygen saturation of 87% on room air. His lung and cardiac exams are normal but there is bluish discoloration of his fingers consistent with cyanosis. A blood gas reveals hypoxemia and hypercapnia, while the CBC suggests polycythemia. With voluntary hyperventilation he is able to restore his blood gases to normal. **Which of the following is the most likely location for the abnormalities seen on his blood gases?**

(A) cerebral cortex
(B) kidney
(C) heart
(D) respiratory center
(E) cerebellum

17. A 63-year-old woman presents to the emergency room with symptoms of dyspnea and coughing up foul-smelling purulent sputum. She has had similar episodes in the past. There are no other constitutional symptoms and she denies excessive alcohol intake. On physical examination, the blood pressure is 138/86 mm Hg, pulse 88 beats/min, respiratory rate 18 breaths/min, and temperature 37.5°C. She appears chronically ill with clubbing of the fingers. Heart sounds are normal, JVP is measured at 4 cm, and there are inspiratory crackles heard at the lung bases posteriorly. There is no hepatosplenomegaly or any palpable lymph nodes. CXR shows scaring in the left lower lobe, which on chest CT scan is identified as cystic changes with airway dilatation and bronchial wall thickening. **Which of the following is the most appropriate initial next step in management?**

(A) antibiotics and postural drainage
(B) oral steroids
(C) radiotherapy
(D) inhaled bronchodilators
(E) anti-tuberculous medications

18. A 32-year-old man presents to the clinic with symptoms of wheezing, cough, and shortness of breath. The symptoms started gradually at first but are worse now and interfering with his daily activities. He cannot identify any triggers and has no family or childhood history of asthma or eczema. On examination, he appears well and the pertinent findings are bilateral expiratory wheezes on auscultation, and the rest of the physical is normal. Further evaluation with pulmonary function tests reveals a reduced FEV1/FVC ratio that corrects with the administration of inhaled salbutamol. **Which of the following statements about a diagnosis of idiosyncratic asthma is correct?**

(A) known antigenic stimulus
(B) adult onset
(C) history of atopy
(D) positive skin tests
(E) high immunoglobulin E (IgE) levels

19. A 20-year-old African-American woman presents to the clinic for assessment of mild shortness of breath on exertion and joint discomfort in her knees, wrists, and ankles. She also complains of a fever and a red tender rash on her shins. Her past medical history is negative and she is not taking any medications.

On physical examination, the pertinent findings are hepatosplenomegaly, generalized lymphadenopathy, and tender erythematous nodules on her shins. She also has "red eyes" but reports no pain or visual changes. A CXR shows bilateral symmetric hilar adenopathy and clear lung fields. During bronchoscopy a transbronchial biopsy is performed and it reveals noncaseating granulomas. **Which of the following is the most likely cause for the eye lesion?**

(A) uveitis
(B) diabetic complications
(C) steroids
(D) congenital origin
(E) infectious infiltration

20. A 74-year-old man presents to the emergency department with new symptoms of blood tinged sputum. For the past week he has noticed streaks of blood in his chronic daily sputum production. He reports no fever or chills, but has lost 10 lb in the past 6 months involuntarily. His past medical history is significant for hypertension, dyslipidemia, and a 40 pack year history of smoking.

On physical examination, he has bilateral expiratory wheezes, and there is clubbing of his fingers. No lymph nodes are detected and the remaining examination is normal. A CXR reveals a left hilar mass. **Which of the following suggests that the tumor is a small cell lung cancer?**

(A) syndrome of inappropriate antidiuretic hormone (SIADH) secretion
(B) acanthosis nigricans
(C) Cushing syndrome
(D) leukemoid reaction
(E) Stevens–Johnson syndrome

21. A 66-year-old man presents to the emergency room with symptoms of feeling unwell and a low-grade fever with cough for several weeks. He has a history of chronic alcoholism and reports drinking heavily for the past month, including episodes of passing out.

On physical examination, he looks unwell but not in any distress. His temperature is 38.5°C, blood pressure 128/76 mm Hg, pulse 100 beats/min, and respirations of 18 breaths/min. The heart sounds are normal and there are crackles in the left lower base. A CXR reveals a left lower lobe infiltrate and air-filled cavity consistent with a lung abscess. **Which of the following is the most appropriate antibiotic therapy?**

(A) penicillin

(B) cloxacillin

(C) ceftriaxone

(D) metronidazole

(E) clindamycin

22. A 44-year-old woman presents to the emergency department with symptoms of increased shortness of breath and nonproductive coughing. She has had asthma since childhood and uses her medications as directed. There are no identified triggers for her asthma, and she has not required ventilatory support during previous exacerbations. Recently, she reports having a "cold" and since then noticed that her peak flow readings are decreasing and she is using her salbutamol puffer more frequently for rescue therapy. On examination, she is in moderate respiratory distress, respirations 25/min, oxygen saturation of 90% on room air, and there are bilateral expiratory wheezes on lung auscultation. Her blood gas indicates a P_{CO_2} of 50 mm Hg. **Which of the following is the most likely mechanism for her carbon dioxide retention?**

(A) impaired lung diffusion

(B) right-to-left shunt

(C) hyperventilation

(D) ventilation–perfusion ratio inequality

(E) increased dead-space ventilation

23. A 53-year-old man presents for evaluation of progressive shortness of breath. His symptoms are insidious in onset and he reports no cough, sputum, or chest discomfort. His past medical history is significant for well-controlled hypertension and type 2 diabetes. He is a lifetime nonsmoker and has no history of occupational exposure to inhaled organic or inorganic particles. Pulmonary function tests reveal a restrictive defect, and a high-resolution CT suggests pulmonary fibrosis. **Which of the following is the most likely role of transbronchial biopsy in this condition?**

(A) assess disease severity

(B) assess possible bronchiolar narrowing

(C) diagnose specific causes of interstitial lung disease

(D) determine degree of inflammation

(E) diagnose possible cancer

24. A 28-year-old man presents to the emergency room complaining of coughing up blood and sputum. He provides a history of recurrent pneumonias and a chronic cough productive of foul-smelling purulent sputum. He has no other past medical history and is a lifetime nonsmoker. On physical examination, there are no oral lesions, heart sounds are normal, and wet inspiratory crackles are heard at the lung bases posteriorly. He also has clubbing of his fingers, but there is no hepatosplenomegaly or any palpable lymph nodes. CXR show fibrosis and pulmonary infiltrates in the right lower lung. **Which of the following is the most appropriate initial diagnostic test?**

(A) chest CT scan

(B) bronchoscopy

(C) bronchography

(D) open thoracotomy

(E) bronchoalveolar lavage (BAL)

25. A 64-year-old woman is admitted to the hospital with right lobar pneumonia and sepsis syndrome. She becomes progressively more short of breath and hypoxemic requiring intubation and mechanical ventilation. Her repeat CXR in the intensive care unit now shows diffuse pulmonary infiltrates and a diagnosis of acute

respiratory distress syndrome (ARDS) is made. **Which of the following mechanisms is the most likely cause for the early "exudative" phase of ARDS?**

(A) increased lung compliance
(B) increased interstitial fibrosis
(C) increased vascular permeability to fluid and proteins
(D) decreased pulmonary perfusion
(E) decreased ventilatory dead space

26. A 23-year-old man is experiencing a flare of his asthma. He is using his salbutamol inhaler more frequently than usual and despite increasing his inhaled steroids he is still short of breath. Previously, his asthma was considered mild with no severe exacerbations requiring oral steroids or hospitalization. With the current flare, he is experiencing recurrent episodes of bronchial obstruction, fever, malaise, and expectoration of brownish mucous plugs. On examination, there is bilateral wheezing. The heart, abdomen, neurologic, and skin exams are normal. A CXR reveals upper lobe pulmonary infiltrates; the eosinophil count is 3000/mL, and serum precipitating antibodies to *Aspergillus* are positive. **Which of the following is the most likely diagnosis?**

(A) ascaris infestation
(B) allergic bronchopulmonary aspergillosis
(C) Churg–Strauss allergic granulomatosis
(D) Löeffler syndrome
(E) hypereosinophilic syndrome

27. A 66-year-old man has progressive shortness of breath due to COPD. He is currently able to do his activities of daily living, but has trouble walking more than 1 block. His physical examination reveals hyperinflation, increased resonance to percussion, and bilateral expiratory wheezes. He is on appropriate medical therapy for his stage of COPD. **Which of the following is also indicated in the management of this condition?**

(A) meningococcal vaccination
(B) yearly influenza vaccination

(C) weight reduction if obese
(D) *Haemophilus influenzae B* vaccination
(E) pneumococcal vaccination

28. A 45-year-old woman is seen in the clinic for assessment of severe symptoms of epigastric and abdominal pain after eating. A trial of acid suppression therapy with proton pump inhibitors (PPI) only partially improved her symptoms. She is referred for elective outpatient upper endoscopy, which is positive for a small duodenal ulcer. Two hours after the procedure she complains of shortness of breath and severe anterior chest discomfort, which is made worse with deep inspiration. On examination, she looks unwell, blood pressure is 150/90 mm Hg, pulse 110/min, and lungs are clear. Heart sounds are normal but there is an extra "crunching"-type sound that is intermittently heard. A CXR demonstrates air surrounding the heart. **Which of the following is the most likely diagnosis?**

(A) acute pericarditis
(B) acute cardiac ischemia
(C) acute mediastinitis
(D) aortic dissection
(E) pneumothorax

29. A 55-year-old woman presents to the emergency room with symptoms of chest pain and is admitted to the coronary care unit with acute coronary syndrome. She again develops chest discomfort and rapidly deteriorates due to hypoxemia and needs intubation and ventilation. Her CXR is compatible with acute "flash" pulmonary edema. Her Po_2 on the blood gas prior to intubation was 44 mm Hg, and now while breathing 100% oxygen on the ventilator her repeat blood gas reveals a Po_2 of 95 mm Hg. **Hypoxemia while receiving 100% oxygen indicates which of the following problems?**

(A) ventilation–perfusion mismatch
(B) shunt-type physiology
(C) hypoventilation
(D) impaired diffusion
(E) interstitial lung disease

30. A 31-year-old man presents to the clinic for evaluation of worsening shortness of breath on exertion. He has severe kyphoscoliosis due to cerebral palsy. He reports no other symptoms of chest discomfort, fever, chills, cough, or sputum production. On physical examination, he is not in distress; he has a severe scoliosis to the left; and decreased air entry to that side. His right lung is clear, the JVP is at 3 cm, and heart sounds are normal. Pulmonary function tests are performed. **Which of the following is the most likely abnormality to be seen on the pulmonary function tests?**

    (A) increased total lung capacity (TLC)
    (B) increased functional residual capacity (FRC)
    (C) decreased TLC
    (D) increased compliance
    (E) increased vital capacity (VC)

31. A 67-year-old woman presents to the clinic complaining of increasing shortness of breath on exertion. She has no prior cardiac or pulmonary history, and reports no symptoms of chest discomfort, cough, sputum production, orthopnea or peripheral edema. Her physical examination including vital signs, cardiac and pulmonary examinations are completely normal. Her CXR, ECG, and CBC are also normal. She then undergoes pulmonary function tests to evaluate her symptoms of dyspnea. The most prominent finding is a reduction of the ratio of FEV1/FVC with no reversibility when given inhaled salbutamol. **Which of the following is the most likely diagnosis?**

    (A) COPD
    (B) ankylosing spondylitis
    (C) pickwickian syndrome
    (D) scleroderma of the chest wall
    (E) lobar pneumonia

32. A 35-year old man who works as a pipe fitter presents to the clinic seeking advice and information about asbestos. He is concerned about asbestos exposure at his most recent job site, where they are retro fitting an old building with new pipes. The asbestos on the job site was just discovered last week, but he and his coworkers have been working in the building for the past month. He clinically feels well and reports no respiratory symptoms; his physical examination is normal. **Which of the following statements concerning asbestosis is correct?**

    (A) the type of asbestos fiber is crucial in determining whether asbestos-related lung disease occurs
    (B) moderate rather than severe obstruction to airflow is characteristic of asbestosis
    (C) mesothelioma is the common malignancy associated with asbestosis
    (D) pleural effusions are invariably associated with malignancy in asbestosis
    (E) short-term (ie, 1–2 years) exposure can result in serious sequelae decades later

33. A 52-year-old man develops sudden-onset shortness of breath on postoperative day 4 after a hemicolectomy for colon cancer. His surgery went well with no operative complications. He reports no cough, sputum, or pleuritic chest pain. His blood pressure is 155/90 mm Hg, pulse 100/min, temperature 37.8°C, lungs are clear, and the heart sounds normal. He has bilateral pedal edema, but no discomfort in his legs. His CXR and ECG are normal. A chest CT (PE protocol) with contrast reveals multiple thrombi in his right upper and middle lobe arteries. **Which of the following statements concerning the management of this condition is most likely correct?**

    (A) continuous IV heparin or subcutaneous low-molecular-weight heparin (LMWH) therapy is indicated
    (B) urgent thrombolytic therapy is indicated
    (C) urgent inferior vena cava (IVC) filter insertion is indicated
    (D) urgent thrombectomy of the clots is indicated
    (E) confirmation of the diagnosis with bilateral ultrasound leg Doppler

34. A 50-year-old man presents to the clinic complaining of excessive daytime sleepiness and a history of snoring. One week ago, he fell asleep

while driving his car and got into a minor accident. On examination, he is obese (body mass index [BMI] >30) and his blood pressure is 160/90 mm Hg. His lungs are clear and the heart sounds are distant. **Which of the following is the most likely explanation for the symptoms associated with this condition?**

(A) related to cardiac dysfunction

(B) neuropsychiatric and behavioral

(C) pulmonary

(D) gastrointestinal (GI)

(E) musculoskeletal

35. A 75-year-old man presents to the clinic for follow-up assessment of his COPD. He has a 45 pack/year history of smoking and quit 1 year ago. At his last visit he complained of worsening dyspnea symptoms despite being on a long acting bronchodilator and tiotropium. Pulmonary function tests (PFTs), a blood gas on room air and CXR were ordered to evaluate his worsening symptoms. The PFTs confirm severe air flow obstruction that is nonreversible and the CXR shows hyperinflation but no other pulmonary pathology. His ABG reveals a pO2 of 52 mm Hg, and a pCO2 of 45 mm Hg. **Which of the following statements concerning hypoxemia in COPD is correct?**

(A) erythrocytosis is an appropriate compensation for hypoxemia, and phlebotomy will worsen symptoms

(B) continuous oxygen therapy is effective in producing symptomatic and hemodynamic improvement in severe hypoxia

(C) a PO_2 of <60 mm Hg is an indication for continuous oxygen therapy

(D) a PO_2 of 65 mm Hg or below is an indication for supplemental oxygen during air travel

(E) continuous supplemental oxygen improves functional ability but does not alter the natural history of obstructive airways disease with severe hypoxemia

36. A 58-year-old steam pipe worker presents with a vague ache in the left chest and mild dyspnea of several months' duration. There is dullness on percussion of the left chest associated with diminished breath sounds. His CXR is shown in Figure 12–1. Which of the following is the most likely diagnosis?

Figure 12–1.

(A) pleural metastases

(B) Paget disease

(C) mesothelioma and asbestosis

(D) pleural effusion

(E) multiple myeloma

37. A 27-year-old man presents to clinic for assessment of new left-sided chest pain and feeling unwell. He describes developing a new cough with some blood-tinged sputum, fever, and chills of 2 days' duration. His past medical history is negative, and he reports smoking about 1 pack a day. On physical examination, the pertinent findings are dullness and crackles in the left lower chest. His CXR is shown in Figure 12–2. **Which of the following is the most likely diagnosis?**

Figure 12–2.

(A) pneumonia, left lower lobe
(B) atelectasis, left lower lobe
(C) PE
(D) tuberculosis
(E) sarcoidosis

38. A 40-year-old man is seen for an insurance assessment. He has no past medical history and feels well. His compete physical examination is normal. His biochemistry, complete blood count (CBC), ECG, and urinalysis are also normal. His CXR is abnormal and presented in Figure 12–3. **Which of the following is the most likely diagnosis?**

Figure 12–3.

(A) hamartoma of the lung
(B) tuberculous granuloma of the left apex
(C) osteochondroma of the left fourth rib
(D) bronchogenic carcinoma
(E) pulmonary metastases

39. A 21-year-old man is seen in the clinic for assessment of a nonproductive cough, shortness of breath, and chest pain which changes with breathing. He also complains of pain in the left arm. On physical examination, there is tenderness over the left shoulder, heart sounds are normal, and the lungs are clear. A CXR reveals a lytic lesion in the left humerus and reticulonodular opacities in the upper and middle lobes (Figure 12–4). The eosinophil count is normal. **Which of the following is the most appropriate initial diagnostic test?**

(A) lung biopsy
(B) humerus bone biopsy
(C) CT scan of chest
(D) bronchoscopy
(E) pulmonary function tests

Figure 12–4.

(A) emphysema
(B) lobar pneumonia
(C) chronic bronchitis
(D) acute bronchitis
(E) CHF

41. A 33-year-old woman, who is otherwise well, presents to the emergency department with symptoms of recurrent episodes of hemoptysis. She has no fever, weight loss, cough, or sputum production. She is not experiencing any dyspnea or chest discomfort and is not taking any medications. She works in an office setting, reports no travel history, and her family history is negative for lung disorders or bleeding diathesis. Her vital signs, oxygen saturation, and physical examination are entirely normal. The CXR, biochemistry, CBC, and coagulation profile are also normal. **Which of the following is the most appropriate initial diagnostic test?**

(A) echocardiogram
(B) gallium scan
(C) CT scan of chest
(D) bronchoscopy
(E) pulmonary function tests

40. 65-year-old man presents to the clinic complaining of severe dyspnea and associated cough with sputum production. The symptoms started insidiously, and are more noticeable lately. Exertion makes the dyspnea worse. There is no chest discomfort, or heart failure symptoms. His past medical history is significant for type 2 diabetes, hypertension, and dyslipidemia. On physical examination, the vital signs are normal, his oxygen saturation is 97% on room air and his cardiac examination is normal. The lungs are clear on auscultation. CXR, ECG, and CBC are normal. His pulmonary function tests are shown in Table 12–1. **Which of the following is the most likely diagnosis?**

42. An 83-year-old man with Parkinson disease presents with low-grade fever and cough for several weeks. Lately, he has been experiencing more rigidity and difficulty with his walking. He is on a levodopa/carbidopa combination for treatment for the past 5 years. On examination, his gait is shuffling and slow. He has a tremor in his left hand at rest, and there is cogwheel rigidity of the forearm. There are crackles in the left lower lung field. CXR reveals a lung abscess in the left lower lobe. **Which of the following is the most likely bacteriologic diagnosis for the lung abscess?**

(A) oropharyngeal flora
(B) tuberculosis
(C) *Staphylococcus aureus*
(D) *Pseudomonas aeruginosa*
(E) *Candida albicans*

TABLE 12–1. PULMONARY FUNCTION STUDIES

FEV1	60% predicted
FVC	110% predicted
FEV1/FVC	60%
TLC	120% predicted
RV	130% predicted
DCO	60% predicted

Abbreviations: FEV1—forced expiratory volume in 1 second; FVC—forced vital capacity; TLC—total lung capacity; RV—residual volume; DCO—diffusing capacity for carbon monoxide.

43. A 69-year-old woman presents to the emergency room complaining of chest discomfort and shortness of breath. The symptoms started suddenly 1 day ago. She has no prior history of chest pain, cardiac, or pulmonary conditions. She recently returned on an overnight flight from Europe. On physical examination, she is comfortable, blood pressure 130/80 mm Hg, pulse 90/min, respirations 18/min, and oxygen saturation 97%. The heart and lungs are normal on auscultation, and there is no edema or leg tenderness on palpation. A CXR and ECG are normal but a quantitative (ELISA) D-dimer assay is positive. **Which of the following statements regarding the D-dimer assay is correct?**

    (A) it is sensitive but not specific
    (B) it is specific but not sensitive
    (C) it is neither specific nor sensitive
    (D) a negative result suggests myocardial ischemia
    (E) it is both sensitive and specific

Figure 12–5.

44. A 24-year-old African-American woman presents with mild dyspnea on exertion. Her symptoms have come on gradually and she reports no pleuritic chest pain, hemoptysis, or sputum production. There is also no history of wheezing, nocturnal or early morning coughing, and she does not smoke. Her past medical history is negative and is not taking any medications. On physical examination, there is generalized lymphadenopathy, the heart sounds are normal and the lungs are clear on auscultation. A CXR shows bilateral symmetric hilar adenopathy and reticulonodular changes in both lungs (See Figure 12–5). She has a restrictive lung disease pattern on pulmonary function testing. **Which of the following is the most likely diagnosis?**

    (A) Hodgkin disease
    (B) tuberculosis
    (C) rheumatic fever
    (D) sarcoidosis
    (E) rheumatoid arthritis (RA)

45. A 30-year-old man presents with coughing up blood and sputum. There is no associated dyspnea, fever, or pleuritic chest pain. His past medical history is significant for recurrent pneumonias and a chronic cough productive of foul-smelling purulent sputum. The sputum production is usually worse when lying down and in the morning. He quit smoking 5 years ago and started when he was 18 years old. On physical examination, he appears chronically ill with clubbing of the fingers. Wet inspiratory crackles are heard at the lung bases posteriorly. CXR shows scaring in the right lower lobe, which on chest CT scan is identified as airway dilatation, bronchial wall thickening, and grapelike cysts. **Which of the following is the most likely diagnosis?** (See Figure 12–6.)

    (A) bronchiectasis
    (B) chronic bronchitis
    (C) disseminated pulmonary tuberculosis
    (D) pulmonary neoplasm
    (E) chronic obstructive emphysema

Figure 12–6.

130/90 mm Hg, and pulse 80/min. Examination of the chest reveals decreased fremitus, dullness to percussion, and absent breath sounds in the left lower lung. There is also a tracheal shift towards the left side.

47. A 72-year-old man with COPD develops acute shortness of breath and presents to the hospital. He appears uncomfortable: blood pressure is 120/90 mm Hg, pulse 100/min, oxygen saturation 85% on room air. On examination of the chest, there is absent fremitus, absent breath sounds, and hyperresonant percussion of the right lung. The trachea is shifted to the left.

48. A 45-year-old woman comes to the emergency department because of increased shortness of breath. Examination of the chest reveals decreased fremitus, low diaphragms, and prolonged expiration phase.

49. A 24-year old woman notices increasing shortness of breath after recent treatment for right lower lobe pneumonia. She has no fever, cough, or sputum production. On examination, the pertinent findings are decreased fremitus, dullness on percussion, and absent breath sounds of the right lower lung. In addition, the trachea has shifted to the left.

50. A 61-year-old man is not feeling well because of shortness of breath and left-sided chest pains that increase with breathing. His examination reveals increased fremitus, dull to percussion, and bronchophony on the left side. His heart sounds are normal.

DIRECTIONS (Questions 46 through 55): The following group of numbered items is preceded by a list of lettered options. For each question, select the one lettered option that is most closely associated with it. Each lettered option may be used once, multiple times, or not at all.

Questions 46 through 50: For each patient with abnormal pulmonary physical findings, select the most likely diagnosis.

(A) acute asthmatic attack
(B) complete pneumothorax
(C) large pleural effusion
(D) atelectasis
(E) lobar pneumonia

46. A 64-year-old woman is admitted to the hospital after the acute onset of left-sided weakness. She has had a large right cerebral stroke and is confined to bed. On the fifth hospital day, her oxygen saturation is noted to be reduced to 90% on room air. She feels fine, the neurologic weakness is unchanged, blood pressure is

Questions 51 through 55: For each patient with lung cancer, select the most likely cell type based on clinical description.

(A) squamous cell carcinoma
(B) adenocarcinoma
(C) large cell carcinoma
(D) small cell carcinoma
(E) bronchioloalveolar carcinoma

51. A 66-year-old man with a 40-pack-per-year history of smoking is investigated for hemoptysis. CXR reveals a central 3-cm mass near the left bronchus. His serum biochemistry is abnormal for elevated calcium, but there is no boney metastasis on the bone scan. Biopsy of the mass is positive for a type of lung cancer associated with paraneoplastic hypercalcemia.

52. A 55-year-old woman presents with symptoms of fever, chills, and colored sputum production. She is a former 40-pack-per-year smoker. Her CXR is abnormal for a 2-cm right hilar mass and right lower lobe infiltrate. She is started on antibiotics and a biopsy of the hilar mass is positive for a type of lung cancer responsive to cytotoxic chemotherapy.

53. A 71-year-old man is having an elective left total knee replacement, when a routine preoperative CXR finds a solitary lung mass. He has no other symptoms related to the lung mass. His surgery is cancelled and a biopsy of the lung mass is positive for a type of cancer that can potentially be cured by surgery.

54. A 58-year-old woman has a witnessed generalized seizure. She has no prior history of seizures, and her only new symptoms are weight loss and anorexia. She looks unwell and cachectic, and the remaining examination is normal. Her serum sodium is 112 mEq/L, serum osmolality is 260 mOsm/kg, and the urine osmolality is 420 mOsm/kg. Her CXR is abnormal for a large left hilar mass. She has a 30-pack-per-year history of smoking. Biopsy of the mass is positive for a lung cancer most commonly associated with ectopic endocrine syndromes.

55. A 58-year-old man comes to the emergency department because of left shoulder pain radiating down his left arm. His only risk factor for cardiac disease is hypertension and a 30-pack-per-year smoking history. On examination, his blood pressure is 150/90 mm Hg in both arms, pulse 100/min, and heart sounds are normal. He also has ptosis of his left eyelid and a left pupil that is smaller than the right. ECG is normal, and a CXR shows a large left apical mass with first and second rib destruction. A biopsy of the mass is consistent with lung cancer most commonly associated with Pancoast syndrome.

Answers and Explanations

1. **(C)** Hypersensitivity pneumonitis is an inflammatory disorder of the lungs involving alveolar walls and terminal airways that is caused by repeated exposure to organic agents. In this example of "farmer's lung," the inhalation of antigens present in moldy hay such as thermophilic actinomyces or *Aspergillus* species are the causative agents. When exposure to moldy hay is stopped, symptoms and signs of farmer's lung all tend to abate and complete recovery usually follows. In acute syndromes, the presentation is 4–8 hours after exposure. Symptoms include fever, chills, malaise, cough, and dyspnea without wheezing. The rate of disease depends on rainfall (which promotes fungal growth) and agricultural practices related to turning and stacking hay. In acute and subacute presentations, removing exposure to the antigen will result in complete recovery. COPD and bronchiectasis are less likely given the absence of prior smoking exposure or lung injury, and both of these disorders usually do have an associated pulmonary infiltrate on CXR unless there is an concomitant lung infection. Asthma can causing wheezing symptoms, and even have mold or dust as triggers but again there is no infiltrate seen on the CXR. *(Fauci, Chapter 249)*

2. **(C)** COPD is defined as a disease state that is characterized by airflow limitation that is not fully reversible. Emphysema and chronic bronchitis are closely related, and the term COPD is often used to encompass both. Chronic bronchitis is a clinical syndrome defined as excessive tracheobronchial mucous production severe enough to cause productive cough for at least 3 months of the year for at least 2 consecutive years. Emphysema is defined as the distention of air spaces distal to the terminale bronchiole, with destruction of alveolar septa. It is primarily a histologic diagnosis. Smoking is the usual antecedent for COPD. *(Fauci, Chapter 254)*

3. **(B)** Tranquilizers and sedatives should be avoided in prolonged asthma attacks. Bronchodilators, fluids, aminophylline, and steroids may be used. In acute situations, IV glucocorticoids are frequently used. Results of therapy should be monitored in an objective manner, with peak expiratory flow rates or FEV1. In acute asthmatic attacks, hypocarbia is usual on blood gas analysis. Normal or elevated $PaCO_2$ is a bad sign and requires intensive monitoring and aggressive treatment. *(Fauci, Chapter 248)*

4. **(E)** Allergic bronchopulmonary aspergillus usually requires long-term treatment with glucocorticoids. The major diagnostic criteria are bronchial asthma, pulmonary infiltrates, eosinophilia greater than 1000, immediate wheal and flare response to *Aspergillus fumigans*, serum precipitins to *A fumigans*, elevated serum IgE, and central bronchiectasis. *(Fauci, Chapter 197)*

5. **(C)** Glucocorticoids is the treatment of choice of sarcoidosis, but numerous other agents have been used. Relatively asymptomatic patients often require no treatment. Steroids are used with ocular, CNS, or other serious complications. Although 50% of patients are left with permanent organ impairment, these are usually not symptomatic or significant. Only in 15–20% of cases does the disease remain active or recur. *(Fauci, Chapter 322)*

6. **(D)** The PCO2 rises in some patients with an acute exacerbation of COPD due to ventilation–perfusion mismatch and respiratory muscle fatigue. The administration of oxygen may result in a small increase in PCO2 in some patients. This should not prevent the administration of O2 to patients since hypoxemia is not well tolerated. Studies show that administration of O2 to COPD patients with hypercapnia does not reduce minute ventilation. Hypoxic drive plays a small role in patients with COPD. Causes of the chronic hypoventilation syndrome include impaired respiratory drive (eg, prolonged hypoxia, central nervous system [CNS] disease), neuromuscular disorders (eg, motor neuron disease, myasthenia gravis), or impaired ventilatory apparatus (eg, kyphoscoliosis, COPD). *(Fauci, Chapter 255)*

7. **(C)** The ventilation–perfusion lung scan is most valuable in ruling out a PE. If properly performed early in the course of symptoms, a normal scan rules out the diagnosis. High-probability scans are usually considered enough evidence of PE to warrant definitive treatment. Intermediate- or low-probability scans may require further investigation depending on the prior probability of disease. More recent data suggest that a normal high-resolution chest CT with contrast rules out clinically significant PE and is replacing perfusion scanning since the lung images may provide an alternate diagnosis for the patient's symptoms. *(Fauci, Chapter 256)*

8. **(C)** Cardiac catheterization is useful to exclude an underlying cardiac shunt as the cause of the pulmonary hypertension. In primary pulmonary hypertension, the pulmonary capillary wedge pressure is normal but the pulmonary systolic and diastolic pressures are elevated. Open lung biopsy is not required. Pulmonary angiography is usually performed only if a lung scan suggests thromboembolic disease. *(Fauci, Chapter 244)*

9. **(D)** Hypoventilation always causes both hypoxemia and hypercapnia. If the hypoventilation syndrome is caused exclusively by impaired respiratory drive (eg, drug overdose), then the alveolar-arterial PaO_2 gradient remains normal. Often, hypoventilation results from more than one disorder in the respiratory system (eg, COPD plus metabolic alkalosis secondary to diuretics and glucocorticoids). *(Fauci, Chapter 246)*

10. **(C)** Chronic bronchitis is a clinical diagnosis defined by the presence of chronic productive cough for 3 months in each of 2 successive years in a patient in whom other causes of chronic cough have been excluded. Emphysema is a pathologic term describing the abnormal permanent enlargement of airspaces distal to the terminal bronchioles, accompanied by destruction of their walls without obvious fibrosis. Emphysema may be noted in patients with COPD. *(Fauci, Chapter 254)*

11. **(A)** In most circumstances, treatment for pulmonary embolism is anticoagulation to prevent further pulmonary emboli. However, in patients with hemodynamic instability primary therapy for the embolus with thrombolysis may be considered. Evidence of right ventricular hypokinesis on echocardiogram can be an indication for such primary therapy. *(Fauci, Chapter 256)*

12. **(B)** Neurogenic tumors are the most common posterior mediastinal masses. Other posterior mediastinal masses include meningoceles, meningomyeloceles, gastroenteric cysts, and esophageal diverticula. Common anterior mediastinal masses include thymomas, lymphomas, teratomas, and thyroid masses. Middle mediastinal masses include vascular lesions, lymph nodes, and pleuropericardial and bronchogenic cysts. *(Fauci, Chapter 257)*

13. **(A)** Most people have two MM genes and a resultant alpha1-antitrypsin level in excess of 2.5 g/L. Homozygotes with ZZ or SS genotypes have severe alpha1-antitrypsin deficiency and develop severe panacinar emphysema in the third or fourth decade of life. Smoking is an important cofactor in the development of disease. Heterozygotes (MZ or MS) have intermediate levels of alpha1-antitrypsin (ie, genetic expression is that of an autosomal codominant

allele). This heterozygous state is common (5–14% of general population), but it is unclear whether it is associated with lung function abnormalities. *(Fauci, Chapter 304)*

14. **(A)** Ankylosing spondylitis (AS) is characterized by bilateral upper lobe fibrosis, which may be complicated by fibrocavitary disease. The pulmonary involvement is rare and is usually very slowly progressive. The cavities can be colonized by *Aspergillus*. Airflow obstruction is not a usual feature of AS and suggests an alternate diagnosis such as asthma or COPD. Hilar adenopathy, pleural effusions, and chronic PE are also not characteristic of AS. *(Fauci, Chapter 318)*

15. **(D)** Death is usually the result of either intractable right heart failure or sudden death. The natural history of the disease is unclear because the disease is asymptomatic for a long period. Survival from diagnosis is dependent on the functional class of the patient. Functional class IV dyspnea suggests a mean survival of only 6 months. Patients with PPH are also at increased risk of venothromboembolic disease and current guidelines recommend chronic anticoagulation with warfarin. Left ventricular failure and myocardial infarction are not usual causes of death in patients with PPH. *(Fauci, Chapter 244)*

16. **(D)** The primary pathology is likely to be located in the respiratory center. Cyanosis, especially when asleep, is caused by a combination of polycythemia and hypoxia. The symptoms of alveolar hypoventilation are caused by both hypercarbia and hypoxemia. *(Fauci, Chapter 246)*

17. **(A)** Antibiotics and postural drainage is the appropriate initial therapy for this patient with bronchiectasis. The choice of antimicrobial agents is guided by the sputum culture, but amoxicillin, TMP/SMX, or levofloxacin can be used for empiric therapy. The general principles of therapy include eliminating underlying problems, improved clearance of secretions, control of infections, and reversal of airflow obstruction. Oral steroids are not considered for the treatment of bronchiectasis unless there is another indication. *(Fauci, Chapter 252)*

18. **(B)** Idiosyncratic asthma is more likely to have its onset in adult life. A significant portion of asthmatics have no known personal or family history of atopy and have normal IgE levels. Upper respiratory infections can serve as triggers for idiosyncratic asthma. *(Fauci, Chapter 248)*

19. **(A)** Acute granulomatous uveitis may be the initial manifestation of sarcoidosis. It can cause blindness. About 25% of patients with sarcoid have eye involvement—three-quarters have anterior uveitis and one-quarter have posterior uveitis. Involvement of lacrimal glands can lead to dry, sore eyes. *(Fauci, Chapter 322)*

20. **(A)** SIADH is more characteristic of small cell lung cancer. Paraneoplastic syndromes are classified as metabolic, neuromuscular, connective tissue, dermatologic, and vascular. Acanthosis nigricans and other cutaneous manifestations (eg, dermatomyositis) are rare (<1%). Clubbing is common and occurs in up to 30% of non-small cell lung cancers. The various endocrine syndromes occur in 12% of cases. At times, paraneoplastic syndromes may be the presenting finding in lung cancer or be the first sign of recurrence, most occur with non-small cell lung cancer. Stevens–Johnson syndrome usually follows drug allergy and is not a paraneoplastic syndrome. *(Fauci, Chapter 85)*

21. **(E)** Traditionally, penicillin was the treatment of choice for anaerobic lung disease, but because of the emergence of beta-lactamase-producing organisms it is no longer the first choice. However, clindamycin, or metronidazole plus either third-generation cephalosporin (ceftriaxone) or fluoroquinolone (levofloxacin) have a better spectrum of activity against oral anaerobes, Gram negatives, and *Streptococcus pneumoniae* for the treatment of lung abscess. *(Fauci, Chapter 252)*

22. **(D)** Disorders of the airways such as asthma or COPD can cause an increased $PaCO_2$ because of severe ventilation–perfusion mismatching

despite normal or increased minute ventilation volume. Carbon dioxide retention is seen in right-to-left shunt only with exercise and is uncommon in impaired diffusion syndromes. *(Fauci, Chapter 248)*

23. **(C)** Transbronchial biopsy helps differentiate idiopathic pulmonary fibrosis (IPF) from similar syndromes with specific treatments. These include chronic hypersensitivity pneumonitis, cryptogenic organizing pneumonia, and sarcoidosis. *(Fauci, Chapter 255)*

24. **(A)** CT scan can confirm the diagnosis and define the extent of bronchiectasis. Occasionally, advanced cases of saccular bronchiectasis can be diagnosed by routine CXR. Open thoracotomy is usually not necessary to make the diagnosis of bronchiectasis, and a BAL is performed only if cultures are required. *(Fauci, Chapter 252)*

25. **(C)** The increased vascular permeability is the hallmark of the disease. Diagnostic criteria include acute onset, $PaO_2/FiO_2 \leq 200$ mm Hg (regardless of positive end-expiratory pressure [PEEP] level), bilateral infiltrate on frontal CXR, and pulmonary artery occlusion pressure $\leq$ 18 mm Hg (or if not measured, no evidence of left atrial hypertension). *(Fauci, Chapter 262)*

26. **(B)** Allergic bronchopulmonary aspergillosis (in asthmatics) is the most likely diagnosis in this patient. Other causes of pulmonary infiltrates and eosinophilia include parasitic reactions, drugs, idiopathic causes which includes Löeffler syndrome (benign, acute eosinophilic pneumonia), chronic eosinophilic pneumonia, hypereosinophilic syndrome, and Churg–Strauss allergic granulomatosis. *(Fauci, Chapter 249)*

27. **(B)** Yearly influenza vaccination is indicated for patients with COPD. Evidence for pneumococcal vaccination is not definitive but some advocate giving it as well. There is no role for vaccination with *H influenzae B* or meningococcus in patients with COPD. Dietary support to prevent malnutrition and improve muscle

strength can be helpful. Exercise programs seem to provide subjective improvement as well. Obviously, stopping smoking is crucial. *(Fauci, Chapter 254)*

28. **(C)** Acute mediastinitis is a rare complication of upper endoscopy. It can also result from trauma to the trachea or esophagus, or dissection of the retroperitoneum. Clinical presentation may include substernal chest pain, subcutaneous emphysema, and Hamman signs, a crunching or clicking noise synchronous with the heartbeat. *(Fauci, Chapter 257)*

29. **(B)** Hypoxemia while receiving 100% oxygen indicates right-to-left shunt. Shunts permit circulation of blood that never passes through the ventilated lung. Shunting can occur within the lung (atelectasis, vascular abnormalities) or outside the lung (congenital cardiac malformations). The hypoxemia of ventilation–perfusion mismatch is more easily correctable by 100% oxygen. *(Fauci, Chapter 246)*

30. **(C)** Bony deformities of the chest can lead to respiratory failure with raised PCO_2, as well as recurrent pulmonary infection. Most patients develop a restrictive lung disease pattern with decreased compliance, reduced TLC and VC. In addition, because of the reduced compliance, the resting position of the lung changes such that FRC is reduced. Finally, the net effect is an increase in the work of breathing. The pattern on pulmonary function testing is usually that of a restrictive pattern. *(Fauci, Chapter 246)*

31. **(A)** In COPD the FEV1 and VC are reduced, but the FEV1 is reduced more because of high airway resistance resulting in a decreased FEV1/FVC ratio. The hallmark of COPD is airway obstruction (FEV1/FVC <70%) that is not reversible with salbutamol. In predominant emphysema, diffusing capacity is more profoundly decreased than in predominant bronchitis. *(Fauci, Chapter 254)*

32. **(E)** All forms of asbestos fiber have been associated with lung disease. Restrictive, not obstructive, disease is characteristic. Lung cancer, either

squamous cell or adenocarcinoma, is the most common malignancy and the risk is greatly increased by smoking. Benign pleural effusions can occur in both symptomatic and asymptomatic individuals. Reports of mesothelioma 30–35 years after brief exposure to asbestos emphasize the importance of a complete occupational/environmental history. *(Fauci, Chapter 250)*

33. **(A)** PE is an important postoperative complication, which requires urgent treatment. This man is hemodynamically stable and treatment consists of anticoagulation to prevent another PE or propagation of the clot. Thrombolytics are not indicated unless there is severe hemodynamic compromise, and especially in him since he has had recent surgery. The efficacy of IV heparin and LMWH is the same, and can be used with caution in the postoperative setting if there is no ongoing bleeding from the operative site. IVC filter would only be indicated if the patient could not be anticoagulated for some absolute contraindication. The thrust of management is therefore prevention. *(Fauci, Chapter 256)*

34. **(B)** The description of a middle-aged man with daytime sleepiness, obesity, hypertension, and snoring suggests obstructive sleep apnea. Although nasal continuous positive airway pressure is effective treatment, simple oxygen therapy is not. Stopping sedative medications and avoiding alcohol improves symptoms. Restless sleep and sudden death have been described as part of the syndrome and surgery (uvulopalatopharyngoplasty or tracheostomy) has been used in severe cases. A wide variety of symptoms can occur, but neuropsychiatric and behavioral manifestations secondary to sleep disturbance are the most common. *(Fauci, Chapter 259)*

35. **(B)** Continuous oxygen supplementation improves symptoms, prolongs life and decreasing hospitalizations in COPD patients with hypoxemia. In prolonged air travel, even those with Po_2 in the mid 70s should be considered for oxygen therapy. A Po_2 below 55 mm Hg is an indication for oxygen therapy, but between 55 and 60 mm Hg, associated evidence of right heart dysfunction should also be present before therapy is commenced. *(Fauci, Chapter 254)*

36. **(C)** In asbestosis, there is moderate pleural thickening, with scalloped margins from apex to base. There is a similar finding in the mediastinal and diaphragmatic pleura. Furthermore, there is a plaque of pleural calcification in the base. The association of asbestosis with mesothelioma has long been known. As the neoplasm progresses, it may envelop the thorax. *(Fauci, Chapter 250)*

37. **(A)** The diagnosis is pneumonia. There is consolidation of the left lower lobe. The increased density, presence of air bronchogram, and the silhouetting of the left diaphragm point to a parenchymal lesion. Pneumococcal infection, as in this patient, is still the most common etiology, although other bacterial infections such as *Klebsiella*, *Streptococcus*, or, *Staphylococcus* is often encountered. Viral and arthropod-borne diseases are also seen. *(Fauci, Chapter 251)*

38. **(B)** There is a calcified nodule in the left apex, due to prior tuberculous infection. This may be from reactivation of tuberculosis, where its preference for the apicoposterior segment is well known, or it is also possible that it may be a calcified Ghon lesion from primary infection. Bronchogenic carcinoma and pulmonary metastasis are less likely given that the patient is completely well without any constitutional symptoms. A hamartoma of the lung can present as a solitary pulmonary nodule but it is not calcified. *(Fauci, Chapter 85)*

39. **(C)** The next most appropriate test would be a better definition of the lung findings with a high-resolution CT scan. The other more invasive investigations may be more appropriate after the CT. Primary pulmonary Langerhans cell histiocytosis (PLCH), also called eosinophilic granuloma of the lung, pulmonary Langerhans cell granulomatosis, and pulmonary histiocytosis X, is an uncommon interstitial lung disease that primarily affects young adults. There is a coarse, reticular pattern in the

whole lung, somewhat more prominent in the upper lobes, suggesting a honeycomb appearance. It is the density here that is abnormal and not the lucency. *(Fauci, Chapter 255)*

40. **(A)** The reduced FEV1/FVC ratio confirms that the patient has air-flow obstruction, and the increased RV and TLC are characteristic of "gas trapping" that occurs in patients with COPD. Finally, the decreased DCO suggests destruction of lung tissue as seen in emphysema. In chronic bronchitis the DCO is usually normal. *(Fauci, Chapter 254)*

41. **(C)** The most appropriate next test would be a lung CT to demonstrate a lesion responsible for the hemoptysis. The other tests are invasive and/or not appropriate for identifying the source of bleeding. *(Fauci, Chapter 34)*

42. **(A)** Most lung abscesses and all anaerobic abscesses involve the normal flora of the oropharynx. Septic embolic usually contain *S aureus*. Factors that predispose to Gram-negative colonization of the oropharynx include hospitalization, debility, severe underlying diseases, alcoholism, diabetes, and advanced age. Impaired consciousness, neurologic disease, swallowing disorders, and nasogastric or endotracheal tubes all increase the likelihood of aspiration. *(Fauci, Chapter 252)*

43. **(A)** A negative D-dimer level rules out thromboembolic disease in patients with intermediate or low pretest probability for DVT/PE. When done by the enzyme-linked immunosorbent assay (ELISA) technique, it is relatively sensitive (ie, a negative result helps rule out DVT or PE). When done by the latex agglutination method (qualitative assay), it is neither specific nor sensitive enough to guide therapy. *(Fauci, Chapter 256)*

44. **(D)** Sarcoidosis is the most likely diagnosis. Granulomatous inflammatory changes of sarcoidosis may occur in almost any organ. About 90% of patients with sarcoid will have an abnormal CXR at some point. *(Fauci, Chapter 322)*

45. **(A)** Bronchiectasis is defined as a permanent abnormal dilatation of large bronchi due to destruction of the wall. It is a consequence of inflammation, usually an infection. Other causes include toxins or immune response. Persistent cough and purulent sputum production are the hallmark symptoms. *(Fauci, Chapter 252)*

46. **(D)**

47. **(B)**

48. **(A)**

49. **(C)**

50. **(E)** Careful physical examination can be very useful in diagnosing many common pulmonary disorders. Atelectasis and large pleural effusions both can present with decreased fremitus, dullness or flatness to percussion, and absent breath sounds. In atelectasis, tracheal shift, if present, is toward the affected side, and the opposite for a large pleural effusion. Asthma's most typical manifestations are prolonged expiration and diffuse wheezing. However, impaired expansion, decreased fremitus, hyperresonance, and low diaphragms can also be found. A complete pneumothorax results in absent fremitus, hyperresonance or tympany, and absent breath sounds. Lobar pneumonia is characterized by consolidation with increased fremitus, dullness, and auscultatory findings of bronchial breathing, bronchophony, pectoriloquy, and crackles. *(Fauci, Chapter 245)*

51. **(A)** Hypercalcemia may be due to metastatic destruction of bone, ectopic formation of parathyroid hormone, or formation of other osteolytic substances. *(Fauci, Chapter 85)*

52. **(D)** Combination chemotherapy has produced promising results in lung cancer, particularly of the small cell anaplastic type. Alkylating agents and anthracyclines are active among other agents. *(Fauci, Chapter 85)*

53. **(A, or B, or C, or E are correct)** Early stage non-small cell lung cancer can be cured by surgery. However, 70% present with disseminated disease. *(Fauci, Chapter 85)*

54. **(D)** The most commonly encountered syndromes are SIADH, Cushing syndrome, and gynecomastia. *(Fauci, Chapter 85)*

55. **(A)** Pancoast syndrome (or superior sulcus syndrome) is found in apical lung tumors, usually epidermoid. Shoulder pain secondary to involvement of the eighth cervical and first and second thoracic nerves is characteristic. Horner syndrome frequently coexists. *(Fauci, Chapter 85)*

CHAPTER 13

Clinical Pharmacology
Questions

DIRECTIONS (Questions 1 through 42): For each of the questions in this section select the one lettered answer that is the best response in each case.

1. A 72-year-old man presents to the clinic for routine follow up of his hypertension. He has essential hypertension for the past 22 years and is currently prescribed ramipril 10 mg once a day. Over the past 2 visits his blood pressure has been elevated above targets and at today's visit it is 155/94 in both arms (after resting in a quiet room for 15 minutes). He confirms adherence to his medications and salt restriction. You decide to prescribe hydrochlorothiazide in addition to the ramipril for his hypertension. **Which of the following is the most likely symptomatic side effect?**

   (A) increased serum potassium
   (B) metabolic acidosis
   (C) sexual impotence
   (D) respiratory alkalosis
   (E) hypernatremia

2. A 73-year-old man presents to the clinic complaining of "heartburn" after meals. The symptoms are not brought on by exertion, and there are no characteristics suggestive of angina. On physical examination, the heart sounds are normal, the lungs are clear, and the abdomen is soft with no masses or hepatomegaly. His ECG is normal and a clinical diagnosis of gastroesophageal reflux is made. To help relieve his symptoms he is prescribed a trial of ranitidine. **Which of the following is the most likely effect of this medication?**

   (A) stimulates acid secretion
   (B) acts on H1 receptors
   (C) acts on the columnar epithelium of the esophagus
   (D) increases bicarbonate production
   (E) decreases basal acid secretion

3. A 58-year-old man with a lung lesion develops hyponatremia (Na 127 mEq/L). He appears euvolemic clinically and the urine electrolytes reveal a high Na (>20 mmol/L) and high osmolality. **Which of the following is the most likely mechanism for the low serum sodium?**

   (A) increased permeability of the proximal renal tubule to water
   (B) increased permeability of the distal renal tubule to water
   (C) decreased glomerular filtration rate
   (D) increased sodium excretion
   (E) active reabsorption of water from the loop of Henle

4. A 38-year-old woman presents to the clinic with new symptoms of palpitations, weight loss, and heat intolerance. On physical examination, she has a mild tremor of her out stretched hands, an enlarged thyroid, and resting tachycardia (heart rate 110/min). Biochemical tests confirm the diagnosis and she is started on methimazole. **Which of the following is the most likely mechanism of this drug?**

   (A) inhibition of iodine uptake
   (B) inhibition of thyroidal organic binding and coupling reactions
   (C) lowering serum calcium
   (D) adrenal suppression
   (E) the same mechanism as perchlorate

5. A 69-year-old man presents to the clinic for follow-up assessment of his hypertension. His blood pressure is poorly controlled on hydrochlorothiazide and metoprolol. Compliance with medications and salt restriction is reviewed with the patient and he is also prescribed long acting nifedipine for optimal control of his blood pressure. **Which of the following is the mechanism of action for this medication?**

(A) beta-adrenergic stimulation
(B) interfering with calcium flux
(C) inhibition of angiotensin 1
(D) alpha-adrenergic blockade
(E) direct smooth muscle relaxation

6. A 48-year-old man presents to the emergency room complaining of fever, cough, and purulent sputum production. His chest x-ray (CXR) reveals a right middle lobe infiltrate and he is started on intravenous (IV) antibiotics after sputum and blood cultures are obtained. The following day his sputum cultures grow *Streptococcus pneumoniae*, which is sensitive to penicillin. He is better now so you step him down to oral treatment with amoxicillin rather than penicillin. **Which of the following is the most likely reason why oral amoxicillin is preferred over penicillin?**

(A) penicillin is not effective orally
(B) amoxicillin is not inactivated by penicillinase
(C) amoxicillin is better absorbed orally
(D) amoxicillin is not effective against coliform organisms and therefore has a narrower spectrum
(E) amoxicillin is not allergenic

7. A 69-year-old man is in the hospital recovering from a hemicolectomy for colon cancer. On post-op day 4 his creatinine is noted to be elevated and he is diagnosed with acute kidney injury due to hypovolemia and poor renal perfusion. **Which of the following drugs requires a major adjustment in dosage?**

(A) levofloxacin
(B) ceftriaxone

(C) amphotericin B
(D) clindamycin
(E) ampicillin

8. **Which of the following are mechanisms of action for thiocyanate and perchlorate?**

(A) inhibit thyroglobulin release
(B) increase basal metabolic rate (BMR)
(C) inhibit iodide transport
(D) inhibit thyroid organic binding
(E) increase thyroxin synthesis

9. A 63-year-old woman with hypertension is seen in follow-up. Her blood pressure is still elevated above target on hydrochlorothiazide. You discuss with her the addition of a second agent and reinforce the importance of lifestyle management. She is started on a beta-blocker. **Which of the following conditions require caution in prescribing this medication?**

(A) migraine headaches
(B) hypertrophic cardiomyopathy (HOCM)
(C) Marfan syndrome
(D) atrioventricular (AV) node dysfunction
(E) intermittent claudication

10. A 69-year-old woman, on routine lab testing, is noted to have a macrocytic anemia with hypersegmented neutrophils. Further history reveals that she has poor dietary habits and suffers from chronic alcoholism. **Which of the following is the most appropriate diagnostic test?**

(A) red blood cell folate level
(B) plasma folate levels
(C) bone marrow
(D) Schilling test
(E) therapeutic trial

11. A 69-year-old man is given a multivitamin containing vitamin B_{12}. He feels well, reports no symptoms, and his physical examination is normal. His CBC is completely normal. **Which of the following is most characteristic of vitamin B_{12} absorption?**

(A) totally dependent on the intrinsic factor

(B) best in the duodenum

(C) improved in folic acid deficiency

(D) best in the distal ileum

(E) prevented by antiparietal cell antibodies

12. A 19-year-old man is brought to the emergency room by his friends because he has taken an overdose of lysergic acid diethylamide (LSD). **Which of the following clinical findings would most likely be seen in this individual?**

(A) pupillary dilatation

(B) pupillary constriction

(C) bradycardia

(D) blindness

(E) deafness

13. A 15-year-old boy presents to the clinic for evaluation of facial acne. Prior treatment attempts with topical therapy have not worked. He is prescribed tetracycline to help clear up the acne. **Which of the following is the most common side effect of tetracycline?**

(A) neutropenia

(B) allergic reactions

(C) hepatitis

(D) gastrointestinal (GI) symptoms

(E) polyuria

14. A 79-year-old man is taking quinidine for paroxysmal atrial fibrillation. He has now developed thrombocytopenia. **Which of the following is the most likely mechanism for this syndrome?**

(A) it is due to bone marrow suppression

(B) it is due to sequestration in the spleen

(C) it is due to intravascular destruction of platelets

(D) it is immunologically mediated

(E) there is cross-reactivity with penicillin

15. A 28-year-old woman with bipolar disorder is taking lithium to control her symptoms. A test of her lithium level reveals a value of 2.3 mEq/L (normal range 0.6–1.25 mEq/L). **Which of the following side effects is most likely to occur?**

(A) mania

(B) depression

(C) tremor

(D) hyponatremia

(E) leukopenia

16. A 69-year-old man with coronary artery disease is experiencing symptoms of angina on exertion. While awaiting further investigations he is prescribed nitroglycerin to help treat the symptoms. **Which of the following is the most likely effect of this medication?**

(A) constricting the coronary arteries

(B) increasing cardiac venous return

(C) increasing cardiac output

(D) constricting peripheral veins and capillaries

(E) decreasing cardiac work

17. A 74-year-old man reports having multiple gouty attacks of his left big toe. He is symptom free currently and is prescribed allopurinol for gout prophylaxis. **Which of the following is the most likely mechanism of action for this medication?**

(A) increasing uric acid production

(B) blocking excretion of uric acid by renal tubular mechanism

(C) inhibiting xanthine oxidase

(D) diminishing inflammation of acute gouty arthritis

(E) stabilizing lysozymes

18. A 29-year-old pregnant woman presents to the clinic complaining of unilateral right leg swelling. She is in the third trimester of an otherwise uncomplicated pregnancy. An ultrasound of the right leg reveals a deep vein thrombosis (DVT) in the leg. **Which of the following statements regarding heparin therapy is correct?**

    (A) is active by mouth
    (B) affects hepatic synthesis of factors
    (C) is monitored by prothrombin time (PT)
    (D) is contraindicated in pregnancy
    (E) may be neutralized by protamine

19. A 19-year-old college student reports smoking cannabis on a social basis. **Which of the following clinical findings is most likely to be seen an hour after inhalation?**

    (A) a decrease in heart rate
    (B) an increase in intraocular pressure
    (C) prolonged reaction time
    (D) peripheral vasoconstriction
    (E) an increase in intelligence quotient (IQ)

20. An 83-year-old woman with chronic heart failure (HF), due to grade IV left ventricular function (ejection fraction <20%), is seen in the clinic for routine follow-up. She takes 80 mg/day of furosemide as part of her treatment, in addition to ramipril and carvedilol. **Which of the following metabolic abnormalities is most likely to be seen while she is taking these medications?**

    (A) metabolic acidosis
    (B) respiratory alkalosis
    (C) metabolic alkalosis
    (D) hyperkalemia
    (E) hypernatremia

21. Three teenaged high school students at the local school develop meningitis. A classmate of theirs is concerned and comes to the clinic for assessment and treatment. **Which of the following is the most appropriate next step in management?**

    (A) penicillin
    (B) sulfonamides

    (C) only reassurance and observation
    (D) rifampin
    (E) doxycycline

22. A 68-year-old woman presents to the clinic with symptoms and signs of CHF. **Which of the following is a contraindication to use furosemide?**

    (A) has hypoalbuminemia
    (B) is oliguric
    (C) has acidosis
    (D) had a rash with trimethoprim-sulfamethoxazole
    (E) is on anticoagulants

23. A 43-year-old woman with breast cancer is being treated with doxorubicin. **Which of the following is a limitation to therapy with doxorubicin?**

    (A) neurologic toxicity
    (B) severe nausea
    (C) cystitis
    (D) neutropenia
    (E) heart failure

24. A 23-year-old homeless man is found to have consumed alcohol adulterated with methanol. He is started on treatment effective for minimizing the toxicity to methanol. **Which of the following is the most likely explanation for the benefit of this treatment?**

    (A) enhances renal excretion of methanol
    (B) prevents biotransformation of methanol
    (C) combines to form a nontoxic polymer
    (D) changes the toxin's volume of distribution
    (E) sedates the patient, thus preventing neurologic damage from methanol

25. A 69-year-old man with heart failure and paroxysmal atrial fibrillation is prescribed amiodarone for maintenance of sinus rhythm. **Which of the following is a known characteristic of amiodarone?**

    (A) excellent oral absorption
    (B) a short half-life

(C) an active metabolite

(D) few drug interactions

(E) a small volume of distribution

26. A 33-year-woman is found unresponsive in her apartment and brought to the emergency room. Her toxin screen is positive for barbiturates and alcohol. **Which of the following features of barbiturate-induced coma is most likely correct?**

(A) requires at least 20–30 times the full sedative dose

(B) is increasing in frequency

(C) is characterized by an initial period of hyperventilation

(D) causes death by depression of the cardiovascular system

(E) causes death by pulmonary complications

27. **Which of the following is a stimulus for insulin secretion?**

(A) hypoxia

(B) hypothermia

(C) severe burns

(D) beta2-adrenergic receptor antagonists

(E) ketones

28. **Which of the following is the most deleterious effect of epinephrine infusion on cardiac function?**

(A) increased heart rate

(B) increased stroke volume

(C) increased cardiac output

(D) arrhythmias

(E) increased coronary blood flow

29. **Which of the following is the most striking difference in the cardiac actions of epinephrine and norepinephrine?**

(A) heart rate

(B) stroke volume

(C) cardiac output

(D) arrhythmias

(E) coronary blood flow

30. **Which of the following statements concerning the relative effects of epinephrine and norepinephrine infusion on peripheral circulation is correct?**

(A) both drugs increase total peripheral resistance

(B) neither drug increases total peripheral resistance

(C) neither drug increases renal blood flow

(D) both drugs increase cutaneous blood flow

(E) both drugs increase muscle blood flow

31. **Which of the following statements concerning the use of isoproterenol and dobutamine for shock is correct?**

(A) isoproterenol is preferred because of its short half-life

(B) neither drug will potentiate cardiac ischemia

(C) dobutamine has a more prominent inotropic effect than chronotropic effect compared with isoproterenol

(D) neither drug affects smooth muscle

(E) isoproterenol raises blood pressure more than dobutamine

32. **Which of the following is the most likely reason why beta2-selective adrenergic agonists are preferred to nonselective beta-adrenergic agonists in the treatment of asthma?**

(A) relax bronchial smooth muscle, and thus decrease airway resistance

(B) improve mucociliary function

(C) suppress the release of leukotrienes and histamine from mast cells in lung

(D) decrease microvascular permeability

(E) have fewer side effects

33. Which of the following statements concerning innate tolerance to alcohol is correct?

(A) it develops over many years of even moderate drinking

(B) high levels of innate tolerance protect against the development of alcoholism

(C) this is likely a result of polygenic inheritance

(D) pharmacokinetic factors are not involved

(E) it is not a factor in the development of alcoholism

34. Which of the following is the most likely reason for pharmacokinetic tolerance?

(A) changes in absorption

(B) changes in distribution

(C) changes specific to that drug

(D) changes in metabolism

(E) renal adaptation

35. Which of the following is an example of learned tolerance?

(A) avoiding alcohol when feeling unsteady

(B) drinking alcohol only with food

(C) walking a straight line when intoxicated

(D) not driving when drunk

(E) using vitamins to prevent alcohol damage

36. Which of the following best describes sensitization to a drug?

(A) an allergic response

(B) a purely behavioral effect

(C) a shift to the right of a dose response curve

(D) reverse tolerance

(E) a response to an acute binge

37. The administration of which of the following drugs is most likely to result in sensitization?

(A) heroin

(B) cocaine

(C) tobacco

(D) alcohol

(E) diazepam

38. Which of the following drugs is most likely to result in addiction among those who have ever used it?

(A) alcohol

(B) tobacco

(C) cocaine

(D) heroin

(E) cannabis

39. Which of the following is a symptom of withdrawal from prolonged moderate dose benzodiazepine usage?

(A) delirium

(B) somnolence

(C) seizures

(D) decreased hearing

(E) anxiety and agitation

40. Which of the following features concerning heroin withdrawal is correct?

(A) it is frequently life-threatening

(B) it starts about 24 hours after the last dose

(C) pupillary constriction is present

(D) irritability and restlessness

(E) blood pressure is lowered

41. Which of the following opioid analgesics is most likely to cause central nervous system (CNS) disturbance?

(A) heroin

(B) morphine

(C) meperidine

(D) fentanyl

(E) codeine

42. Which of the following is the most likely reason why fentanyl does not disturb cardiovascular stability as much as morphine?

(A) is water soluble

(B) is lipid soluble

(C) does not stimulate histamine release

(D) is long acting

(E) is not as potent as morphine

DIRECTIONS (Questions 43 through 65): The following group of numbered items is preceded by a list of lettered options. For each question, select the one lettered option that is most closely associated with it. Each lettered option may be used once, multiple times, or not at all.

Questions 43 through 47: For each patient with an acid-peptic disorder, select the mechanism of action of the prescribed medication.

(A) neutralizes gastric acid

(B) works by binding to cysteine

(C) inhibits gastrin release

(D) irreversible H1-receptor blockade

(E) synthetic analogue of prostaglandin E1

(F) reversibly competes with histamine for binding to the H2 receptor on parietal cells

(G) prevents hydrolysis of mucosal proteins by pepsin

(H) can enhance gastric secretion

(I) inhibition of the gastric H/K, adenosine triphosphatase (ATPase) pump

43. A 27-year-old woman occasionally uses calcium carbonate (Tums) for "heartburn" symptoms after a large meal.

44. A 56-year-old man has intermittent symptoms of burning-type epigastric discomfort. The symptoms are not related to exertion and a recent cardiac evaluation is normal. He is felt to have gastroesophageal reflux disease (GERD) and is prescribed ranitidine for symptom relief.

45. A 76-year-old woman with urosepsis becomes hypotensive and needs admission to the intensive care unit (ICU) for inotropic medications, mechanical ventilation, and monitoring. She is prescribed sucralfate for the prophylaxis of gastric stress ulcers.

46. A 46-year-old man with rheumatoid arthritis (RA) takes naproxen (nonsteroidal anti-inflammatory drug [NSAID]) for the treatment of his joints inflammation and discomfort. He is prescribed

misoprostol for NSAID-induced gastric ulcer prophylaxis.

47. A 43-year-old man presents with presyncope and a history of very dark black stools starting 2 days ago. He also reports having nonspecific abdominal discomfort for the past month. Upper endoscopy reveals a duodenal ulcer, and biopsies are positive for *Helicobacter pylori*. He is prescribed omeprazole as part of "triple therapy" for the eradication of *H pylori*.

Questions 48 through 52: For each patient with a toxic ingestion or exposure, select the most likely clinical effect.

(A) combines with cytochromes and catalase to block hydrogen and electron transport, thus producing tissue asphyxia

(B) methemoglobinemia

(C) vertigo, hyperventilation, tinnitus, and deafness

(D) bone-marrow depression

(E) acute hepatic insufficiency

(F) severe renal injury

48. A 43-year-old man works in a factory where industrial solvents are frequently used to clean the equipment.

49. A 75-year-old woman with rheumatoid arthritis (RA) takes aspirin for symptom control. She usually adjusts the dose of her own medications depending on how she is feeling.

50. A young child ingests silver polish by accident. The local poison control center states that cyanide is a common ingredient of silver polish.

51. A troubled youth has a long history of gasoline sniffing.

52. A 45-year-old man with chronic alcoholism ingests antifreeze.

Questions 53 through 56: For each patient with an arrhythmia, select the most appropriate treatment.

(A) digitalis

(B) verapamil

(C) diltiazem

(D) beta-blockers

(E) adenosine

(F) quinidine

(G) flecainide

(H) propafenone

(I) nonsynchronized electric defibrillation

(J) sotalol

(K) procainamide

(L) disopyramide

(M) amiodarone

53. A 37-year-old woman presents with palpitations and light-headedness. She has a history of palpitations and previously was told that she has "Wolff–Parkinson–White" (WPW) syndrome. Her blood pressure is 110/80 mm Hg and pulse 150 beats/min. Her lungs are clear and heart sounds are normal. The electrocardiogram (ECG) reveals a regular wide complex tachycardia at 150 beats/min and no P waves are visible.

54. A 67-year-old man is brought to the hospital because of a witnessed syncopal event. His past medical history is significant for depression and he is taking amitriptyline. The past few days he has felt unwell from the "flu" and has been vomiting. His potassium is 2.4 mEq/L. While in the emergency room, he has another syncopal event and the monitor records polymorphic VT with increased QT interval (torsades de pointes).

55. A 64-year-old man presents with increased shortness of breath. He has a past history of chronic obstructive pulmonary disease (COPD) and recently developed increased cough and sputum production but no fever or chills. He appears in mild respiratory distress, respirations are 26/min, pulse 120 beats/min, blood pressure 145/84 mm Hg, and oxygen saturation 90%. He has bilateral expiratory wheezes.

His ECG reveals multifocal atrial tachycardia (MAT) (discrete P waves with at least three different morphologies).

56. A 23-year-old woman presents with palpitations to the emergency room. The symptoms have been going on for 1 hour. There is no prior history of cardiac disease or family history of arrhythmias or sudden cardiac death. Her pulse is 170 beats/min, blood pressure 115/80 mm Hg, and respirations 16/min. The lungs are clear and heart sounds are normal. The ECG reveals a narrow complex regular tachycardia at 170/min, and no P waves are visible.

Questions 57 through 60: Match the chemotherapeutic agent with the disease it is most often used in.

(A) Hodgkin disease

(B) acute lymphocytic leukemia

(C) multiple myeloma

(D) chronic lymphocytic leukemia

(E) chronic granulocytic leukemia

(F) malignant melanoma

(G) colon cancer

(H) hairy cell leukemia

(I) prostate cancer

(J) Kaposi sarcoma

57. Melphalan.

58. Methotrexate.

59. Bleomycin.

60. Flutamide.

Questions 61 and 62: For each patient on a specific medication, select the most likely side effects to occur.

(A) sensory loss

(B) prolonged QT interval

(C) Parkinsonism-like symptoms

(D) action tremor

(E) insomnia

61. A 74-year-old woman with Alzheimer disease is treated with haloperidol.

62. A 69-year-old woman being treated for dysrhythmias with quinidine

Questions 63 through 65: For each patient with a clinical symptom, select the most appropriate medication.

    (A) albuterol
    (B) ethanol
    (C) amitriptyline
    (D) NSAIDs
    (E) propranolol

63. A 29-year-old woman presents with increasing shortness of breath and coughing. She had asthma as a child but has not required any treatment for the past 10 years. On examination, she has expiratory wheezes. Which of the above may cause bronchodilation?

64. A 69-year-old man suffers from heartburn. Lately he has been experiencing more severe symptoms than usual including waking up at night with epigastric discomfort. His clinical examination is normal. Which of the above may increase gastric secretion?

65. A 79-year-old woman complains of dry mouth. She reports no other symptoms and cannot recall the medications she is currently taking. Which of the above may be a factor?

Answers and Explanations

1. **(C)** The most common symptomatic side effect in men is impotence, and it should be specifically looked for. The most serious complications relate to fluid and electrolyte imbalance and include hyponatremia, hypokalemia, volume contraction, and metabolic alkalosis. *(Brunton, p. 849)*

2. **(E)** Ranitidine is an H2-blocker that reversibly competes with histamine for binding to H2 receptors on gastric parietal cells. Its effect is to decrease basal acid secretion, but it also has a significant effect on stimulated (eg, food, hypoglycemia, vagal stimulation) acid production. The other items listed are not effects of ranitidine. *(Brunton, p. 971)*

3. **(B)** The mediator of hyponatremia is likely antidiuretic hormone (ADH). Although controlling water permeability is the main function under ADH control, there is some evidence that ADH influences sodium transport in the cortical collecting duct. ADH can also act as a neurotransmitter. Autonomic effects of ADH in the CNS include bradycardia, increase in respiratory rate, suppression of fever, and alteration of sleep patterns. *(Brunton, pp. 778–779)*

4. **(B)** Methimazole is an effective treatment for hyperthyroidism. Methimazole interferes with thyroid function mainly by inhibition of thyroidal organic binding and coupling reactions. In contrast to other agents such as perchlorate, the action of thioamides is not prevented by large doses of iodide. *(Brunton, pp. 1527–1528)*

5. **(B)** Nifedipine is a synthetic agent that is a potent systemic vasodilator for the treatment of hypertension. At doses used clinically, nifedipine does not block transmission through the AV node. The vasodilatation can result in a reflex increase in heart rate. It has no effects on alpha or beta-receptors, and it does not inhibit angiotensin 1. *(Brunton, pp. 832–834)*

6. **(C)** Polar side chains added to penicillin molecules made these compounds acid stable, and therefore have improved oral absorption as compared to penicillin V. Intake of food prior to ingestion of ampicillin will decrease absorption. In cases of severe renal impairment, the dose should be adjusted downward. Penicillinase-producing organisms will inactivate amoxicillin, and penicillin is an effective oral agent but the oral bioavailability of amoxicillin is better and therefore usually chosen over penicillin. *(Brunton, p. 1139)*

7. **(A)** Most of the fluoroquinolones are renally excreted, and therefore require dose adjustment in renal failure. Exceptions are moxifloxacin and pefloxacin, which are metabolized by the liver. The other antibiotics do not require any adjustment for renal failure. Ampicillin needs to be adjusted only with severe renal failure. *(Brunton, p. 1121)*

8. **(C)** Because of their toxicity, neither drug is widely used in treatment, but both are effective in inhibiting iodide transport. They work by preventing the thyroid gland from concentrating iodide. Thiocyanate is produced following enzymatic hydrolysis of certain plant glycosides (eg, cabbage), and may be a contributing factor to endemic goiter in certain parts of the world where iodide intake is low. *(Brunton, pp. 1530–1531)*

9. **(D)** If pre-existing AV conduction defects are present (either by disease or use of other drugs), significant and symptomatic bradyarrhythmias can occur when beta-blocker are prescribed. Beta-blockers are frequently used in the treatment of hypertrophic cardiomyopathy and for migraine prophylaxis and might prevent aortic dilatation in Marfan syndrome. It rarely can cause clinical problems in patients with claudication (the unopposed alpha effect can cause vasoconstriction and worsening symptoms) *(Brunton, pp. 287–288)*

10. **(A)** Folate deficiency can be secondary to small bowel disease, alcoholism, inadequate intake, disease states with high cell turnover (hemolytic anemia), drugs (methotrexate), and pregnancy. The concentration of folate in plasma changes rapidly with changes in food intake, so the diagnosis of anemia secondary to folate deficiency is made more reliable by measuring red blood cell folate. A Schilling test is used to establish the cause of vitamin B_{12} deficiency, and a bone-marrow test is not indicated until B_{12} and folate deficiencies have been ruled out as the cause of the macrocytic anemia. *(Brunton, p. 1460)*

11. **(D)** Vitamin B_{12} absorption is best in the distal ileum. Receptors for the intrinsic factor are present in the distal ileum, but mass action absorption also occurs with large doses. However, the oral route is still felt to be unreliable if hematologic or neurologic effects are present. The Schilling test, with and without intrinsic factor, can help diagnose the exact cause of B_{12} deficiency. *(Brunton, pp. 1454–1455)*

12. **(A)** Sympathomimetic effects such as pupillary dilatation, piloerection, hyperthermia, and tachycardia are common in an overdosage of LSD. Other symptoms include dizziness, weakness, drowsiness, nausea, and paresthesias. The hallucinogenic effects can last for hours and are mainly visual. *(Brunton, pp. 624–625)*

13. **(D)** GI symptoms are the major side effects of tetracycline. Stomatitis, glossitis, and diarrhea are seen and may be related to superinfections. Hepatic toxicity has been reported but is rare except in massive doses or during pregnancy. Tetracyclines can cause discoloration of teeth in children and in fetuses of mothers given the drug during pregnancy. *(Brunton, p. 1178)*

14. **(D)** Thrombocytopenia usually occurs after weeks or months of therapy. It is due to formation of drug-platelet complexes that evoke a circulating antibody. Thrombocytopenia and bleeding can be severe but resolve rapidly on discontinuing the drug. The antibody is long-lasting, and reintroduction of quinidine, even in a small dose, can rapidly cause thrombocytopenia. Other hypersensitivity reactions to quinidine include hepatitis, bone-marrow suppression, and a lupus syndrome. The most common side effects of quinidine are gastrointestinal and include nausea, vomiting, and diarrhea. *(Brunton, pp. 928–929)*

15. **(C)** Lithium is used primarily for bipolar affective disorder, either to treat mania or prevent recurrences of the bipolar disorder. It has also been used in severe unipolar depression. Acute intoxication can result in vomiting, diarrhea, tremor, ataxia, coma, and convulsions. Leukocytosis is also a side effect of lithium therapy. Polyuria and polydipsia secondary to acquired nephrogenic diabetes insipidus is a common side effect and results in hypernatremia. Both acute and chronic intoxication can be lethal. The toxic and therapeutic levels of lithium are very close, and patients on lithium require close medical observation, including measurement of serum lithium levels. *(Brunton, pp. 487–488)*

16. **(E)** The benefit of nitroglycerin is probably due to diminution in cardiac output and work of the heart. Nitroglycerin generally dilates most veins and arteries, and this result in both a decreased preload and a decreased afterload for the heart. This leads to decreased myocardial oxygen requirements. Although coronary artery dilation also occurs, it is probably not as important in relieving anginal pain. *(Brunton, pp. 827–828)*

17. **(C)** Allopurinol effectively blocks uric acid production by inhibiting xanthine oxidase.

Allopurinol is indicated in patients with a history of uric acid calculi of the urinary tract. In addition, it is often used in patients with malignancy (eg, leukemia, lymphoma), particularly when chemotherapy or radiation therapy is being used. *(Brunton, pp. 708–709)*

18. **(E)** Heparin can be neutralized by the administration of protamine. Heparin must be given parenterally (usually intravenously or subcutaneously) to be active, and its activity is monitored by the partial thromboplastin time (PTT), not the PT. It is safer than oral anticoagulants in pregnancy and does not deplete clotting factors as its mode of action. Rather, it potentiates the effect of antithrombin III on the clotting cascade. When low-molecular-weight heparin is used, it has a more predictable pharmacokinetic profile which allows for a weight-adjusted dosage without laboratory follow up. *(Brunton, pp. 1471–1474)*

19. **(C)** All the possible therapeutic effects of cannabis are accompanied by psychoactive effects, which include impaired cognition and perception, prolonged reaction time, and impaired memory and learning. The most common therapeutic use of cannabis is as an antiemetic during cancer chemotherapy. It might have some analgesic and anticonvulsant properties. Its ability to lower intraocular pressure has not been therapeutically useful in glaucoma. *(Brunton, pp. 622–623)*

20. **(C)** In addition to dehydration, metabolic alkalosis, and hypokalemia result from the use of furosemide. Loop diuretics such as furosemide act primarily to inhibit electrolyte reabsorption in the thick ascending limb of the loop of Henle. The degree of diuresis is greater than in other classes of diuretics. Despite being on the ACE-inhibitor (ramipril), hypokalemia still occurs in patients with HF taking this medication combination. *(Brunton, pp. 752–753)*

21. **(D)** This is likely an outbreak of meningitis secondary to *Neisseria meningitidis*. The first line of drugs used for treatment of acute disease includes ceftriaxone. For prophylaxis, rifampin is the preferred agent. The other options are not used for the prophylaxis of *N meningitidis* *(Brunton, pp. 1208–1209)*

22. **(D)** Furosemide is related to sulfonamide, and severe allergic reactions can occur. Furosemide is effective despite gross electrolyte disturbances or hypoalbuminemia. Excretion of large volumes of bicarbonate-poor urine leads to alkalosis, so an acidosis is not a contradiction in severe fluid and electrolyte depletion; a trial in oliguric states is often appropriate. *(Brunton, pp. 752–753)*

23. **(E)** Cardiomyopathy is characteristic of these drugs and is characterized by arrhythmias and cumulative dose-related HF. Anthracyclines include daunorubicin and doxorubicin. The major site of metabolism is the liver, and the mechanism of action includes inhibition of deoxyribonucleic acid (DNA)-dependent ribonucleic acid (RNA) metabolism. *(Brunton, pp. 1358–1359)*

24. **(B)** Ethanol is the standard antidote for methanol. It inhibits the conversion of methanol to its toxic metabolite, formic acid, by alcohol dehydrogenase. *(Brunton, pp. 592–593, 599–600)*

25. **(C)** With prolonged treatment, the active *N*-desethyl derivative of amiodarone accumulates in plasma, and its concentration may exceed that of the parent compound. Amiodarone is poorly (approximately 30%) absorbed and there is marked interindividual variability. The half-life is long, 25–60 days, presumably because it is extensively bound to tissues, resulting in a large volume of distribution and a reservoir of drug. Complicating the use of amiodarone is multiple drug interactions and toxicities including liver, thyroid, and lung. *(Brunton, pp. 920–921)*

26. **(E)** Most deaths from barbiturate-induced coma are caused by pulmonary complications (atelectasis, edema, bronchopneumonia) or renal failure. Hypoventilation is characteristic, and only 10 times the full reactive dose can cause severe poisoning. This low toxic-therapeutic ratio is one reason why barbiturate use (hence barbiturate coma) is declining. *(Brunton, pp. 414–420)*

27. **(E)** Ketones, glucose amino acids, and fatty acids promote insulin secretion. Stimulation of alpha2-adrenergic receptors inhibits insulin secretion, whereas beta2-adrenergic receptor stimulation enhances release of insulin. As a result, beta2-adrenergic receptor antagonists decrease insulin levels. Activation of the autonomic nervous system (hypoxia, hypothermia, severe burns, surgery) will also suppress insulin secretion. *(Brunton, pp. 1615–1616)*

28. **(D)** All the changes listed are correct, but the increased automaticity of the heart with the development of ventricular premature beats (or more serious ventricular arrhythmias) is the most prominent change. *(Brunton, pp. 243–245)*

29. **(C)** Epinephrine results in a more rapid heart rate and more powerful systolic contraction resulting in increased cardiac output. Norepinephrine results in an unchanged or even decreased cardiac output. *(Brunton, pp. 244–248)*

30. **(C)** Both epinephrine and norepinephrine decrease renal blood flow. Epinephrine decreases total peripheral resistance whereas norepinephrine increases total peripheral resistance. Both drugs decrease cutaneous blood flow and only epinephrine increases muscle blood flow. *(Brunton, p. 244)*

31. **(C)** The preferential effect of dobutamine on contractility makes it useful in low cardiac output states. Both drugs are very short-acting, can potentiate cardiac ischemia, and affect smooth muscle. Unlike isoproterenol, dobutamine frequently increases blood pressure quite significantly, thus requiring dosage adjustment. *(Brunton, pp. 250–251)*

32. **(E)** Most of the side effects from the use of beta-adrenergic agonists in asthma come from stimulation of the beta1-receptors in the heart. Thus, beta$_2$-selective agonists, which act primarily in the lung, are safer to use. Both selective and nonselective beta-agonists will decrease airway resistance. This is their major therapeutic effect. The effects on mucociliary transit, mast cells, and microvascular permeability occur with both nonselective and selective agonists, but the clinical importance of these effects is unclear. *(Brunton, pp. 251–253)*

33. **(C)** It is felt that innate tolerance is a polygenic characteristic. Frequently, variation in pharmacokinetic variables (absorption, metabolism, excretion), which can be inherited, are the cause of different levels of innate tolerance. Those who have high levels of innate tolerance are more likely to become addicted to alcohol. There is a higher concordance rate for alcoholism among identical twins than fraternal twins, but it is not 100%. *(Brunton, pp. 601–602)*

34. **(D)** The most common cause of pharmacokinetic tolerance is an increase in the metabolism of the drug. Since these same enzymes can then metabolize other drugs, this kind of tolerance is not necessarily specific to the drug that induced it. *(Brunton, pp. 609–611)*

35. **(C)** Learned tolerance refers to the reduction of the effect of a drug due to compensatory mechanisms that are learned. An example is walking a straight line despite the motor impairment caused by alcohol. This likely represents both acquisition of motor skills and the learned awareness of one's deficit; thus the person walks more carefully. *(Brunton, p. 610)*

36. **(D)** Sensitization is the reverse of tolerance. It refers to an increase in effect of the drug with repetition of the same dose. It does not occur during an acute binge. The dose response curve would be shifted to the left. *(Brunton, p. 611)*

37. **(B)** Cocaine and amphetamines are the drugs most likely to cause sensitization. It is poorly studied in humans, but it is thought that stimulant psychosis results from sensitization after prolonged use. *(Brunton, p. 611)*

38. **(B)** Almost one-third of people who have tried tobacco become addicted. In comparison, about 15% become addicted to alcohol. Heroin is also highly addictive (23% of users become addicted), but since so few people even try heroin, the addiction rate in society as a whole is quite low (0.4%). *(Brunton, pp. 608–609)*

39. **(E)** Muscle cramps, anxiety, insomnia, and dizziness are among the common side effects of withdrawal from moderate dose usage. Withdrawal seizures and delirium occur usually in withdrawal from high dosage. Withdrawal should be done gradually, often over many months. *(Brunton, pp. 614–615)*

40. **(D)** Craving for opioids, restlessness, irritability, and anxiety are common symptoms of heroin withdrawal. Piloerection, pupillary dilatation, sweating, tachycardia, and blood pressure elevation are frequently seen signs of heroin withdrawal. It starts within 6–12 hours of the last dose and is quite unpleasant, but not life-threatening. *(Brunton, pp. 618–619)*

41. **(C)** Meperidine has a half-life of 3 hours, but it has an active metabolite, normeperidine, which has a half-life of 15–20 hours. Therefore, accumulation of normeperidine with toxicity is common. The drug should not be used for prolonged periods (over 48 hours), and probably should not be used at all in those susceptible to delirium (eg, the elderly). *(Brunton, p. 570)*

42. **(C)** Morphine releases histamine and can cause cardiovascular instability. Fentanyl does not release histamine, and causes only mild decreases in heart rate and blood pressure. Fentanyl, a lipid-soluble drug, has an elimination half-life between 3 and 4 hours. It is 100 times more potent than morphine. *(Brunton, p. 571)*

43. **(A)** Although doctors seldom prescribe antacids because of the availability of superior medications, patients still use them extensively. As well as neutralizing acid, calcium carbonate enhances secretion in the stomach. The release of CO_2 from bicarbonate can result in belching, nausea, and abdominal distension. Belching can exacerbate gastroesophageal reflex. *(Brunton, pp. 974–975)*

44. **(F)** Ranitidine inhibits acid production by reversibly competing with histamine for binding to H2 receptors on parietal cells. Ranitidine's most prominent effect is on basal acid secretion, but it still significantly suppresses stimulated (feeding, gastrin, etc.) acid production. *(Brunton, pp. 971–972)*

45. **(G)** After the mucosa is damaged by acid, further damage is caused by pepsin-mediated hydrolysis of mucosal proteins. Sucralfate, in an acid environment, forms a sticky protective gel over epithelial tissues and ulcer craters to prevent further damage by pepsin. This viscous layer can inhibit absorption of many drugs, so patients should wait for at least 2 hours after taking other medications before taking sucralfate. *(Brunton, pp. 973–974)*

46. **(E)** Prostaglandins have two effects on gastric mucosa: they inhibit acid secretion by binding to the EP3 receptor on parietal cells, and they have a cytoprotective effect by stimulating mucin and bicarbonate secretion and local mucosal blood flow. Misoprostol is a synthetic prostaglandin analogue, and has both an acid suppression and cytoprotective effect. *(Brunton, p. 973)*

47. **(I)** Omeprazole is a potent suppressor of acid secretion by the parietal cell. It inhibits the H, K-ATPase pump (proton pump) and reduces daily basal and stimulated acid secretion by 80%–95%. Proton pump blockers are part of the regimen for the eradication of *H pylori*. *(Brunton, pp. 969–970)*

48. **(E)** In chronically poisoned patients, neurologic symptoms and evidence of liver damage may develop. Many industrial solvents are chlorinated hydrocarbons and have been implicated in several deaths. Carbon tetrachloride was once used widely for medical purposes and as a cleaning agent. It has been replaced by safer alternatives. Hepatotoxicity of these compounds is exacerbated by concurrent ethanol ingestion. In lethal cases, death is usually due to deep narcosis, aspiration of vomitus, or cardiac arrhythmias. *(Brunton, pp. 625–626)*

49. **(C)** Salicylates are associated with vertigo, hyperventilation, tinnitus, and deafness. Excretion of salicylates is renal, and in the presence of normal renal function, about 50% will be excreted in 24 hours. Severe toxicity can

cause severe acid-base abnormalities. It can be difficult to diagnose when the toxicity is secondary to a therapeutic regimen. *(Brunton, pp. 691–692)*

50. **(A)** Cyanide is contained in silver polish, insecticides, rodenticides, and some plants. Inhalation of hydrogen cyanide may cause death within a minute; oral doses act more slowly, requiring several minutes to hours. Cyanide combines with cytochromes and catalase to produce tissue asphyxia. The treatment for cyanide poisoning includes the administration of IV sodium thiosulfate, which hastens the transformation of the cyanide to thiocyanate, which is excreted in the urine. *(Brunton, p. 885)*

51. **(D)** Benzene is associated with bone-marrow depression. Benzene is present to some extent in most gasolines, and poisoning may result from ingestion or vapors. Acute benzene poisoning can cause severe CNS symptoms such as blurred vision, tremors, shallow and rapid respiration, ventricular irregularities, paralysis, and loss of consciousness. *(Brunton, pp. 625–626)*

52. **(F)** Ethylene glycol is widely used as antifreeze. It causes CNS depression and renal toxicity characterized by oxalate crystals in the tubules. As in methanol poisoning, ethanol is used as a competitive substance for alcohol dehydrogenase to decrease the rate of formation of toxic metabolites. *(Brunton, pp. 599–600)*

53. **(K)** Digitalis and verapamil decrease the refractoriness of the accessory pathways in Wolff–Parkinson–White syndrome (WPW) and the ventricular rate can exceed 300/min. This can be life-threatening and is treated with IV procainamide or cardioversion. *(Fauci, Chapter 226)*

54. **(I)** Numerous cardiac and noncardiac medications can cause torsades de pointes. Although it has been described with amiodarone, this is quite rare. The arrhythmia can result in sudden death. Unstable forms of this arrhythmia are treated with cardioversion. *(Fauci, Chapter 226)*

55. **(B)** MAT usually occurs in the setting of advanced lung disease. Treatment involves withdrawing theophylline and improving lung function. There may be some role for treatment with verapamil. *(Fauci, Chapter 226)*

56. **(E)** Adenosine is the agent of first choice for the termination of AV nodal or AV reentrant tachycardias that are not terminated by vagal maneuvers such as carotid sinus massage. IV beta-blockers and calcium channel blockers are second choice. Digitalis IV acts too slowly and is not recommended for this type of arrhythmia. *(Fauci, Chapter 226)*

57. **(C)** Melphalan is an alkylating agent of the nitrogen mustard type. Although not curative therapy, it is particularly useful in the management of multiple myeloma, breast cancer, and ovarian cancer. *(Brunton, p. 1328)*

58. **(B)** Methotrexate is classified as an antimetabolite, and is a folic acid analogue. It is used in the treatment of acute lymphocytic leukemia. Other tumors where methotrexate has an effect include osteogenic sarcoma, mycosis fungoides, and lung cancer. *(Brunton, pp. 1338–1339)*

59. **(A)** Bleomycin, a naturally occurring antibiotic, is useful in Hodgkin disease, non-Hodgkin lymphoma, and cancers of the testes, head and neck, skin, esophagus, lungs, and genitourinary tract. *(Brunton, pp. 1361–1362)*

60. **(I)** Flutamide is an antiandrogen that is useful in prostate cancer. Leuprolide, a gonadotropin-releasing hormone analogue, and various estrogen compounds are the other hormonal-type agents used in prostate cancer therapy. *(Brunton, p. 1388)*

61. **(C)** Parkinsonism-like symptoms can occur with haloperidol (phenothiazine) use and disappear when it is withdrawn. Dystonic movements involving the mouth, tongue, and shoulder girdle are also a side effect of phenothiazines. As well as having useful antipsychotic effects, phenothiazines are useful as antiemetics and antinausea agents. They can also potentiate the effects of sedatives, analgesics,

and general anesthetics. Some phenothiazines are intrinsically sedating, but none of them commonly interfere with sleep. *(Brunton, pp. 477–480)*

62. **(B)** The slowed repolarization can result in a prolonged QT interval. Life-threatening polymorphic ventricular tachycardias (torsades de pointes) can be provoked by quinidine. It is rarely used in modern practice. The increased refractory period accounts for the effect on tachycardia. Similar effects are seen with procainamide. *(Brunton, pp. 928–929)*

63. **(A)** Ephedrine, isoproterenol, and albuterol are beta-adrenergic agonists and cause bronchodilatation. Ipratropium bromide also results in bronchodilatation by its anticholinergic effect.

In susceptible individuals, the beta2-adrenergic blocking effect of propranolol can cause life-threatening bronchoconstriction. The other medications listed have no effect on bronchial airways. *(Brunton, pp. 195, 719–720)*

64. **(B)** Alcohol may increase secretion by stimulating gastrin and histamine release. Caffeine and other methylxanthines can also stimulate acid production. Vagal cholinergic stimulation is a major stimulus for gastric secretion. *(Brunton, pp. 727–728)*

65. **(C)** Xerostomia (dry mouth) can result from the anticholinergic side effects of taking amitriptyline. The other medications on the list are not usually known to cause a dry mouth. *(Brunton, pp. 446–447)*

CHAPTER 14

Comprehensive Practice Exam
Questions

DIRECTIONS (Questions 1 through 95): For each of the questions in this section select the one lettered answer that is the best response in each case.

1. A 28-year-old man presents to the clinic for evaluation of painful urination and cloudy-color penile discharge. The symptoms started 2 days ago and are not associated with any other symptoms. His past medical history is not significant and he is not on any medications.

   His physical examination is completely normal except for a purulent discharge that can be expressed from his penis. A swab of the fluid reveals Gram-negative diplococci within neutrophils. **Which of the following is the most appropriate treatment?**

   (A) intramuscular ceftriaxone plus oral doxycycline
   (B) oral penicillin G
   (C) intramuscular penicillin V
   (D) intramuscular ampicillin and oral penicillin V
   (E) intravenous (IV) tobramycin

2. An 84-year-old woman is presenting for the first time to your practice for an annual visit and assessment. Her past medical history is significant for Type 2 diabetes, hypertension, and dyslipidemia. Her medications include aspirin, metformin, ramipril, and atorvastatin.

   On physical examination the pertinent findings are a blood pressure of 156/86 mm Hg, and a heart rate 88/min. The cardiac exam is normal except for an S4 and 1+ pedal edema, the lungs are clear, and her screening neurologic assessment is normal. **Which of the following is a better characteristic feature of geriatric patients compared to younger patients?**

   (A) medical problems are less complex
   (B) they spend less money on housing
   (C) homeostenosis is impaired
   (D) hepatic enzyme deterioration is a result of aging
   (E) senile dementia is a result of aging

3. A 72-year-old man is brought to the clinic by his daughter because she is concerned about his memory. A careful history, mini mental status, and physical examination confirm your suspicions of the patient having Alzheimer disease. **Which of the following investigations is included in the initial work up for reversible causes of dementia?**

   (A) electroencephalogram (EEG)
   (B) urine tests for heavy metals
   (C) thyroid function tests
   (D) red blood cell (RBC) folate
   (E) urinary and plasma amino acids

4. A 74-year-old woman presents to the emergency department complaining of palpitations. The symptoms started suddenly 2 hours ago and are not associated with any shortness of breath or chest discomfort. Her past medical history is only significant for hypertension and prior hysterectomy for uterine fibroids.

On physical examination, the blood pressure is 122/83 mm Hg, and the heart rate is 118 beat/min with an irregular rhythm. The cardiac exam reveals a JVP at 3 cm, irregular S1 and normal S2 with no S3 or murmurs. The lungs are clear on auscultation and the remaining exam is normal. Her ECG shows atrial fibrillation with a ventricular rate of 120 beats/min. Her thyroid-stimulating hormone (TSH) level is very low. **Which of the following cardiac findings might also be seen in this condition?**

(A) aortic regurgitation
(B) hypotension
(C) soft S_1
(D) systolic murmurs
(E) soft S_2

5. A 74-year-old woman presents to the clinic for evaluation of increasing back pain and malaise. The symptoms are insidious in onset and she reports no history of recent trauma to the back. Her past medical history is significant for hypertension and breast cancer which was diagnosed 7 years ago and treated with surgery and adjuvant therapy.

On physical examination, the pertinent findings are percussion tenderness over the lower spine. An x-ray of the lumbar spine reveals lytic lesions compatible with metastatic bone disease, and her serum calcium level is elevated. **Which of the following mediators is least likely to be involved?**

(A) interleukin-6 (IL-6)
(B) ectopic parathyroid hormone (PTH)
(C) tumor necrosis factor (TNF)
(D) interleukin-1 (IL-1)
(E) prostaglandins

6. A 30-year-old woman develops acute onset of erythema nodosum, fever, malaise, and anorexia. The chest x-ray (CXR) reveals bilateral hilar lymphadenopathy and a left paratracheal lymph node. **Which of the following is the most likely diagnosis?**

(A) acquired immune deficiency syndrome (AIDS)
(B) rheumatic fever
(C) sarcoidosis
(D) tuberculosis
(E) bronchogenic carcinoma

7. **Which of the following imaging techniques is best able to measure regional brain substrate uptake and metabolic kinetics?**

(A) magnetic resonance imaging (MRI)
(B) computed tomography (CT)
(C) positron emission tomography (PET)
(D) serial thallium scintigrams
(E) Doppler ultrasound

8. A 47-year-old man presents to the emergency room with symptoms of fever, chills, and lightheadedness. He was previously well until the day of presentation and has no significant past medical history.

On examination he appears unwell, the blood pressure is 87/66 mm Hg, and sitting brings on a lightheaded feeling. The heart rate is 110 beats/min, temperature 38.5°C, and O2 saturation 96% on room air. The only pertinent finding is a generalized erythematous macular rash over his torso and lower limbs. He is started on empiric antibiotics and given intravenous fluids to support his blood pressure. Over the next day, he develops gangrene on his left leg and requires transfer to the intensive care unit. **Which of the following is the most likely organism?**

(A) *Corynebacterium diphtheriae*
(B) *Streptococcus* group C
(C) *Neisseria gonorrhoeae*
(D) *Streptococcus* group A
(E) *Salmonella enteritidis*

9. A 56-year-old woman presents to the hospital because of symptoms of dyspnea, blurry vision, and headaches. The symptoms started that morning and are getting worse. Her past medical history is significant for hypertension and osteoarthritis. She stopped taking her anti-hypertensive medications 3 months ago because of side effects.

On examination, her blood pressure is 210/130 mm Hg, heart rate 100 beats/min, and oxygen saturation 95%. Her fundi reveal retinal hemorrhages and papilledema. The heart sounds are normal expect for an S4, and the lungs have lower lobe crackles. **Which of the following is the most appropriate agent to reduce her blood pressure?**

(A) IV hydralazine
(B) IV labetalol
(C) oral methyldopa
(D) IV nitroprusside
(E) sublingual nifedipine

10. A 56-year-old man complains of increased thirst and increased urinary volume and frequency. He has also noticed new symptoms of constipation and generalized aches and pains. He has no significant past medical problems and his physical examination is normal.

Initial investigations consist of a normal complete blood count (CBC) fasting blood glucose and urinalysis. His sodium, urea, and creatinine are normal, but calcium is 12.4 mg/dL (8.4–10.2 mg/dL). Further testing reveals an elevated PTH level. **Which of the following is the most likely mechanism for the polyuria in this condition?**

(A) direct effect of PTH on the kidney
(B) hypercalcemia-induced renal tubular acidosis (RTA)
(C) hypercalcemia-induced chronic renal failure
(D) hypercalcemia-induced defect in renal concentrating ability (nephrogenic diabetes insipidus)
(E) hypercalcemia-induced defect in renal glucose handling

11. A 13-year-old boy is brought to the clinic by his mother because she has noticed periods when he seems to be unresponsive, associated with blinking of his eyes. These episodes are momentary, and he seems normal thereafter. His past health history is unremarkable and the physical examination is completely normal. **Which of the following is the most effective treatment?**

(A) phenytoin
(B) carbamazepine
(C) phenobarbital
(D) gabapentin
(E) ethosuximide

12. A 76-year-old man is seen in clinic for assessment of persistent lymph node enlargement. He is otherwise feeling well, and has no fever, weight loss or night sweats. On physical examination, there is generalized lymphadenopathy in his right axilla and cervical lymph node chains. The nodes are 1–2 cm in size, nontender, and mobile. The remaining examination is normal. **Which of the following lymphoid malignancies is invariably of B-cell origin?**

(A) chronic lymphocytic leukemia (CLL)
(B) hairy cell leukemia
(C) Burkitt lymphoma
(D) mycosis fungoides
(E) angioimmunoblastic lymphadenopathy

13. A 28-year-old woman with human immunodeficiency virus (HIV) infection has progressed to developing AIDS. She contracted the virus from sharing needles while doing intravenous drugs. Since being diagnosed with HIV she has declined antiviral therapy and does not have regular medical follow-up. **Which of the following conditions is considered an AIDS-defining illness?**

(A) antibodies to HIV
(B) palpable lymphadenopathy
(C) Kaposi sarcoma
(D) oral candidiasis (thrush)
(E) herpes zoster (shingles)

14. A 22-year-old woman is evaluated for symptoms of chronic diarrhea, weight loss, and abdominal pain. The diarrhea is nonbloody, watery, and unformed stools 4–5 times a day. Her appetite and caloric intake are normal and she in not trying to lose weight. There is no prior history of bowel trouble, her past medical history is negative and she is not taking any medications. She reports no travel history or sick contacts and her family history is negative for bowel disorders.

On physical examination, her weight is 53 kg, and her abdomen is soft and nontender with normal bowel sounds. The remaining examination is normal. Stool cultures for infectious agents are negative. She undergoes a colonoscopy and biopsy which is diagnostic. **Which of the following is more characteristic of ulcerative colitis when compared to Crohn disease?**

(A) segmental involvement

(B) granulomas

(C) lymph node involvement

(D) rectal bleeding

(E) palpable abdominal mass

15. A 28-year-old pregnant woman (34 weeks) presents to the emergency department with symptoms of sudden onset dyspnea and tachycardia. There is no associated chest discomfort, cough, fever, or sputum production. A few days prior to presentation, she noticed unilateral swelling in her left leg, which she attributed to the pregnancy. The pregnancy was uncomplicated up to this point, and her only medication is a multivitamin. She has no prior history of cardiac or respiratory diseases.

On physical examination, the blood pressure is 104/76 mm Hg, heart rate 110/min, respiratory rate 20/min, and O2 saturation of 99% on room air. The JVP is 6 cm, heart sounds are normal with a 2/6 systolic ejection murmur over the left sternal border, the lungs are clear to auscultation and there is swelling in the left calf greater than the right calf. **Which of the following is the most likely diagnosis?**

(A) primary pulmonary hypertension

(B) pulmonary embolism

(C) myocardial infarction

(D) paroxysmal supraventricular tachycardia (PSVT)

(E) lobar pneumonia

16. A 60-year-old homeless man is brought to the emergency because of new symptoms of falling down, confusion, and double vision. He is only able to provide a limited history, and contact with a social worker at a nearby shelter confirms these are new symptoms for him. His past medical history is significant for chronic alcoholism with previous admissions for treatment of alcohol withdrawal. The patient reports heavy alcohol consumption for the past month.

On physical examination, he appears disheveled with multiple bruises, and the vital signs are normal. Pertinent findings are an enlarged (16 cm) and tender liver, with no palpable spleen or clinical evidence of ascites. The extraocular movements are abnormal and reproduce his double vision (bilateral sixth nerve palsy), motor strength in all limbs is normal, and reflexes are symmetric and 2+. His gait is wide based and ataxic. **Which of the following is the most appropriate treatment?**

(A) thiamine

(B) lecithin

(C) vitamin D

(D) phenytoin

(E) diazepam

17. A 58-year-old woman with metastatic breast cancer presents to the emergency room complaining of increased thirst, back pain, and frequent urination. Her physical examination is normal except for clinical signs of volume depletion. Initial laboratory investigations reveal a calcium level of 13.4 mg/dL.

She is given intravenous normal saline to replace the volume deficit and treatment with calcitonin is considered. **Which of the following is most characteristic of calcitonin?**

(A) it increases bone resorption

(B) it decreases renal calcium clearance

(C) it is produced by hepatocytes

(D) it raises blood phosphate

(E) it binds to osteoclasts

18. A 15-year-old boy presents to the clinic feeling unwell 2 weeks after a severe sore throat. He complains of pain and swelling in his elbows and knees, and the onset of a new rash on his chest and abdomen. Prior to this he was otherwise well.

    On physical examination, the vital signs are normal, and cardiac auscultation reveals a new holosystolic murmur over the apex radiating to the axilla. There is a maculo-papular rash over his chest and abdomen that is nontender on palpation. The elbows, knees, and wrists are tender on joint palpation and movement. **Which of the following might also be seen on further examination?**

    (A) chronic arthritis
    (B) involvement of spinal joints
    (C) subcutaneous nodules
    (D) erythema nodosum
    (E) meningeal irritation

19. A 38-year-old woman is seen in follow up for on-going symptoms of dyspnea and fatigue. She has developed a dilated cardiomyopathy after an episode of viral myocarditis 3 months ago, and despite appropriate medications for the treatment of heart failure she continues to have NYHA Class 4 symptoms. In the past month, she has had 2 admissions to hospital for decompensated heart failure. Her cardiologist is considering a referral to a heart transplant program for evaluation given her on-going difficulties and poor functional status. **Which of the following is the most important factor in selecting a patient as a potential heart transplant recipient?**

    (A) absence of long-standing pulmonary hypertension
    (B) survival on mechanical assistance devices
    (C) availability of a human lymphocyte antigen (HLA)-compatible donor
    (D) age under 20 years
    (E) ventricular ejection fraction <20%

20. A 72-year-old woman has an elevated WBC count on routine testing. The manual differential of the WBC notes an increased number of mature lymphocytes. She reports no recent illnesses or infectious symptoms, and her past medical history is significant for hypertension, osteoarthritis, chronic stable angina, and dyslipidemia. She is taking appropriate medications for these conditions and has no change in symptoms or medications. Her physical examination is normal. **Which of the following features best characterizes CLL?**

    (A) usually a T-cell disorder
    (B) a disease of children
    (C) responsive to splenectomy
    (D) frequently asymptomatic
    (E) most common in Asians

21. A 69-year-old man is brought to the emergency department for new symptoms of confusion and sleep disturbance. He is not able to provide any history but his partner notes that he has cirrhosis due to chronic alcoholism. She states that he has maintained abstinence from alcohol for the past 3 months. His medications include nadolol, furosemide, spironolactone, and lactulose.

    On examination, he looks jaundiced, the blood pressure is 102/78 mm Hg supine, and 86/64 mm Hg standing with an increase in heart rate from 72 to 100 beats/min. He is afebrile and the oxygen saturation is 98% on room air. The abdomen is soft; there is a palpable spleen tip and no evidence of ascites. He is not oriented to place or time and moves all four limbs on command. A digital rectal exam reveals dark black stool. **Which of the following is the most likely cause?**

    (A) spontaneous bacterial peritonitis (SBP)
    (B) spironolactone
    (C) nadolol
    (D) gastrointestinal (GI) bleeding
    (E) stroke

22. A 27-year-old man is found to have an abnormal urinalysis on routine testing. He has no past medical history of renal disease and is completely asymptomatic. The urinalysis reveals 3+ proteinuria and hematuria, and microscopy confirms the presence of rbc casts. His blood pressure is 152/94 mm Hg, pulse 88/min, and the remaining physical examination is normal. **Which of the following is the most likely diagnosis?**

    (A) diabetes mellitus (DM)
    (B) amyloidosis
    (C) immunoglobulin A (IgA) nephropathy (Berger disease)
    (D) focal glomerulosclerosis
    (E) thalassemia minor

23. A 63-year-old man presents to the clinic for reassessment of on-going symptoms of dyspnea on exertion. He has a 60-pack-per-year history of smoking and has been previously diagnosed as having emphysema. He now reports improvement in his dyspnea symptoms and is doing well since being prescribed tiotropium at his last visit.

    On physical examination, his blood pressure is 136/88 mm Hg, pulse 76/min, respiratory rate 14/min, and oxygen saturation 96% on room air. His cardiac exam is normal and there is normal air entry into the lungs and no expiratory wheezes. **Which of the following features is most characteristic of this diagnosis?**

    (A) mild dyspnea
    (B) copious purulent sputum
    (C) hematocrit over 55%
    (D) severe pulmonary hypertension at rest
    (E) decreasing diffusing capacity

24. A 26-year-old man with a recent diagnosis of rheumatoid arthritis (RA) presents to the clinic complaining of muscle weakness in his hands. He is taking prednisone 20 mg/day and methotrexate 10 mg once a week for the treatment of his RA. On examination, he has multiple active joints in his hands and wrists. Strength in the hand muscles and wrist flexors and extensors is reduced (graded 4 out of 5). Strength in his legs is normal. **Which of the following features is characteristic of muscle weakness in RA?**

    (A) occurring after several months of pain and immobility
    (B) showing a neutrophilic infiltrate on muscle biopsy
    (C) secondary to vasculitis
    (D) showing heavy mononuclear cell infiltrate on muscle biopsy
    (E) showing type II fiber atrophy and muscle fiber necrosis on muscle biopsy

25. An 18-year-old woman has a low hemoglobin value of 10.5 g/dL on routine CBC testing. The red cells are microcytic, but the WBC and platelet counts are normal. She has an adequate intake of iron-containing foods, her menstrual flow is normal, and there is no other history of blood loss. Her physical examination is completely normal, and iron studies reveal a normal ferritin level. She states that other members in her family have also been told they are anemic and given a diagnosis of alpha-thalassemia. **Formation of which of the following hemoglobins is increased in alpha-thalassemia?**

    (A) H
    (B) A
    (C) F
    (D) A2
    (E) C

26. A 67-year old-woman presents to the clinic for evaluation of numbness in her feet. The symptoms started gradually and are more noticeable now. There is no weakness in her feet or difficulty walking. Her past medical history is significant for Type 2 diabetes for the past 10 years and she currently takes metformin and glyburide. Physical examination confirms sensory loss in the feet to touch and vibration. **Which of the following is most characteristic of diabetic neuropathy?**

    (A) it is usually bilateral
    (B) pain is not a feature
    (C) it most commonly affects the brain

(D) it spares the autonomic system

(E) it does not improve with meticulous control of blood glucose

27. A 57-year-old man, previously asymptomatic and on no medications, develops a painful left big toe. There is no history of trauma to the toe. It is so painful that even the weight of the bed sheets on the toe is excruciating. On examination, there is a swollen red toe, with limited range of motion. There are no other active joints. **Which of the following medications is relatively contraindicated?**

(A) indomethacin

(B) colchicine

(C) ibuprofen

(D) allopurinol

(E) naproxen

28. A 73-year-old woman is brought to the hospital with new symptoms of right-sided weakness and difficulty talking. The symptoms started 12 hours ago and have gradually become worse over the course of the day. She reports no headache, nausea, vomiting, or fever/chills. Her past medical history is significant for hypertension and dyslipidemia.

The pertinent findings on examination are right face, arm and leg weakness, as well as sensory loss on the right side. She also has difficulty naming simple objects like a pen or glass, and her speech is incomprehensible. She is admitted to the hospital with a clinical diagnosis of right-sided hemiparesis and expressive aphasia. A CT scan of the brain reveals a stroke in the right middle cerebral artery territory. **Which of the following is the most common cause of ischemic stroke?**

(A) cerebral hemorrhage

(B) cerebral embolism

(C) arteritis

(D) dissecting aneurysm

(E) hemorrhage into atherosclerosis

29. A 20-year-old man presents to the hospital with new symptoms of blood in his urine. There is no associated abdominal pain, back pain, or dysuria. He also notes new swelling in his feet and around his eyes. Prior to the onset of these symptoms he was well with no prior health history.

On physical examination, his blood pressure is 146/88 mm Hg, pulse 68/min, and respiratory rate 12/min. There is periorbital and pedal edema, the JVP is at 3 cm, heart sounds are normal with no murmurs or rubs, and the lungs are clear on auscultation. The remaining examination is normal. **Which of the following is the most likely diagnosis?**

(A) nephrotic syndrome

(B) multiple myeloma

(C) diabetic nephropathy

(D) nephrolithiasis

(E) acute glomerulonephritis

30. A 36-year-old man is evaluated for persistent abdominal symptoms starting over 3 months ago. He has tried a 1-month trial of omeprazole with limited improvement in his symptoms. A diagnostic upper endoscopy reveals a duodenal ulcer with no active bleeding. **Which of the following is the most common symptom of duodenal ulcer?**

(A) epigastric pain

(B) nausea

(C) melena

(D) anorexia

(E) midback pain

31. An elderly patient is receiving a blood transfusion for anemia due to myelodysplastic syndrome (MDS). He was diagnosed with MDS 2 years ago and over the past 6 months has required blood transfusions every 6 weeks for symptomatic anemia. His past medical history also includes hypertension, Type 2 diabetes, and coronary artery disease. Half way through the transfusion of the second unit of packed red blood cells he develops tachypnea, lumbar pain, tachycardia, and nausea. **Which of the following is the most likely explanation?**

    (A) anxiety
    (B) fluid overload
    (C) hemolysis
    (D) pulmonary embolism
    (E) acute leukemia

32. A 23-year-old pregnant woman (14 weeks' gestation) presents to the clinic complaining of excessive sweating and palpitations. She also notes minimal weight gain in the past 3 weeks, feeling tremulous at times and loose frequent bowel movements. Up until now her pregnancy has been uncomplicated, and she has no prior health issues.

    On examination she appears flushed, her blood pressure is 94/62 mm Hg, pulse 110/min, and there is a fine tremor in her outstretched fingers. Her thyroid is diffusely enlarged and nontender on palpation. Biochemical tests reveal a low TSH, and elevated T4 (thyroxine) level. **Which of the following treatments is contraindicated?**

    (A) thyroid surgery
    (B) propylthiouracil (PTU)
    (C) drugs that cross the placenta
    (D) radioactive iodine
    (E) glucocorticoids

33. A 78-year-old woman is brought to the clinic by her daughter because she is concerned about her mother's mood. The patient's husband of 48 years passed away 6 months ago after a lengthy illness due to metastatic colon cancer. Since then she reports having a poor appetite, decreased interest in activities, and frequent

thoughts about dying. She is started on nortriptyline to help improve her mood and functional status. **Which of the following is the most common side effect of nortriptyline?**

    (A) impaired cardiac contractility
    (B) heart block
    (C) weight loss
    (D) anticholinergic side effects
    (E) diarrhea

34. A 23-year-old woman is found to have a systolic murmur during routine clinical examination. She has no prior history of heart disease or murmurs and feels fine when she is exercising at the gym. An echocardiogram reveals that she has mitral valve prolapse. **Which of the following is most characteristic of mitral valve prolapse?**

    (A) a pansystolic murmur
    (B) usually a benign course
    (C) sudden death
    (D) infective endocarditis
    (E) highest incidence in men over age 50

35. A 14-year-old boy presents to the hospital with severe leg swelling that started 2 weeks ago. He also notes feeling tired and having little energy to play sports with his friends. His past medical history is negative and he is not taking any medications.

    On examination, his blood pressure is 163/96 mm Hg, and there is pedal edema up to his knees, as well as periorbital edema. His remaining clinical exam is normal. A urinalysis is positive for 3+ proteinuria and on 24-hour urine collection the total protein excretion is 5.4 grams/day. He undergoes a renal biopsy and there are no changes seen on light microscopy, but electron microscopy shows foot process fusion and no deposits on the membranes. **Which of the following is the most likely diagnosis?**

    (A) mesangial proliferative glomerulonephritis
    (B) minimal change disease
    (C) focal glomerulosclerosis

(D) membranous glomerulonephritis

(E) Goodpasture syndrome

36. A 65-year-old man presents to the emergency room complaining of intermittent hemoptysis for the past 1 week. He describes no chest pain, fever, cough, or chronic sputum production. He smokes 1 pack of cigarettes a day and has done so for the past 35 years. There are no risk factors for DVT or PE, and he is not taking any medications.

On physical examination, his vital signs are normal, JVP is at 2 cm, heart sounds are normal, and the chest is clear on auscultation. There are no palpable lymph nodes and the remaining examination is normal. His sputum cytology is positive for malignant cells, but the CXR and CT chest are normal. **Which of the following is the next best step in management?**

(A) annual CXR

(B) unilateral pneumonectomy

(C) blind percutaneous needle biopsies

(D) bronchoscopic brushings and biopsies

(E) mediastinoscopy and biopsy

37. A 34-year-old man presents with dyspnea and increasing peripheral edema. He recently had a "flu-like" illness with intermittent sharp left-sided chest pain. On examination, his jugular venous pressure (JVP) is elevated at 8 cm, heart sounds are soft, and the blood pressure (BP) is 104/76 mm Hg with a 20 mm Hg decrease in systolic arterial pressure during slow inspiration. **Which of the following is the most likely diagnosis?**

(A) cardiac tamponade

(B) pulmonary hypertension

(C) ventricular septal defect

(D) coarctation of the aorta

(E) malignant hypertension

38. A 45-year-old man develops end-stage renal disease due to diabetic nephropathy. He undergoes a renal transplant with a kidney donated from his sister. **Which of the following immune suppression therapies are usually used to prevent rejection in renal transplant patients?**

(A) splenectomy and irradiation

(B) plasmapheresis and steroids

(C) cyclosporine and steroids

(D) azathioprine and plasmapheresis

(E) steroids and thymectomy

39. A 42-year-old woman presents to the emergency department for evaluation of new onset double vision and weakness in her right leg. There is no headache, fever, or sensory loss symptoms. About 2 years ago she had developed left eye pain and visual loss that resolved spontaneously.

On physical examination, the vital signs are normal, there is impaired right eye movement on lateral gaze, and weakness in the left leg graded 4–/5. The tone in the leg is also increased and the plantar response is up going in the left foot. A MRI of the brain shows multiple areas of demyelination in the white matter. **Which of the following is the most likely diagnosis?**

(A) cerebral emboli

(B) subclavian steal syndrome

(C) Guillain–Barré syndrome

(D) recurrent transient ischemic attacks (TIAs)

(E) multiple sclerosis

40. A 16-year-old female presents to the hospital for evaluation of abdominal pain, discomfort in multiple joints, and a skin rash. The symptoms started 2 days ago and she has no significant past medical history.

On examination, the abdomen is tender, but there is no rigidity or rebound tenderness. There are multiple palpable purpuric lesions on her skin, and there are no acute joints. Laboratory investigation reveals a normal CBC, but an abnormal urinalysis with hematuria and proteinuria. **Which of the following is the most likely diagnosis?**

(A) hemolytic-uremic syndrome

(B) thrombotic thrombocytopenic purpura

(C) heavy metal poisoning

(D) subacute bacterial endocarditis (SBE)

(E) Henoch–Schönlein purpura (HSP)

41. A 74-year-old postmenopausal woman is found to have mild hypercalcemia on routine electrolyte testing. She reports no symptoms of bone pain or hypercalcemia and otherwise feels well. Her PTH level is slightly elevated and consistent with a diagnosis of primary hyperparathyroidism. She has multiple medical comorbidities and decides against having parathyroid resection surgery. **Which of the following treatments might she benefit from?**

    (A) estrogen therapy
    (B) androgen therapy
    (C) calcium therapy
    (D) radioiodine therapy
    (E) oral bisphosphonate therapy

42. A 23-year-old man of African descent presents to the emergency room complaining of fever and chills. He recently returned from a trip to East Africa where he was visiting friends and relatives. While there he visited urban and rural areas. He did not take any prophylaxis for travel-related illnesses. A thick and thin blood film is diagnostic for the infectious agent causing his symptoms. He is started on appropriate therapy, but soon after develops anemia due to hemolysis. **Which of the following is the most likely diagnosis?**

    (A) fulminant malaria
    (B) paroxysmal nocturnal hemoglobinuria
    (C) hereditary spherocytosis
    (D) glucose-6-phosphatase dehydrogenase (G6PD) deficiency
    (E) microangiopathic hemolysis

43. A 20-year-old woman presents to the clinic for evaluation of new symptoms of cough and yellow sputum production. She also reports feeling feverish and having intermittent right-sided chest pain on deep breathing. On physical examination, she appears well and the pertinent findings are dullness on percussion in the right lower lobe and inspiratory crackles on auscultation of the lungs. A chest x-ray confirms there is a right lower lobe infiltrate. **Which of the following is the most appropriate treatment of community-acquired pneumonia?**

    (A) carbenicillin
    (B) tobramycin
    (C) levofloxacin
    (D) methicillin
    (E) tetracycline

44. A 60-year-old man presents with symptoms of polyuria and nocturia. Investigations reveal a normal fasting glucose and calcium level. His urine electrolytes suggest a renal transport defect. **Which of the following is the most likely cause for his symptoms?**

    (A) acute nephritis
    (B) acute renal failure (ARF)
    (C) renal tubular defects
    (D) nephrolithiasis
    (E) systolic hypertension

45. A 62-year-old man is experiencing severe epigastric discomfort for the past month. The symptoms are made worse with eating and there is no relationship to activity. He has no risk factors for atherosclerosis and his past medical history is negative. The physical examination is entirely normal. An ECG is normal even when the patient is experiencing symptoms and the pain is felt to be noncardiac in origin. An upper endoscopy is performed and it reveals severe erosive esophagitis and he is started on pantoprazole for treatment. **Which of the following is the mechanism of action of this therapy?**

    (A) binds to the ulcer bed
    (B) antagonizes H2 receptors
    (C) inhibits acetylcholine
    (D) stimulates mucin secretion
    (E) inhibits parietal cell proton pump

46. A 70-year-old woman, previously in good health, is found to have an asymptomatic monoclonal immunoglobulin peak on serum electrophoresis. Her physical examination is normal, as is her CBC, electrolytes, renal function and calcium level. A skeletal survey does not reveal any osteolytic lesions and a bone-marrow aspirate reveals 5% plasma cells.

Which of the following is the most likely diagnosis?

(A) monoclonal gammopathy of uncertain significance (MGUS)

(B) multiple myeloma

(C) Waldenström macroglobulinemia

(D) amyloidosis

(E) non-Hodgkin lymphoma

47.   A 30-year-old woman presents to the clinic complaining of dry mouth and eyes. The symptoms started gradually but now are becoming more bothersome. She has no significant past medical history and her only medication is the oral contraceptive pill. On physical examination, the vital signs are normal. The eyes and mouth appear normal but there is symmetric enlargement of the parotid glands. The remaining examination is normal. Testing of her serum is positive for Ro/SS-A autoantibodies. **Which of the following is the most likely diagnosis?**

(A) ankylosing spondylitis

(B) mixed connective tissue disease

(C) systemic sclerosis

(D) thrombotic thrombocytopenic purpura

(E) Sjögren syndrome

48.   A 24-year-old man is brought to the emergency room with a gun-shot wound to his chest. The emergency medical service has already given him 4 liters of normal saline via 2 large-bore IVs but his blood pressure still remains low at 74/45 mm Hg. He likely has ongoing internal bleeding as a result of his injuries and an emergency transfusion with unmatched blood is requested to stabilize his clinical status. **Which of the following is considered suitable for unmatched blood transfusion?**

(A) blood type AB

(B) polycythemic individual

(C) a sibling of the recipient

(D) blood type O

(E) Lewis A positive

49.   A 37-year-old woman presents with shortness of breath on exertion. She has a past history of rheumatic fever as a child. On cardiac auscultation, there is a loud S1 and a mid-to-late low-pitched diastolic murmur. You suspect she has mitral stenosis. **Which of the following findings is most likely to be seen on the CXR in someone with mitral stenosis?**

(A) general enlargement of the heart

(B) Kerley B lines

(C) attenuation of pulmonary arteries

(D) straightening of the left heart border

(E) diffuse modulation of the lower lung fields

50.   A 25-year-old woman presents to the clinic complaining of symptoms of fatigue and weakness. The symptoms are worse near the end of the day and she finds it difficult to continue working as a bank teller. She has no prior health issues and is not taking any medications. Her sleep patterns are unchanged and she feels refreshed in the morning.

On examination, there is diplopia and ptosis noted in the extraocular muscle with prolonged upward gaze. In addition, repetitive muscle exercises of her hands with open and close maneuvers causes hand grip weakness. The remaining neurological examination is normal. **Which of the following is the most likely diagnosis?**

(A) myasthenia gravis

(B) multiple sclerosis

(C) TIAs

(D) muscular dystrophy

(E) cerebral palsy

51. A 45-year-old-woman is seen in the clinic requesting mammography for breast cancer screening. She reports no breast lumps, skin changes, or nipple discharge. Her past medical history is only significant for 2 prior pregnancies that were uncomplicated and resulted in the birth of 2 healthy children at term. Her clinical examination is normal. **Which of the following women have the highest risk of developing breast cancer?**

    (A) cousins of breast cancer patients
    (B) those receiving CXRs as children
    (C) those with late-onset menarche
    (D) multiparous
    (E) those who have already had one breast cancer

52. A 16-year-old man is having recurrent bouts of pneumonia. After his third episode in the past 12 months, further investigations are carried out to look for a potential cause. His results indicate that he has cystic fibrosis (CF). **Which of the following is correct for patients with CF diagnosed as an adult?**

    (A) the reproductive system is not involved
    (B) heatstroke occurs
    (C) pulmonary hypertension is avoided
    (D) GI disease is mild
    (E) hypersplenism is prominent

53. A 25-year-old is seen in the clinic for assessment of an incidental finding on a CXR of a 2-cm solitary pulmonary nodule in the left lower lobe. He feels well and reports no dyspnea, chest pain, or constitutional symptoms. He does not smoke and has never had a previous CXR. The physical examination is completely normal. The nodule has a "popcorn ball"-type calcification pattern. **Which of following is the most appropriate next step in management?**

    (A) left lower lobe resection
    (B) serial CXRs
    (C) needle aspiration biopsy
    (D) left pneumonectomy
    (E) mediastinoscopy

54. A 60-year-old man presents to the emergency department with chest pain described as retrosternal chest pressure radiating to the jaw. The symptoms started at rest and coming and going, but never lasting more than 15 minutes. He has a prior history of hypertension and smokes 1 pack/day. He is currently chest-pain free and on physical examination the blood pressure is 156/88 mmHg, pulse 88/min, and O2 saturation 98%. The heart and lung examination is normal.

    His ECG shows ST-segment depression in leads V1 to V4 that is new, and the first set of cardiac enzymes is negative. He is diagnosed with unstable angina pectoris, admitted to a monitored unit, and started on low molecular weight heparin, aspirin, nitroglycerin, and beta-adrenergic blockers. He continues to have ongoing chest pain symptoms. **Which of the following is the most appropriate next step in management?**

    (A) IV streptokinase
    (B) coronary angiography
    (C) exercise testing
    (D) oral aspirin
    (E) antihypertensive therapy

55. A 34-year-old man presents to the emergency room with increasing shortness of breath. He has a past medical history of asthma that is previously well controlled but 2 weeks ago he developed a "cold" and has noticed increased coughing and shortness of breath ever since. He reports no fevers, chills, or sputum production. He is now using his salbutamol inhaler for rescue therapy 6 times a day and feels unwell. His physical examination is normal except for wheezing on expiration. A CXR is normal and he is prescribed prednisone 30 mg once a day for one week. **Which of the following is the major effect of glucocorticoids in asthma?**

    (A) anti-inflammatory
    (B) bronchodilatory
    (C) sedative
    (D) mucus dissolving
    (E) antibacterial

56. A 56-year-old man is seen in the clinic for symptoms of new onset pedal and periorbital edema. His past medical history is negative except for an appendectomy as a child. He has no associated symptoms other than discomfort related to the pedal edema. He is on no medications and the physical examination confirms pedal and periorbital edema. His cardiac exam, including JVP is normal and the lungs are clear to auscultation. A 24-hour urine collection is consistent with nephrotic range proteinuria. He undergoes a kidney biopsy, and the renal lesion is consistent with a diagnosis of focal and segmental glomerulosclerosis (FSGS). **Which of the following changes are most likely to be seen on immunofluorescence studies of the renal biopsy in FSGS?**

(A) nodular deposits of immunoglobulin M (IgM) and complement 3 (C3)
(B) linear deposits of immunoglobulin G (IgG)
(C) nothing
(D) granular deposits of IgG and complement 4 (C4)
(E) extensive fibrin strands

57. A 26-year-old woman complains of burning retrosternal chest pain, radiating to the sides of the chest that is aggravated by bending forward. **Which of the following structures is this pain most likely to arise from?**

(A) heart
(B) lumbar spine
(C) intercostal nerves
(D) pancreas
(E) esophagus

58. A 34-year-old woman presents to the clinic complaining of intermittent discomfort in her hands. She notices that in the winter months or while washing in cold water her hands turn pale and then eventually warm up and regain color. She has also noticed symptoms of dry eyes and dry mouth lately. Her physical examination is completely normal. Serologic testing for scleroderma is positive. **Which of the following is the most appropriate management for her Raynaud phenomenon?**

(A) amphetamines
(B) ergotamines
(C) beta-blocking drugs
(D) warm clothing
(E) surgical sympathectomy

59. A 9-year-old boy presents to the clinic for evaluation of easy bruising. Investigations confirm the diagnosis of hemophilia A. **Which of the following is the most common presentation of hemophilia A?**

(A) hematuria
(B) melena
(C) hemarthrosis
(D) pressure neuropathy
(E) intracerebral hemorrhage

60. Three weeks after surgery to implant a mechanical aortic valve, a 70-year-old man develops chest pain, fever, and leukocytosis. On examination, the JVP is increased, there is a mechanical S2 sound, and a pericardial friction rub. **Which of the following is the most likely diagnosis?**

(A) infection in the aortic valve
(B) postpericardiotomy syndrome
(C) cytomegalovirus (CMV) infection
(D) pulmonary embolism
(E) acute myocardial infarction

61. A 73-year-old-woman presents to the clinic complaining of fatigue and feeling unwell. She notes the symptoms are worse on exertion, but denies any chest pain or shortness of breath. Her past medical history is significant for hypertension and type 2 diabetes. Both conditions are well controlled on her current medications. On physical examination, the vital signs are—blood pressure 135/80 mm Hg, pulse 72/min, and respiratory rate 10/min. The lungs are clear on auscultation and the heart sounds are normal. A CBC reveals a hemoglobin value of 9.5 g/dL and a MCV 105 μm^3. **Which of the following typically causes a macrocytic anemia?**

    (A) vegan diet
    (B) iron deficiency
    (C) thalassemia
    (D) chronic inflammation
    (E) sideroblastic anemia

62. An 18-year-old woman develops weakness, weight gain, amenorrhea, abdominal striae, and behavioral abnormalities. Physical examination reveals lateral visual field loss. **Which of the following is the most likely diagnosis?**

    (A) a functional pituitary tumor
    (B) adrenal hyperplasia
    (C) anorexia nervosa with bulimia
    (D) glioblastoma multiforme
    (E) multiple sclerosis

63. A 64-year-old man with Type 2 diabetes has his fasting lipid profile measured. **Which of the following is the most common pattern of dyslipidemia in Type 2 diabetes?**

    (A) increased triglycerides only
    (B) increased low-density lipoprotein (LDL) only
    (C) increased high-density lipoprotein (HDL) only
    (D) decreased triglycerides and increased HDL
    (E) increased triglycerides and decreased HDL

64. A previously asymptomatic 62-year-old woman presents with sudden onset of severe midback pain. X-rays reveal an anterior compression fracture of T10. Other vertebral bodies show decreased mineral density and prominent vertical striations. **Which of the following is the most likely diagnosis?**

    (A) multiple myeloma
    (B) metastatic breast cancer
    (C) vitamin D deficiency
    (D) osteoporosis
    (E) Paget disease of bone

65. A 70-year-old man, with no evidence of heart disease, develops transient right arm and leg weakness, which resolves within 1 hour. CT scan of the brain is normal and carotid ultrasound Doppler reveals 60% stenosis of left carotid artery. **Which of the following is the most appropriate treatment for this patient?**

    (A) carotid endarterectomy
    (B) aspirin
    (C) beta-blockers
    (D) nonsteroidal anti-inflammatory drugs (NSAIDs)
    (E) calcium channel antagonists

66. A 60-year-old woman being investigated for menorrhagia is found on history to have lethargy, constipation, cold intolerance, and muscle stiffness. **Which of the following is the most likely diagnosis?**

    (A) uterine carcinoma
    (B) systemic lupus
    (C) hypothyroidism
    (D) severe iron deficiency
    (E) hypercalcemia

67. A 20-year-old patient with asymptomatic lymphadenopathy in the right supraclavicular area is found to have nodular sclerosing Hodgkin disease on biopsy. There is no other evidence of disease on his imaging tests. **Which of the following is the most appropriate next step in management?**

(A) combination chemotherapy with MOPP (mechlorethamine, vincristine [Oncovin], procarbazine, prednisone)

(B) wide surgical excision following radiotherapy

(C) combination chemotherapy with ABVD (adriamycin [doxorubicin], bleomycin, vinblastine, dacarbazine)

(D) radiotherapy alone

(E) observation until symptoms occur

68. A 45-year-old man presents to the emergency department with weakness, fever, weight loss, and abdominal pain. On examination, he is hypertensive, the heart sounds are normal, and lungs are clear. While being investigated, he has a focal seizure. Laboratory studies show a high erythrocyte sedimentation rate (ESR), anemia, acute kidney injury, and a positive test for hepatitis B surface antigen. **Which of the following is the most likely diagnosis?**

(A) polyarteritis nodosa (PAN)

(B) acute hepatitis B

(C) SBE

(D) multiple staphylococcal abscesses

(E) chronic active hepatitis

69. Patients with AIDS can develop chorioretinitis with blindness, enteritis with intractable diarrhea, interstitial pneumonitis, and adrenalitis. **Which of the following infections is the most likely cause of these illnesses?**

(A) cryptosporidium

(B) herpes zoster

(C) *Toxoplasma*

(D) pneumocystis carinii pneumonia

(E) CMV

70. A 45-year-old man presents to the emergency department with new onset of jaundice. He has no prior history of liver or gallbladder disease. An ultrasound of the liver reveals that the cause of his jaundice is due to extra-hepatic biliary obstruction. **Which of the following is most likely correct concerning his jaundice?**

(A) negative urine bilirubin

(B) marked increase in conjugated bilirubin

(C) normal unconjugated bilirubin

(D) painless jaundice

(E) decrease in glucuronyl transferase

71. A 19-year-old man presents to the clinic because he is concerned about a pigmented skin lesion. **Which of the following characteristics suggests a dysplastic nevus (atypical mole) rather than a benign acquired nevus?**

(A) uniform tan color

(B) located on buttock

(C) 4 mm in diameter

(D) 20 similar lesions on body

(E) located on back

72. A 73-year-old man is brought to the emergency department because of decreased urine output for the past 2 days. **Which of the following urine values distinguishes prerenal azotemia from other causes of acute kidney injury?**

(A) urine osmolality <400

(B) brown granular casts

(C) urine creatinine <20

(D) a high fractional excretion of filtered sodium

(E) urine sodium of <20

73. A 27-year-old-man is brought to the emergency room because he is feeling unwell, and endorses symptoms of chest discomfort and shortness of breath. He has experienced similar symptoms in the past during times of stress, but this is the first presentation to the emergency room. His past medical history is negative and he is not taking any medications or recreational drugs.

On physical examination, he looks well, blood pressure is 157/88 mm Hg, pulse 110/min, and respiratory rate 22/min. The lungs are clear on auscultation, the heart sounds are normal, and there is no pericardial or pleural rub. His ECG, CXR, and cardiac enzymes are normal, and his symptoms are attributed to anxiety. **Which of the following blood gas results is most likely seen in a patient with hyperventilation due to anxiety?**

(A) increased PCO_2

(B) decreased PO_2

(C) decreased pH

(D) decreased PCO_2

(E) increased PO_2

74. A 57-year-old woman presents to the hospital with a 2-hour history of retrosternal chest pain and dyspnea. Her electrocardiogram (ECG) reveals an acute myocardial infarction pattern. **Which of the following ECG patterns is consistent with that interpretation?**

(A) tall P waves

(B) prominent U waves

(C) small QRS complex

(D) elevated ST segments

(E) widened QRS complex

75. A 34-year-old man is brought to the emergency room by his family because of extreme lethargy. After further questioning, he admits to taking a large number of phenobarbital tablets. **Which of the following is the most appropriate next step in management?**

(A) acidification of urine to pH 3.0

(B) repetitive administration of activated charcoal

(C) ipecac to induce vomiting

(D) hemoperfusion

(E) hemodialysis

76. A 45-year-old man was exposed to high levels of radiation after an accident at a nuclear reactor 5 years ago. **Which of the following illnesses is he at greatest risk of developing?**

(A) aplastic anemia

(B) radiation dermatitis

(C) lung cancer

(D) multiple myeloma

(E) leukemia

77. A 67-year-old-woman presents to the clinic complaining of feeling lightheaded every time she stands up. Her past medical history is significant for hypertension, gout, and increased cholesterol. She reports no symptoms of chest discomfort, shortness of breath, or palpitations. She cannot recall her medications but thinks one of them is a "water pill." Her physical examination is normal except for a postural drop in blood pressure which reproduces her symptoms. **Which of the following diuretics will continue to induce significant diuresis after return of blood volume to normal levels?**

(A) hydrochlorothiazide

(B) spironolactone

(C) triamterene

(D) furosemide

(E) metolazone

78. A 34-year-old man with HIV is taking isoniazid (INH) and rifampin for the treatment of tuberculosis. He has finished 4 months of therapy without any complications but now complains of numbness in his feet. Clinical examination confirms a symmetric peripheral neuropathy. **Which of the following statements is correct regarding the polyneuropathy that occurs in association with INH treatment?**

(A) acute

(B) demyelinating

(C) pure sensory

(D) vitamin sensitive

(E) pure motor

79. A 28-year-old-man is seen in the clinic complaining of intermittent bouts of joint discomfort involving his knees. The pain first started about 3 months ago and waxes and wanes. His past medical history is negative and he is not taking any medications. About 1 year ago he recalls having a febrile illness with muscle aches and pains. The illness resolved on its own but he did notice a round flat red rash on his abdomen around the same time.

    His physical examination is entirely normal, and there is no evidence of any active joints. Further history reveals that he went camping in the Northeastern United States last year prior to the onset of his symptoms. **Which of the following is the most likely diagnosis?**

    (A) RA
    (B) Lyme disease
    (C) syphilis
    (D) PAN
    (E) systemic lupus erythematosus (SLE)

80. **Which of the following statements concerning women's health issues is correct?**

    (A) breast cancer is the leading cause of death in American women
    (B) men benefit more from thrombolytic therapy than women
    (C) the mortality from acute myocardial infarction is greater in women than men
    (D) estrogen therapy decreases mortality in postmenopausal women primarily by its ability to prevent osteoporosis-related fractures
    (E) immune-related disorders are less common in women

81. A 28-year-old-woman is seen in clinic for routine follow-up of her pregnancy at 32 weeks' gestation. She feels well and reports no new symptoms. This is her first pregnancy and she has no past medical history. Her only medication is a multivitamin.

    On physical examination, her vital signs are blood pressure 156/92 mm Hg, pulse 88/min, and respiratory rate 16/min. Her visual acuity is normal and she has no periorbital edema. The heart and lung examination is normal and there is 1+ pedal edema. Her liver edge is not tender, the fundus is palpable above the umbilicus, and the neurologic examination including reflexes is normal. **Which of the following statements concerning hypertension during pregnancy is correct?**

    (A) preeclampsia becomes manifest during the end of the middle trimester
    (B) angiotensin-converting enzyme (ACE) inhibitors are useful antihypertensives in pregnant women
    (C) pregnancy increases the risk for future renal impairment in women with essential hypertension
    (D) alpha-methyldopa is a useful antihypertensive in pregnant women
    (E) gestational hypertension infrequently recurs in subsequent pregnancies

82. A 31-year-old-woman is seen in clinic at 36 weeks' gestation because she is concerned about infections that her baby may acquire during pregnancy and birth. This is her first pregnancy and she reports no complications to date. She states that her immunizations are up to date and she is not experiencing any febrile illness or genitourinary symptoms. **Which of the following statements concerning pregnancy and infection is correct?**

    (A) CMV is the most common cause of congenital viral infection
    (B) postpartum infections are the most common cause of maternal mortality in the United States
    (C) *N gonorrhoeae* infection is transmitted to the child only during delivery
    (D) asymptomatic bacteriuria is common but unimportant in pregnant women
    (E) HIV infection in newborns is invariably contracted during the first trimester

83. A 35-year-old man presents with severe left-sided periorbital headaches associated with nasal stuffiness and tearing of the eye. He experiences 3 short-lived attacks a day, usually occurring at the same time of the day for the past 3 weeks. He has had similar headaches a year ago. **Which of the following characteristics about these headaches is correct?**

    (A) are likely tension headaches
    (B) are typical of common migraine (without an aura)
    (C) may be relieved by the vasodilation of alcohol
    (D) usually recur in cycles lasting several months to years
    (E) can be relieved by administration of oxygen

84. A 75-year-old woman presents to the emergency department with a sudden onset of a communication disorder. The symptoms started 4 hours ago and initially her family thought she was intoxicated and confused. On examination, you note that she speaks fluently but in a series of incomprehensible syllables. She also cannot read or repeat sounds or words. **Which of the following is characteristic of this syndrome?**

    (A) unlikely to improve with time
    (B) usually associated with hemiparesis of the dominant side
    (C) usually associated with hemiparesis of the nondominant side
    (D) usually in the distribution of the posterior cerebral artery
    (E) frequently associated with parietal lobe sensory defects

85. A 38-year-old man develops severe retrosternal chest pain radiating to the back and presents to the emergency department. The pain is aggravated by breathing and movement. He has always been in perfect health but did have a mild upper respiratory tract infection 1 week ago. His cardiogram is shown in Figure 14–1. **Which of the following is the most likely cause for his condition?**

    (A) occlusion of left anterior descending artery
    (B) occlusion of circumflex artery
    (C) a viral infection
    (D) dissection of the aortic artery
    (E) pneumococcal infection

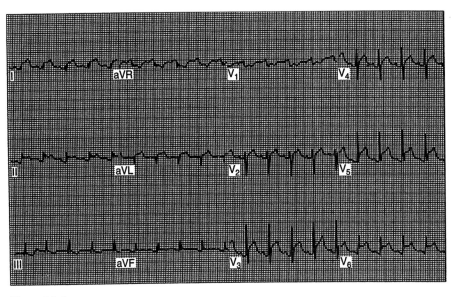

Figure 14–1.

86. A 27-year-old woman presents to the clinic complaining of cough and fever with yellow sputum production. She is a nonsmoker and, although ill, is deemed to not require hospitalization. Her CXR is revealed in Figure 14–2. **Which of the following statements regarding her management is correct?**

Figure 14–2.

(A) a repeat CXR in 2 weeks
(B) a repeat CXR in 6 weeks
(C) antibiotic coverage for *Legionella* infection
(D) antibiotic coverage for *Mycoplasma* infection
(E) antibiotic coverage for Gram-negative infection

87. A 63-year-old man has significant symptoms of shortness of breath for 2 years. The symptoms are worse with exertion such as going up one flight of stairs. He reports no chest pain, or heart failure symptoms. He does endorse a chronic cough with clear sputum production in the morning but no fever, chills, or pleuritic chest pain.

On physical examination, his blood pressure is 137/86 mm Hg, pulse 72/min, respiratory rate 12/min, and oxygen saturation 96% on room air. His JVP and heart sounds are normal, and there is no pedal edema. On chest examination there is an increased anterior–posterior diameter and hyper-resonance to percussion. On auscultation the inspiratory to expiratory ratio is reduced. His CXR is revealed in Figure 14–3. **Which of the following is the most likely diagnosis?**

Figure 14–3.

(A) primary pulmonary hypertension
(B) right ventricular dysfunction
(C) left ventricular dysfunction
(D) emphysema
(E) mitral stenosis

88. A 42-year-old woman presents with fever, weight loss, and malaise. She has lost 10 lb over the past 3 months and is also experiencing non-specific abdominal symptoms. She reports no night sweats, cough, sputum, or shortness of breath symptoms. On physical examination, the blood pressure is 190/100 mm Hg (normal 1 year earlier), heart sounds are normal, the abdomen is soft and nontender and the remaining exam is normal. Her ESR is 105 mm/h, and the urinalysis reveals numerous RBCs. Her abdominal angiogram is revealed in Figure 14–4. **Which of the following is the most likely diagnosis?**

Figure 14–4.

(A) Wegener granulomatosis
(B) rapidly progressive glomerulonephritis
(C) renal artery stenosis
(D) hypernephroma
(E) PAN

89. A 29-year-old man presents to the clinic complaining of back pain for the past several months. It takes him over 2 hours to "loosen up" in the morning. He notes that taking ibuprofen helps relieve the back pain. He has no other joint symptoms and otherwise feels well. His past medical history is negative. On examination, the pertinent finding is decreased range of motion in the lumbar spine on forward flexion. His x-ray is shown in Figure 14–5. **Which of the following is the most likely diagnosis?**

Figure 14–5.

(A) RA
(B) spondylolithiasis
(C) osteomalacia
(D) ankylosing spondylitis
(E) bone involvement with Hodgkin disease

90. A 69-year-old man has had mild arthritis involving many joints for several years. Over 1 or 2 days, he develops severe pain and swelling of his knee. His x-ray reveals calcifications in his articular cartilage. **Which of the following is the most likely diagnosis?**

(A) acute gout
(B) RA
(C) pseudogout
(D) infectious arthritis
(E) torn ligament

91. A 75-year-old man complains of chronic dysphagia to fluids and solids. On occasion, he regurgitates food he has eaten 1 or 2 days before. Last year, he was hospitalized for pneumonia, but he is otherwise well. His barium swallow x-ray is shown in Figure 14–6. **Which of the following is the most appropriate next step in management?**

Figure 14–6.

Figure 14–7.

(A) endoscopic dilatation

(B) myotomy

(C) balloon dilatation of lower esophageal sphincter

(D) surgical excision

(E) vigorous antireflux therapy with surgery if medical management fails

92. A 69-year-old woman is feeling fatigued. Blood work reveals hemoglobin of 9.0 g/dL (14 g/dL 1 year earlier). She has no other symptoms. Her blood film is shown in Figure 14–7. **Which of the following is the most appropriate next diagnostic test?**

(A) serum B_{12} level

(B) hemoglobin electrophoresis

(C) colonoscopy

(D) bone-marrow aspiration

(E) sickle cell preparation

93. A 94-year-old female nursing home resident is referred for evaluation of anemia of 8 g/dL. She has dementia, and adequate documentation of her past medical history is not available. She eats well and is cooperative. Examination reveals evidence of cognitive impairment, primitive reflexes, and a well-healed midline abdominal scar. Her blood film is shown in Figure 14–8. You presume a relationship between the anemia and the previous surgery. **Which of the following surgical procedures is most likely to cause her current anemia?**

(A) gastrectomy

(B) vagotomy and pyloroplasty

(C) cholecystectomy

(D) right hemicolectomy

(E) common bile duct exploration

Figure 14–8.

94. A 42-year-old man suffers a myocardial infarction during coronary angiography. **Which of the following is the approximate risk of this complication?**

(A) 1 in 10,000

(B) 1 in 100

(C) 1 in 100,000

(D) 1 in 1000

(E) unknown

95. An asymptomatic 59-year-old man is treated with oral anticoagulants for chronic atrial fibrillation. When reviewing the benefits of warfarin therapy, he asks about the risks of major bleeding while taking the medication. **Which of the following is the best estimate of the major bleeding complication rate with warfarin anticoagulation?**

(A) 5% per year

(B) 10% per year

(C) 1%–3% per year

(D) unknown

(E) <1% per year

DIRECTIONS (Questions 96 through 108): The following group of numbered items is preceded by a list of lettered options. For each question, select the one lettered option that is most closely associated with it. Each lettered option may be used once, multiple times, or not at all.

Questions 96 through 100: Match the appropriate statement about pharmacology with each of the following medications.

(A) increased sensitivity with aging

(B) decreased sensitivity with aging

(C) altered excretion with aging

(D) altered metabolism with aging

(E) altered distribution with aging

96. Beta-blockers.

97. Nitrazepam.

98. Warfarin.

99. Lithium.

100. Fentanyl.

Questions 101 through 105: For each of the following side effects, select the most likely medication to cause them.

(A) selective serotonin reuptake inhibitors (SSRIs)

(B) mineral oil

(C) diuretics

(D) INH

(E) phenytoin and phenobarbital

(F) salicylates

(G) corticosteroids

(H) L-Dopa

101. Disinterest in food with protein/calorie malnutrition.

102. Zinc deficiency.

103. Vitamin B$_6$ deficiency.

104. Impaired calcium absorption.

105. Altered vitamin D metabolism.

Questions 106 through 108: For each of the following situations, select the most likely sleep disturbance.

(A) sleep more than younger adults

(B) increased arousals during the night

(C) increased slow-wave sleep

(D) sleep improved with alcohol

(E) most common cause of excessive daytime sleepiness in the elderly

106. A common change in sleep as people age.

107. Common in a 73-year-old woman with Alzheimer disease.

108. Sleep apnea syndrome.

DIRECTIONS (Questions 109 through 113): For each of the questions in this section select the one lettered answer that is the best response in each case.

109. A 73-year-old man is brought to the hospital by his family. He is very confused, and collateral history reveals that this is a new finding. Physical examination reveals crackles in his lungs, some abdominal distension, and bilateral asterixis. **Which of the following is the most appropriate initial diagnostic test?**

   (A) CT scan of head
   (B) CT scan of head with enhancement
   (C) CXR
   (D) MRI of head
   (E) spiral CT of chest

110. A 69-year-old woman is brought to the hospital under an order of medical evaluation after she was found confused in an unkempt apartment with 5 cats. Extensive investigation does not reveal a specific cause of confusion in this woman, and the medical service wonders whether the true diagnosis is dementia. **Which of the following cognitive or behavioral impairments is more typical of delirium than dementia?**

   (A) impaired long-term memory
   (B) paranoid behavior
   (C) language impairment
   (D) impaired attention
   (E) fluctuating performance

111. A 77-year-old man is brought to the hospital by his granddaughter for evaluation of confusion. He has no focal findings and his neuro-imaging studies are normal. Further investigations reveal a urinary tract infection, and the man improves somewhat after treatment, but still exhibits poor judgment and bizarre behavior. Pressing the family for information, the intern unearths a history of 8 years of progressive bizarre behavior. The man has undressed himself, made inappropriate sexual comments, has urinated in hallways, and pushed food into his mouth with alarming speed. **Which of the following is the most likely diagnosis?**

   (A) Alzheimer disease
   (B) frontotemporal dementia
   (C) dementia with diffuse Lewy bodies
   (D) vascular dementia
   (E) benign frontal tumor

112. A 68-year-old woman with frontotemporal dementia is being cared for at home by a supportive family. **Which of the following is the most common reason for considering nursing home placement in this individual?**

   (A) inability to perform instrumental activities of daily living (IADLs)
   (B) immobility
   (C) forgetfulness
   (D) intolerable behavior
   (E) incontinence

113. A 69-year-old man has developed memory difficulty and is seen for further evaluation. Complete neurologic assessment is normal except for the mini-mental status examination (MMSE) where he sores 19/30. His laboratory investigations and brain imaging are normal, and there does not appear to be any reversible cause for the memory deficits. His clinical features are most compatible with a diagnosis of Alzheimer disease. **Which of the following pathologic changes are most likely to be seen in the brain of a patient with Alzheimer disease?**

   (A) microangiopathic changes
   (B) lacunar infarcts
   (C) diffuse Lewy bodies
   (D) pigmentary degeneration
   (E) neurofibrillary tangles

Answers and Explanations

1. **(A)** This patient has gonorrhea, and since 1986, increasing penicillin resistance has meant that penicillin/ampicillin are no longer drugs of choice. Alternatives to ceftriaxone include ciprofloxacin, ofloxacin, or cefixime given orally, with 7 days of doxycycline, or a single 1 g dose of azithromycin in case of coinfection with *Chlamydia*. In Asia and the Pacific (as well as in California), quinolones are not considered first-line therapy because of the high rate of resistant organisms. In these locations, ceftriaxone is the drug of choice. In pregnant women, erythromycin replaces doxycycline. Disseminated gonococcal infection should be treated in a hospital with IV antibiotics. *(Fauci, Chapter 137)*

2. **(C)** The impaired physiologic reserve of every organ system is characteristic of aging. The term *homeostenosis* has been used to describe this phenomenon. Decline in most systems starts in the third decade and is gradual and progressive. Decrements in each organ system seem independent of other systems and are influenced by diet, environment, personal habits (eg, exercise), and genetic factors, as well as just chronologic age. At times, it can be difficult to differentiate between age-related physiologic change and age-related diseases. *(Fauci, Chapter 9)*

3. **(C)** Besides hypothyroidism, other tests to rule out reversible causes might include serum electrolytes, B_{12} levels, CBC, Venereal Disease Research Laboratory (VDRL), and CT or MRI. Diagnosis of Alzheimer disease remains a diagnosis of exclusion. However, the insidious and subtle onset, with few focal signs (except for higher mental functioning) and a slowly progressive course are characteristic. Careful attention to the pattern of cognitive defects also improves diagnostic accuracy. The intensity of investigation will depend on numerous factors, including age, presence of atypical findings, and the timing of presentation. There is as yet no definite consensus on the most appropriate plan of investigation. *(Fauci, Chapter 365)*

4. **(D)** This patient has hyperthyroidism. Cardiac complications are more common in the elderly patient and may dominate the clinical presentation. There is often a wide pulse pressure, systolic murmurs, increased intensity of the first heart sound, and cardiomegaly. Sinus tachycardia and atrial fibrillation are the most common arrhythmias. A to-and-fro high-pitched sound in the pulmonic area (Means–Lerman scratch) can mimic a pericardial friction rub. Aortic regurgitation, soft heart sounds, and hypotension are not usual findings in hyperthyroidism. *(Fauci, Chapter 335)*

5. **(B)** Ectopic PTH production in malignancy is quite rare. A whole host of locally produced hormones and cytokines, as well as ectopically produced hormones, are implicated in local osteoclastic hypercalcemia. Parathormone-related protein (PTHrP) is often elevated in malignant hypercalcemia (with or without bony metastases), but not ectopic PTH with is different from PTHrP. *(Fauci, Chapter 96)*

6. **(C)** Sarcoidosis presents as an asymptomatic CXR in at least 10%–20% of cases in the United States, but more frequently in countries where pre-employment CXRs are mandatory. At least

40% of patients present with acute symptoms and hilar lymphadenopathy. Approximately 90% will have an abnormal CXR at some point in their illness. Only a small proportion develops progressive disease. This patient's clinical presentation of hilar adenopathy, fever, and erythema nodosum are only characteristic of sarcoidosis, the other diagnosis are not compatible with this constellation of symptoms. (Fauci, Chapter 322)

7. (C) PET scans use glucose analogues to demonstrate metabolic activity. Functional MRI scans are now being used extensively to assess areas of brain activity. (Fauci, Chapter 362)

8. (D) Streptococcus group A can cause a toxic shock-like syndrome, and has been increasing in frequency in North America. Streptococcal toxic shock-like syndrome was so named because of its similarity to staphylococcal toxic shock syndrome. The illness includes fever, hypotension, renal impairment, and the respiratory distress syndrome. It is usually caused by strains that produce exotoxin. It may be associated with localized infection as well; the most common associated infection is a soft-tissue infection such as necrotizing fasciitis. The mortality is high (up to 30%), usually secondary to shock and respiratory failure. The rapid progression of the disease and its high mortality demand early recognition and aggressive treatment. Management includes fluid resuscitation, pressor agents, mechanical ventilation, antibodies, and, if necrotizing fasciitis is present, surgical débridement. (Fauci, Chapter 130)

9. (D) Nitroprusside is very effective in lowering blood pressure and is easy to titrate and adjust to response. Labetalol is also useful since is can be administered in an oral preparation, but has more contraindications. It is particularly useful in the setting of angina or myocardial infarction. Regardless of which drug is selected, early administration of medications for long-term control is mandatory. (Fauci, Chapter 241)

10. (D) This man has primary hyperparathyroidism. Hypercalcemia induces a tubular

concentrating defect by interfering with ADH-mediated water pore function (aquaporin-2 channel) on distal tubular cells. This results in the polyuria and polydipsia symptoms of diabetes insipidus. Chronic hypercalcemia can also cause renal stones, type 1 (distal) RTA and chronic renal failure but these effects are not directly responsible for the polyuria. PTH has no direct effect on the concentrating ability of the distal tubule. (Fauci, Chapter 347)

11. (E) Ethosuximide and valproic acid are common medications used to treat absence seizures. Side effects of ethosuximide include GI irritation, skin rash, and bone marrow suppression. (Fauci, Chapter 363)

12. (B) Hairy cell leukemia is a B-cell malignancy. Burkitt lymphoma is of T-cell origin 5% of the time. CLL can be of T- or B-cell origin. Mycosis fungoides and angioimmunoblastic lymphadenopathy are of T-cell origin. (Fauci, Chapter 105)

13. (C) The current case definition of AIDS in a patient with HIV infection is done by symptoms and CD4+ T-lymphocyte cell count. Any category C symptoms (eg, cervical cancer, mycobacterium avium infection, CMV retinitis, Kaposi sarcoma, etc) indicates frank AIDS as does a CD4+ T-cell count <200/μL regardless of symptoms. Shingles and thrush are category B symptoms. (Fauci, Chapter 182)

14. (D) Rectal bleeding is more characteristic of ulcerative colitis, as is malignancy with long-standing disease, but both can occur in regional enteritis. Transmural involvement, lymph node involvement, skip lesions, granulomas, and anorectal complications (abscesses, fistulas, fissures) are characteristic of Crohn disease. (Fauci, Chapter 289)

15. (B) Sudden onset of unexplained dyspnea is the most common and often the only symptom of pulmonary embolism. Findings on physical examination may be deceptively normal, but tachycardia is a consistent finding. Pleuritic chest pain and hemoptysis suggest a peripheral embolism adjacent to the pleura.

Myocardial infarction is a rare complication in pregnancy and likely to present with chest pain, and primary pulmonary hypertension while common in young woman would present with the insidious onset of dyspnea on exertion. PSVT has a much faster heart rate, which presents as sudden onset of palpitations. *(Fauci, Chapter 7)*

16. **(A)** The patient has Wernicke encephalopathy and requires treatment with thiamine. A delay of a few hours may permit progression to psychosis. The eye findings in Wernicke encephalopathy include bilateral (but not necessarily symmetrical) abductor weakness or paralysis, horizontal diplopia, strabismus, and nystagmus. The nystagmus is most frequently horizontal or vertical gaze-evoked nystagmus. There is no indication to administer phenytoin for this patient, and while diazepam maybe important for prophylaxis against alcohol withdrawal symptoms, the most important immediate treatment is thiamine. *(Fauci, Chapter 269)*

17. **(E)** Calcitonin is secreted by cells in the thyroid. Calcitonin reduces bone resorption and increases renal calcium clearance. The inhibition of osteoclast-mediated bone resorption and the stimulation of renal calcium clearance are mediated by receptors on osteoclasts and renal tubular cells. Other receptors to calcitonin are present in the brain, GI tract, and immune system. *(Fauci, Chapter 347)*

18. **(C)** Major manifestations of rheumatic fever include carditis, migratory polyarthritis, chorea, erythema marginatum, and subcutaneous nodules. Minor manifestations include arthralgia, fever, elevated acute phase reactants (ESR, C-reactive protein), and prolonged PR interval. The diagnosis is made with 2 major, or 1 major and 2 minor criteria, and evidence of group A streptococcal infection (positive throat culture or rapid streptococcal antigen test, or rising antibody titers). *(Fauci, Chapter 315)*

19. **(A)** The presence of severe pulmonary hypertension can result in intraoperative death and is a contraindication for transplantation. Other important selection criteria for transplantation are body size, ABO match, negative lymphocyte cross-match, and other co-morbid disease states. In the United States, it is estimated that only 2000 potential donor hearts become available each year for 20,000 potential recipients. This means that careful recipient selection is very important. The optimal candidates will have a high likelihood of return to a high level of function, to be mentally vigorous and medically compliant. *(Fauci, Chapter 228)*

20. **(D)** CLL is frequently discovered on routine evaluation of elderly patients and may not require treatment for several years. Splenomegaly, when present, rarely leads to symptoms. It is usually a disorder of B cells and is very indolent in its course. Most therapeutic regimens are designed for symptom control, not cure. Common reasons for treatment include hemolytic anemia, cytopenias, disfiguring lymphadenopathy, symptomatic organomegaly, or systemic symptoms. Chlorambucil is easy to administer, but fludarabine is considerably more effective. It requires IV administration. Maintenance therapy is not helpful. *(Fauci, Chapter 105)*

21. **(D)** GI bleeding is the most common precipitating factor for hepatic encephalopathy. Patients with cirrhosis and portal hypertension are at risk for variceal bleeding. Diuretic therapy by causing hypokalemia, and SBP are other common causes. In this patient the postural hypotension and dark stools suggests that GI bleeding is the likely cause rather than his diuretics or SBP. Narcotics and sedatives are also frequently implicated as precipitants for hepatic encephalopathy. *(Fauci, Chapter 302)*

22. **(C)** Berger disease is characterized by immunoglobulin A (IgA) deposits in the mesangium. It most commonly affects older children and young adults, and is more common in Blacks than in Whites. Macroscopic hematuria may occur with inter-current illness or vigorous exercise. The prognosis is variable but tends to progress slowly. Spontaneous remissions are more common in children than in adults. About 20%–50% of patients develop

end-stage renal disease within 20 years of diagnosis. Other causes of asymptomatic hematuria, with or without proteinuria, include sickle cell disease, Alport syndrome, resolving glomerulonephritis, and thin basement disease. *(Fauci, Chapter 277)*

23. **(E)** Chronic obstructive pulmonary disease (COPD) due to emphysema usually demonstrates severe dyspnea, scanty mucoid sputum, normal hematocrit, and decreased diffusing capacity on pulmonary function testing. Chronic bronchitis is characterized by milder dyspnea, greater sputum production, more frequent hypercarbia and polycythemia, and more evidence of cor pulmonale and pulmonary hypertension. *(Fauci, Chapter 254)*

24. **(E)** Muscle weakness in RA is common and can occur within weeks of onset of RA. It is most apparent in muscles adjacent to involved joints. There is not usually a vasculitis present, although a mononuclear infiltrate may be present. The most common finding on biopsy is type II fiber atrophy and muscle fiber necrosis. *(Fauci, Chapter 314)*

25. **(A)** Alpha-thalassemia involves a decrease in alpha-chain production and leads to the formation of beta-globin tetramers known as hemoglobin H. Individuals normally inherit four alpha-chain genes. The clinical syndrome depends on how many genes are deleted. Deletion of 1 gene results in a silent carrier state. Deletion of all 4 is the most severe and presents as hydrops fetalis. This condition is incompatible with life. *(Fauci, Chapter 99)*

26. **(A)** Diabetic neuropathy usually presents as peripheral polyneuropathy, usually bilateral, and can include symptoms of numbness, paresthesia, severe hyperesthesia, and pain. Impairment of proprioceptive fibers can lead to gait abnormalities and Charcot joints. Mononeuropathy is less common and is often spontaneously reversible. Common syndromes include wrist or foot drop and third, fourth, or sixth cranial nerve palsies. Autonomic neuropathy may cause gastroesophageal dysfunction, bladder dysfunction, and orthostatic hypotension. Randomized controlled trials in Type 1 and 2 diabetes demonstrate that good glycemic control results in lower microvascular complications such as retinopathy or neuropathy. *(Fauci, Chapter 338)*

27. **(D)** Uricosuric drugs and allopurinol have no role in the treatment of acute gouty arthritis. Salicylates are also not used in the treatment of gout. The treatments of choice are colchicine, NSAIDs, and intra-articular steroid injection. Response is best when initiated early in the disease. Colchicine can be given intravenously to avoid GI distress. A short course of systemic corticosteroids is also quite effective therapy. Allopurinol is started only when all inflammation is gone and colchicine prophylaxis has been started. It is not always required. *(Fauci, Chapter 327)*

28. **(B)** The two broad categories of ischemic stroke are embolic and thrombotic. Emboli can originate from an arterial atheroma (eg, common carotid bifurcation) or from the heart. In the latter case, anticoagulants are often indicated. On occasion, emboli occur without obvious source (eg, hypercoagulable states, malignancy, ecclampsia). *(Fauci, Chapter 364)*

29. **(E)** Causes of acute glomerulonephritis include infectious diseases, especially *Streptococcus*, vasculitides, and primary glomerular disease. The acute nephritic syndrome consists of the abrupt onset of hematuria and proteinuria, often accompanied by azotemia and renal salt and water retention. Oliguria may be present. *(Fauci, Chapter 277)*

30. **(A)** The pain may be described as sharp, burning, or gnawing, usually 90 minutes to 3 hours after eating, relieved by food or antacids. The pain frequently awakens the patient at night. Symptoms are usually episodic and recurrent. Periods of remission are usually longer than periods with pain. The ulcer crater can recur or persist in the absence of pain. Only a minority of patients with dyspepsia are found to have an ulcer on endoscopy. *(Fauci, Chapter 1855)*

31. **(C)** Intravascular hemolysis from blood transfusion is usually due to ABO incompatibility, often from human error. Symptoms of intravascular hemolysis include flushing, pain at the infusion site, chest or back pain, restlessness, anxiety, nausea, and diarrhea. Signs include fever and chills, shock, and renal failure. In comatose patients, hemoglobulinuria or bleeding from disseminated intravascular coagulation can be the first sign. Management is supportive. Acute hemolysis can also result from antibodies directed against other RBC antigens such as Rh, Kell, or Duffy. *(Fauci , Chapter 107)*

32. **(D)** Radioactive iodine is contraindicated both in scanning and treatment as it damages the fetal thyroid. Propylthiouracil crosses the placenta, but is safe and effective in pregnancy. The lowest effective dose should be used. Hyperthyroidism is hardest to control in the first trimester and easiest in the third trimester. *(Fauci, Chapter 7)*

33. **(D)** Antihistamine side effects (sedation) and anticholinergic side effects (dry mouth, constipation, urinary hesitancy, blurred vision) are the most common side effects. Orthostasis is probably the most common serious side effect and is difficult to manage. Severe cardiac toxicity is uncommon and diarrhea and weight loss are associated with SSRI antidepressants. *(Fauci, Chapter 386)*

34. **(B)** Reassurance regarding the benign nature of the disease is the mainstay of management. The most common pathogenic mechanism is thought to be excessive or redundant mitral leaflet tissue, with the posterior leaflet more commonly involved. Myxomatous degeneration can also be seen on pathologic examination. Current guidelines do not recommend antibiotic prophylaxis for endocarditis in patients with MVP with or without murmur. *(Fauci, Chapters 118 and 230)*

35. **(B)** In minimal change disease there are little or no changes seen on light microscopy. The disease is most common in children. Spontaneous remission is common in children and is enhanced by steroid therapy. Over 95% of children achieve remission within 8 weeks of institution of prednisone therapy. Therefore, in children with nephrotic syndrome, empiric therapy is frequently employed, rather than initial renal biopsy. Only 50% of adults will remit, and thus biopsy is more frequently required. Relapse is common in both children and adults. *(Fauci, Chapter 277)*

36. **(D)** Over 90% of lesions can be localized by fiberoptic bronchoscope in the sedated, but awake patient and collection of a series of differential brushings and biopsies. When lesions are found, conservative resection is usually performed. Five-year cure rates in such lesions approach 60%, but second primaries are common (5% per patient per year). There is no evidence that screening programs based on sputum examination will decrease mortality. *(Fauci, Chapter 85)*

37. **(A)** The drop in systolic pressure with inspiration is an important clue to cardiac tamponade, called pulsus paradoxus. When severe, the arterial pulse may weaken on palpation during inspiration. Pulsus paradoxus is uncommon in constrictive pericarditis and rare in restrictive cardiomyopathy. It is commonly found in severe asthma as well. *(Fauci, Chapter 232)*

38. **(C)** Cyclosporine A blocks production of interleukin-2 (IL-2) by helper-inducer (CD4+) T cells. It works alone but is more effective in combination with glucocorticoids. The use of cyclosporine has improved 1-year cadaveric survival rates to the 80%–85% range. Side effects include hepatotoxicity, hirsutism, tremor, and gingival hyperplasia, but only the nephrotoxicity presents a serious management problem. *(Fauci, Chapter 276)*

39. **(E)** Typically, multiple sclerosis presents with optic neuritis. There is usually a history of at least 2 episodes of neurologic deficit at more than one site. Other common presenting symptoms include weakness, sensory loss, and paresthesias. *(Fauci, Chapter 375)*

40. **(E)** This patient has HSP; other symptoms include arthralgia and GI symptoms. Renal

biopsy shows immunoglobulin deposits. There is an underlying vasculitis. The prognosis is generally good, although relapses can occur before the final remission. The lack of bloody diarrhea makes this less likely to be hemolytic uremic syndrome, and there are on other clinical features of thrombotic thrombocytopenic purpura such as fever, CNS symptoms, or hemolysis. (*Fauci, Chapter 319*)

41. **(E)** Many experts will elect to follow elderly patients with mild hyperparathyroidism who are asymptomatic and have normal renal function and bone mass. Oral bisphosphonate therapy may be appropriate to preserve bone mass. Estrogen therapy may retard demineralization of the skeleton and may also reduce blood and urinary calcium levels. However, there is insufficient evidence for a formal recommendation. There is no clear consensus on when asymptomatic hyperparathyroidism requires surgery. (*Fauci, Chapter 347*)

42. **(D)** Other drugs, besides antimalarials, that precipitate hemolysis in G6PD deficiency include dapsone, phenacetin, doxorubicin, and nalidixic acid. The disease is sex-linked, and thus most common in males. About 11% of people of African descent have an abnormal allele. Female heterozygotes have a dual population of red cells and, depending on the proportion, may develop symptoms. During hemolysis, older red cells with the lowest enzyme levels are destroyed, and diagnostic tests done at this time may be falsely normal. They should be repeated some time after the hemolysis has resolved. (*Fauci, Chapter 101*)

43. **(C)** Levofloxacin would be effective for most strains of *Streptococcus pneumoniae*, *Legionella pneumophila*, and other likely pathogens. Other commonly used drugs for community-acquired pneumonia are high-dose amoxicillin, cefuroxime, trimethoprim-sulfamethoxazole, and doxycycline. Theoretically, empiric therapy should be guided by knowledge of local resistance patterns. (*Fauci, Chapter 2515*)

44. **(C)** Other clues to renal tubule defects include electrolyte disorders, renal osteodystrophy,

large kidneys, and proteinuria. Categories of tubulointerstitial kidney disease include toxins (exogenous and metabolic), neoplasia, immune diseases, vascular disorders, infections, and hereditary renal diseases. Defects in urinary acidification and concentrating ability are frequently the most troublesome manifestations of tubulointerstitial kidney disease. (*Fauci, Chapter 271*)

45. **(E)** Proton pump inhibitors (eg, omeprazole and lansoprazole) are the most effective treatments for ulcerative esophagitis. Antacids, sucralfate, and H2-blockers are all useful in less severe reflux disease. (*Fauci, Chapter 287*)

46. **(A)** MGUS is vastly more common than multiple myeloma, occurring in 1% of the population over age 50. Patients with MGUS have smaller M components (usually <30 g/L); no urinary Bence Jones protein; <10% bone marrow clonal plasma cells, and no anemia, renal failure, lytic bone lesions, or hypercalcemia. About 25% of patients with MGUS will go on to develop multiple myeloma. This patient's normal investigations and percentage of marrow plasma cells makes the diagnosis MGUS rather than myeloma. (*Fauci, Chapter 106*)

47. **(E)** Sjögren syndrome is an immunologic disorder characterized by progressive destruction of the exocrine glands leading to mucosal dryness. Pathology reveals lymphocytic infiltration. About one-third develop systemic (nonglandular) symptoms. The most common systemic manifestation is arthritis or arthralgia. If vasculitis occurs, purpura, urticaria, skin ulcers, and mononeuropathy are its most common manifestations. (*Fauci, Chapter 317*)

48. **(D)** The type O donor may contain sufficient anti-A or anti-B to destroy some of the patient's RBCs, but this is seldom clinically significant. Generally, however, crystalloid or colloid solutions are sufficient for volume replacement until properly matched blood is available. (*Fauci, Chapter 107*)

49. **(D)** Other early changes in mitral stenosis include prominence of the main pulmonary

arteries and backward displacement of the esophagus. CXR changes are caused by enlargement of the left atrium. Severe disease can cause pulmonary congestion (Kerley B lines) and enlargement of the right ventricle, right atrium, and superior vena cava. *(Fauci, Chapter 230)*

50. **(A)** In myasthenia gravis, the distribution of muscle weakness is characteristic with early involvement of the cranial nerves, especially the lids and extraocular muscles. Women are more frequently affected than men (3:2 ratio), and the age for peak incidence in women is in the third or fourth decade. The other feature is the fatigability of muscle strength with repeated exercise which distinguishes this patient's weakness from muscular dystrophy. *(Fauci, Chapter 381)*

51. **(E)** History of one breast cancer is a risk factor for a second tumor. Risk of breast cancer is increased in women with a family history, early menarche, late menopause, nulliparity, and late age at first pregnancy. Obesity, alcohol, and dietary fat are other possible risk factors. *(Fauci, Chapter 86)*

52. **(D)** Patients with minimal or absent GI symptoms and atypical respiratory symptoms may be diagnosed as adults. This accounts for 7% of cases. Moreover, because of modern therapy, about 36% of CF patients in the United States are over 18 years of age, and 12% are over 30. *(Fauci, Chapter 253)*

53. **(B)** Signs of benignity of a solitary pulmonary nodule are lack of growth over a prolonged period and certain patterns of calcification. "Popcorn" calcification does suggest a benign hamartoma. A search for previous CXRs can provide a definitive diagnosis. In nonsmokers under age 35, 1% of solitary pulmonary nodules are malignant. In this patient, a follow up CXR to demonstrate stability of the lesion is more appropriate than biopsy or resection. *(Fauci, Chapter 85)*

54. **(B)** A period of 24–48 hours is usually allowed to attempt medical therapy. Cardiac catheterization

and angiography may be followed by bypass surgery or angioplasty. For those who do settle down, some form of subsequent risk stratification (eg, exercise ECG) is indicated. *(Fauci, Chapter 238)*

55. **(A)** Glucocorticoids are not bronchodilators, and their major use is in reducing airway inflammation. It is difficult to provide precise recommendations for their use, and a wide range of systemic and inhaled doses are used. *(Fauci, Chapter 248)*

56. **(C)** Immunofluorescence is usually negative. By electron microscopy, focal basement membrane collapse and denudation of epithelial surfaces are noted. The course is generally progressive in adults. It is believed that remission of proteinuria with steroid therapy will improve the prognosis. Cytotoxic drugs and cyclosporine have also been used in treatment. The degree of proteinuria correlates with the likelihood of developing renal failure. The disease recurs rapidly in transplanted kidneys, suggesting a humoral factor in pathogenesis. *(Fauci, Chapter 277)*

57. **(E)** Heartburn is a characteristic symptom of reflux esophagitis and may be associated with regurgitation. Odynophagia and atypical chest pain also occur in esophageal disease. *(Fauci, Chapter 286)*

58. **(D)** For most patients with Raynaud, appropriate clothing and precaution to prevent exposure to cold is required for therapy. Surgical sympathectomy usually provides only temporary improvement and does not prevent progression of the vascular lesion. Nifedipine is now the drug of choice for treating symptoms not responding to local warming measures (gloves, mitts) and avoidance of smoking and cold. Reserpine, alpha-methyldopa, and prazosin may also be useful. *(Fauci, Chapter 243)*

59. **(C)** The most common presentation is hemarthrosis with pain in a weight-bearing joint such as the hip, knee, or ankle. Hematuria is also common. Bleeding can occur at almost any site without prior trauma. *(Fauci, Chapter 110)*

60. **(B)** The principal symptom is the pain of acute pericarditis that usually develops 1–4 weeks following the cardiac surgery but could appear after months. It can also occur after myocardial infarction (Dressler syndrome) or after trauma to the heart (stab wound, blunt trauma). The syndrome can remit and recur for up to 2 years. The acute symptoms usually subside in 1–2 weeks. The clinical symptoms and signs suggest pericarditis is the diagnosis and rule out myocardial infarction, and pulmonary embolism. *(Fauci, Chapter 232)*

61. **(A)** A vegan diet (no meat, eggs, fish, cheese, and other animal products) can result in B12 deficiency. Iron deficiency, thalassemia, chronic inflammation, or sideroblastic anemia do not cause macrocytosis. *(Fauci, Chapter 100)*

62. **(A)** The patient has Cushing syndrome secondary to an adrenocorticotropic hormone (ACTH)-secreting pituitary tumor. Relatively few of such patients have a large pituitary tumor that affects the visual pathways. Over 50% have a microadenoma, which is under 5 mm in diameter. *(Fauci, Chapter 336)*

63. **(E)** Elevated triglycerides are the most common dyslipidemia in DM. However, the LDL particles in DM are more atherogenic than in nondiabetics, even though they are not elevated by DM alone. DM frequently results in lower HDL levels as well. *(Fauci, Chapter 338)*

64. **(D)** The vertebral bodies in osteoporosis may become increasingly biconcave because of weakening of the subchondral plates. This results in "codfish" vertebra. When vertebral collapse occurs, the anterior height of the vertebra is usually decreased. Plain x-rays are insensitive diagnostic tools because up to 30% of bone mass can be lost without any apparent x-ray changes. Dual-energy x-ray absorptiometry (DEXA) and CT scan are more sensitive tests for bone loss, but their exact clinical role has not been clearly established. *(Fauci, Chapter 348)*

65. **(B)** Aspirin is given in low doses such as 80 to 325 mg/day, although the initial studies were done with higher doses. Carotid endarterectomy is the best treatment for stenoses of 70% or more. *(Fauci, Chapter 364)*

66. **(C)** Later symptoms of hypothyroidism include loss of intellectual and motor activity, declining appetite, dry hair and skin, and deepening voice. In the elderly, hypothyroidism can be misdiagnosed as due to aging or to other diseases such as Parkinson disease, Alzheimer disease, or depression. *(Fauci, Chapter 335)*

67. **(D)** Radiation therapy in stage 1A Hodgkin disease has a very high cure rate. Patients must be followed for hypothyroidism. The long-term disease-free survival is 80%. Mantle irradiation can result acutely in transient dry mouth, pharyngitis, fatigue, and weight loss. The most common long-term effect is hypothyroidism (in 30% of cases), but radiation pneumonitis and fibrosis or pericardial disease can occur. Although radiotherapy alone would be acceptable in this case, there is a trend to add chemotherapy as well. *(Fauci, Chapter 105)*

68. **(A)** PAN may be associated with hepatitis B antigenemia in 30% of cases, suggesting immunologic phenomena in the pathogenesis of the disease. Aneurysmal dilatations along involved arteries are characteristic and their presence in small- and medium-sized arteries in renal, hepatic, and visceral vasculature is diagnostic. Biopsy of involved areas can also be diagnostic. *(Fauci, Chapter 319)*

69. **(E)** CMV can also cause neurologic complications from CNS infection. Treatment is with ganciclovir, foscarnet, or cidofovir. Relapse rates are high with both drugs, and therefore maintenance therapy is mandatory. *(Fauci, Chapter 182)*

70. **(B)** Biliary tract obstruction results in elevated conjugated hyperbilirubinemia. Most patients have fever, pain, chills, elevated alkaline phosphatase, as well as increased conjugated bilirubin. Mechanical obstruction is most commonly due to stones, tumors, or strictures. For reasons that are unclear, the serum bilirubin tends to plateau and rarely exceeds levels of 600 mmol/L (25 mg/dL). *(Fauci, Chapter 43)*

71. **(B)** Dysplastic nevi and benign acquired nevi are both most common on sun-exposed areas such as the back. Atypical moles can occur on the scalp, breasts, and buttocks, rare areas for benign acquired nevi. Both lesions are usually associated with similar lesions (10–40 on average for benign nevi, often >100 in the case of dysplastic nevi). Dysplastic nevi are larger (>6 mm) and have irregular pigmentation and borders. *(Fauci, Chapter 83)*

72. **(E)** Prerenal azotemia usually has urine osmolality over 500, urine creatinine over 40, and fractional excretion of sodium <1. The urinary sediment in prerenal azotemia reveals hyaline casts. In intrinsic renal azotemia, heme-granular casts are seen. *(Fauci, Chapter 45)*

73. **(D)** The behavioral respiratory control system of the brain drives the hyperventilation, which leads to decreased P_{CO_2} and increased pH. If alkalemia is present with the hypocarbia, symptoms can be quite significant. They include dizziness, visual impairment, syncope, and seizures secondary to cerebral vasoconstriction; paresthesias, carpopedal spasm, and tetany (secondary to decreased free serum calcium); muscle weakness (secondary to hypophosphatemia); and cardiac arrhythmias (secondary to alkalemia). *(Fauci, Chapter 258)*

74. **(D)** ST segment elevation is the hallmark of acute MI, other early ischemic changes are tall, peaked T waves that then develop into inverted T waves. Q waves develop later once there is transmural muscle injury and infarction. *(Fauci, Chapter 239)*

75. **(B)** Activated charcoal absorbs barbiturates very effectively and is useful in decontamination of the GI tract. Renal elimination of phenobarbital is enhanced by alkalinization of the urine to a pH of 8 with sodium bicarbonate and fluids. Hemodialysis and hemoperfusion are reserved for extreme cases with refracting hypotension. Short-acting barbiturates are metabolized in the liver, so fluid administration and alkalinization are not helpful. *(Fauci, Chapter e35)*

76. **(E)** Exposure to ionizing radiation is more likely to cause cancer if it occurs at an early age. Radiation-induced malignancy tends to occur at the same age as the same malignancy in the general population. This suggests that radiation is not the only factor. *(Fauci, Chapter 374)*

77. **(D)** The loop diuretics inhibit tubular reabsorption of sodium, potassium, and chloride in the loop of Henle and can continue to cause diuresis even during volume contraction. The site of action of furosemide is in the thick ascending limb of the loop of Henle. *(Fauci, Chapter 227)*

78. **(D)** INH acts as a pyridoxine antagonist and causes polyneuropathy in slow acetylators. Both sensory and motor involvement occurs. Treatment with pyridoxine can improve symptoms. *(Fauci, Chapter 376)*

79. **(B)** The first stage of Lyme disease is an acute infection with the spirochete *Borrelia burgdorferi*, usually transmitted by tick bite. It is most common in the summer in rural, wooded areas. About 60% of patients who have not received antibiotic therapy will develop arthritis months later. The typical pattern is intermittent attacks of oligoarthritis lasting weeks to months. The knees are the most common joints involved. The clinical pattern of joint involvement and absence of physical findings rules out RA or SLE. *(Fauci, Chapter 166)*

80. **(C)** The mortality from acute myocardial infarction is greater in women, particularly African-American women. It is unclear whether this correlation is independent of age and disease severity. Ischemic heart disease, not breast cancer, is the leading cause of death in American women. The relative benefit of thrombolytic therapy seems similar in men and women. Estrogen therapy's major effect in decreasing mortality is via its reduction (40%–50%) in deaths due to ischemic heart disease. This has not yet been verified in prospective trials. Estrogen therapy has not been shown to be beneficial in secondary prevention of heart disease in women. Immune-related disorders (RA, lupus, multiple sclerosis,

thyroid disease) are usually more common in women. *(Fauci, Chapter 6)*

81. **(D)** Alpha-methyldopa has been used extensively throughout pregnancy, with no evidence of harm to the fetus. ACE inhibitors are associated with increased fetal loss. Preeclampsia and eclampsia are diseases of the second and third trimester of pregnancy. There is no evidence that pregnancy affects the course of essential hypertension. Gestational hypertension has a high rate of recurrence in subsequent pregnancies. *(Fauci, Chapter 7)*

82. **(A)** CMV is the most common congenital viral infection, affecting 1%–2% of all American newborns. Only a small minority of these infants are abnormal. *N gonorrhoeae* infection can be transmitted in utero, during delivery, or in the postpartum period. Asymptomatic bacteriuria occurs in up to 7% of all pregnancies. Treatment can prevent about 75% of all acute pyelonephritis in pregnancy; thus, screening is warranted. HIV infection is usually transmitted during the perinatal period. Although postpartum infections are a significant cause of maternal mortality, the most important are thromboembolic disease, hypertension, ectopic pregnancy, and hemorrhage. *(Fauci, Chapter 7)*

83. **(E)** This story of daily attacks of periorbital pain with annual recurrence in a man between age 30–50 is typical of cluster headaches. The recurrent bouts last days to weeks. The headaches can be provoked by alcohol and relieved by oxygen administration. Prophylactic treatment, however, is preferred. *(Fauci, Chapter 15)*

84. **(E)** Expressive (Wernicke) aphasia involves disease (most commonly ischemic infarction) in the distribution of the lower division of the middle cerebral artery. It is frequently associated with parietal lobe sensory deficits and hemianopsia; motor disturbance is not part of the syndrome. The condition may improve with time. *(Fauci, Chapter 27)*

85. **(C)** The ECG reveals diffuse ST elevation with characteristic concave upward shape and PR depression in the precordial leads. This is more typical of pericarditis than of myocardial infarction. The presentation, symptoms, and age of the patient are all typical for viral pericarditis. *(Fauci, Chapter 232)*

86. **(B)** Community-acquired pneumonia in previously healthy young people is commonly caused by *S pneumoniae, Mycoplasma,* viruses, or *Chlamydia.* The pattern of dense right upper lobe consolidation in this case strongly suggests a typical bacterial pneumonia, such as *S pneumoniae.* A follow-up CXR in 6 weeks is appropriate to ensure that no underlying abnormality is the cause of the problem. *(Fauci, Chapter 251)*

87. **(D)** The CXR is typical of COPD, with flattened diaphragms, hyperlucent lungs, and increased retrosternal air space. *(Fauci, Chapter 254)*

88. **(E)** Renal, musculoskeletal, and peripheral nerve involvement are the most common manifestations of PAN. Generally, if no tissue is easily available for biopsy, an arteriogram is a better diagnostic test than a blind biopsy. This arteriogram reveals multiple aneurysmal dilatations, the classic finding in PAN. *(Fauci, Chapter 319)*

89. **(D)** The x-ray reveals typical evidence of sacroiliitis, with widening of the joints, sclerosis, and evasions. Similar findings can be seen in psoriatic and enteropathic spondyloarthropathy. *(Fauci, Chapter 318)*

90. **(C)** The articular calcification chondrocalcinosis is typical for pseudogout or calcium pyrophosphate disease (CPPD). The most common joint involved is the knee, but the wrist, shoulder, ankle, elbow, and hand are also frequently involved. Definitive diagnosis depends on finding typical rhomboid-shaped crystals with weak-positive birefringence in the synovial fluid, but chondrocalcinosis in the correct setting allows a presumptive diagnosis. Numerous diseases are associated with CPPD, but the

most common predisposing factor is advancing age. *(Fauci, Chapter 327)*

91. **(B)** The x-ray reveals a Zenker diverticulum. Halitosis, aspiration (perhaps explaining his pneumonia), regurgitation of old meals, and dysphagia are typical symptoms. Surgical treatment involves a cricopharyngeal myotomy. At times, a diverticulectomy is also required. *(Fauci, Chapter 286)*

92. **(C)** The film shows hypochromic, microcytic red cells, suggesting iron deficiency. Although thalassemia can mimic iron deficiency, the normal hemoglobin 1 year earlier makes this unlikely. Anemia of chronic disease is unlikely because there are no signs of such a chronic disease. Thus, blood loss from the GI tract is the most likely cause. *(Fauci, Chapter 98)*

93. **(A)** The macrocytic cells and hypersegmented neutrophil are characteristic of megaloblastic anemia. Vitamin B_{12} and folate deficiency are the most common cause. Lack of intrinsic factor because of gastrectomy will eventually result in B_{12} deficiency. *(Fauci, Chapter 100)*

94. **(D)** Coronary angiography is a relatively safe procedure in the right individual. There are complications associated with this procedure that must be reviewed with the patient while obtaining informed consent. The risk of stroke and myocardial infarction is 1 in 1000 with coronary angiography. Other complications are arrhythmias, allergic reaction to the dye, and renal dysfunction. *(Fauci, Chapter 223)*

95. **(C)** The major bleeding complication rate with long-term warfarin anticoagulation is approximately 1%–3% per year when the target international normalized ratio (INR) is 2–3. *(Fauci, Chapter 112)*

96. **(B)** Beta-adrenergic receptors become less sensitive with advancing age. Higher rates of isoproterenol infusion are required in the elderly to achieve an increased resting heart rate. Clinically, higher doses of propranolol have been shown to be required in the elderly to achieve similar degrees of beta-blockade as in the young. *(Fauci, Chapter 24 1)*

97. **(A)** The response to benzodiazepines is more pronounced in the elderly, even when corrected for pharmacokinetics. Prior impairment is a factor in this response. *(Fauci, Chapter 11)*

98. **(A)** Despite similar pharmacokinetics, the dose of warfarin to provide effective anticoagulation is lower in the elderly. *(Fauci, Chapter 112)*

99. **(E)** The elderly have more body fat and less body water. A water-soluble drug such as lithium will have a considerably smaller volume of distribution. Thus, dosages should be decreased in the elderly to prevent toxicity. *(Fauci, Chapter 9)*

100. **(A)** Failure to correct for the elderly patient's increased sensitivity to narcotics can result in significant toxicity. *(Fauci, Chapter 9)*

101. **(A)** Tricyclic antidepressants and SSRIs are both effective treatments for depression, but their side-effect profiles are different. Tricyclics can promote weight gain while weight loss is more common with SSRIs. *(Fauci, Chapter 385)*

102. **(C)** Diuretics promote urinary losses of magnesium, zinc, and potassium. Zinc deficiency is also seen in liver cirrhosis, Type 2 diabetes, and lung cancer. *(Fauci, Chapter 71)*

103. **(D)** INH can result in pyridoxine (vitamin B_6) deficiency, particularly in malnourished individuals. It is recommended that patients who are elderly, or have DM, poor nutrition, alcoholism, seizure diathesis, or uremia, take pyridoxine while on INH. *(Fauci, Chapter 71)*

104. **(G)** Corticosteroids impair calcium absorption. They are useful in managing hypercalcemia, but bisphosphonates are the usual drug of choice. *(Fauci, Chapter 348)*

105. **(E)** Both phenytoin and phenobarbital can cause altered vitamin D metabolism and can even result in osteomalacia. Calcium absorption

from the gut is also blocked directly. *(Fauci, Chapter 346)*

106. **(B)** Sleep becomes more shallow with the loss of deep stages of sleep, resulting in more frequent arousals. Specific sleep disturbances such as sleep apnea and periodic leg movements increase with advancing age as well. *(Fauci, Chapter 28)*

107. **(B)** Neurodegenerative disorders can cause a change in normal circadian rhythm by causing a breakdown in the temporal organizing of sleep-wake cycling. This alteration in time of sleeping can be very disruptive to family members. The sleep pattern can be polyphasic, with multiple irregularly distributed periods of sleep, rather than one long sleep period at night. This can result in the patient's awakening during the night, which is also very disruptive. *(Fauci, Chapter 28)*

108. **(E)** Sleep apnea syndrome is the most common cause of daytime sleepiness in the elderly. The prevalence (at least in sleep disorder centers) increases with advancing age. Narcolepsy (usually having started earlier in life) and periodic limb movement disorder (restless legs) are other common causes of excessive daytime sleepiness. *(Fauci, Chapter 28)*

109. **(C)** The lack of focal neurologic findings suggests that the confusion is secondary to delirium. Bilateral asterixis is frequently seen in metabolic encephalopathy, particularly in cases of hepatic encephalopathy, hypercapnia, or drug ingestion. In this case, the most urgent investigations would be to rule out pneumonia with respiratory failure. *(Fauci, Chapter 26)*

110. **(E)** Although impaired attention is the hallmark of delirium (along with impaired consciousness), it can also be impaired in dementia. In very mild cognitive impairment, deficits in attention might differentiate delirium from dementia, but in the usual hospitalized patient, fluctuation in performance (particularly with regard to attention and level of consciousness) is probably more helpful. *(Fauci, Chapter 26)*

111. **(B)** The progressive nature of the disorder suggests a degenerative dementia, and the predominance of disinhibited behavior suggests the frontal lobes are involved. Frontal dementias can result from trauma, tumor, or ischemia, but this history suggests a degenerative disorder. Alzheimer's can involve the frontal lobes and mimic a frontal dementia. *(Fauci, Chapter 365)*

112. **(D)** In frontal dementia, and others as well, behavioral disturbances are often the reason for institutionalization. *(Fauci, Chapter 365)*

113. **(E)** Alzheimer disease is the most common cause of dementia in Western countries. Microscopically, there are neuritic plaques containing A-beta-amyloid in the neuronal cytoplasm. These plaques stain silver and are referred to as neurofibrillary tangles (NFT). There is also accumulation of A-beta-amyloid in arterial walls of cerebral blood vessels. *(Fauci, Chapter 365)*

Bibliography

Brunton LL, Lazo JS, Parker KL. *Goodman & Gilman's The Pharmacological Basis of Therapeutics*. 11th ed. New York, NY: McGraw-Hill; 2006.

Fauci AS, Braunwald MD, Kasper DL, et al. *Harrison's Principles of Internal Medicine*. 17th ed. New York; NY: McGraw-Hill; 2008.

Wolff K, Johnson RA. *Fitzpatrick's Color Atlas & Synopsis of Clinical Dermatology*. 6th ed. New York, NY: McGraw-Hill; 2009.

Index